CH00723024

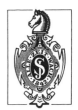

Thomas J. Vogl

# MRI
# of the Head and Neck

Functional Anatomy – Clinical Findings –
Pathology – Imaging

With contributions by
J. Assal  J. Balzer  S. Dresel  D. Eberhard
G. Grevers  M. Juergens  F. Peer  H. Schedel
C. Schmid  W. Steger  C. Wilimzig

With 179 Figures in 422 Separate Illustrations
and 62 Tables

Springer-Verlag
Berlin  Heidelberg  New York
London  Paris  Tokyo
Hong Kong  Barcelona
Budapest

Privatdozent Dr. med. habil. Thomas J. Vogl
Radiologische Klinik Innenstadt
der Radiologischen Universitätsklinik München,
Ziemssenstraße 1, W-8000 München 2, FRG

*Contributors*

J. Assal, J. Balzer, S. Dresel, D. Eberhard, M. Juergens,
F. Peer, H. Schedel, C. Schmid, W. Steger, C. Wilimzig
Radiologische Klinik Innenstadt
der Radiologischen Universitätsklinik München,
Ziemssenstraße 1, W-8000 München 2, FRG

PD Dr. G. Grevers
Klinik und Poliklinik für HNO-Kranke
der Universität München, Klinikum Großhadern,
Marchioninistraße 15, W-8000 München 70, FRG

Revised and enlarged from: T. J. Vogl, Kernspintomographie
der Kopf-Hals-Region. © Springer-Verlag Berlin Heidelberg 1991

ISBN-13:978-3-642-76792-0     e-ISBN-13:978-3-642-76790-6
DOI: 10.1007/978-3-642-76790-6

Library of Congress Cataloging-in-Publication Data.
**Vogl, Thomas J.** ([Kernspintomographie der Kopf-hals-region. English] MRI of the head
and neck : functional anatomy – clinical findings – pathology – imaging / Thomas J. Vogl ;
with contributions by J. Assal ... [et al.]. p.   cm.
"Revised and enlarged from: T. J. Vogl, Kernspintomographie der Kopf-Hals-Region.
Springer-Verlag Berlin Heidelberg 1991" – T. p. verso. Includes bibliographical references
and index.
ISBN-13:978-3-642-76792-0
1. Head – Magnetic resonance imaging. 2. Neck – Magnetic resonance imaging. I. Title.
[DNLM: 1. Head – radiography. 2. Head and Neck Neoplasms-radiography. 3. Magnetic
Resonance Imaging – methods. 4. Neck-radiography.   WE 705 V883k]   RC 936.V64
1992   617.5'107548 – dc20   92-2185

© Springer-Verlag Berlin Heidelberg 1992
Softcover reprint of the hardcover 1st edition 1992

The use of general descriptive names, registered names, trademarks, etc. in this publica-
tion does not imply, even in the absence of a specific statement, that such names are
exempt from the relevant protective laws and regulations and therefore free for general
use.
Product liability: The publishers cannot guarantee the accuracy of any information about
dosage and application contained in this book. In every individual case the user must
check such information by consulting the relevant literature.

Reproduction of the figures: Gustav Dreher GmbH, Stuttgart, FRG

21/3130-5 4 3 2 1 0 – Printed on acid-free paper

To my family, Claudia and Maximilian

# Foreword

Magnetic resonance imaging has changed the face of diagnostic imaging in recent years. After the introduction of MRI, it was soon apparent that this new modality would become indispensable in diagnostic imaging of the head and neck. The complex diseases of this region cannot be slotted into one medical discipline and consequently represent a challenge for many clinical and theoretical specialties. Diagnostic imaging of the head and neck is of particular interest for otolaryngology, oromaxillofacial surgery, and neurosurgery, as well as internal medicine and oncology. This book on the applications of MRI in the head and neck emphasizes and integrates functional anatomy, clinical findings, imaging, and diagnostic strategies. Richly illustrated with MR images and including correlative images obtained using other modalities, it is a comprehensive introduction to head and neck radiology and particularly to the diagnostic applications of MRI in this region.

All areas of the head and neck that are accessible to imaging procedures are thoroughly discussed and outstandingly illustrated. The author has accumulated ten years of experience in this area, in constant close collaboration with colleagues from other specialties. His work has been recognized by many professional associations, and he was awarded the *Deutscher Röntgenpreis* (German Roentgen Prize) for his outstanding contributions to the field.

The organization according to disease entities and the accompanying exhaustive description of the diagnostic possibilities of MRI should result in this book becoming a valued reference source, not only for the radiologist, but for colleagues from other clinical specialties as well.

I trust that this monograph will find a wide readership and that it will contribute to a greater interdisciplinary understanding of the complex diseases of the head and neck.

Munich, April 1992                    Prof. Dr. Dr. h. c. Josef Lissner

# Preface

The diagnostic evaluation of the head and neck has undergone revolutionary changes in the past few years due to the introduction and the refinement of computer tomography and magnetic resonance imaging. The variety of methods available and their increased complexity require new approaches to treatment selection and utilization. Many of these approaches are presented in this volume.

For tumors of the petrous part of the temporal bone and the skull base, the advent of high-resolution CT and MRI has provided radiologists with the unique opportunity to intensify their dialogue with otologic surgeons and neurootologists. The two new modalities have completely replaced polytomography.

However, CT and MRI of the temporal bone, like so many types of radiologic imaging, involve careful physical monitoring if they are to be effective. During the period under review, several technical advances were made, including direct sagittal CT and, in MRI, the introduction of the paramagnetic contrast medium gadolinium diethylenetriamine pentaacetic acid (Gd-DTPA).

The complex pattern of spread of disease in the nasopharynx and paranasal sinuses, usually involving soft tissue and bony structures, requires an imaging method that displays both tissues well. New MRI techniques with their superior soft tissue resolution depict tumor margins in the nasopharynx and related spaces more accurately than does CT. Thus MRI has remarkably improved our ability to diagnose lesions in this area, and with the introduction of Gd-DTPA the superiority of MRI over CT might increase even further.

The radiologist plays an important part in choosing the best diagnostic and therapeutic approach for masses of the salivary glands. The decision is greatly facilitated by the information on location, size, and character of a mass in the submandibular or the parotid glands that is provided by CT, ultrasound, or MRI. Recently published data show that plain MRI is superior to CT in the diagnosis of lesions in the parotid gland by virtue of its better soft tissue contrast and the absence of artifacts from metallic implants.The contrast agent Gd-DTPA helps to differentiate benign and malignant lesions.

Recognition of both bone involvement and extraorbital spread is essential for the correct diagnosis and treatment of orbital tumors. CT, with its high contrast resolution, has generally been considered the radiographic method of choice for imaging these masses and the associated bony changes. Although MRI adds to the information yielded by orbital CT in many fields, it has been slow to replace CT as the preferred imaging modality for orbital disease. Although, with improvements in surface coil imaging and the development of new paramagnetic contrast agents. MRI has evolved into an important tool in orbital evaluation, the full potential of the different MRI techniques has not yet been realized.

The oral cavity, oropharynx, and larynx are relatively accessible to the examining physician. The role of both CT and MRI is to define the extent to which a disease has spread into the surrounding deep soft tissues. MRI is superior to CT for demonstrating soft tissue lesions and especially for identifying malignant tumors such as carcinomas. The problem of noncontrast MRI is the evident overestimation of tumor size in long $T_2$-weighted sequences and the disappointing tumor-fat contrast in these images. Gd-DTPA is useful in increasing the sensitivity of short $T_1$-weighted sequences, improving tumor-fat contrast.

The physician must take care to select techniques that ensure accurate diagnosis of thyroid and parathyroid disease. A wide array of diagnostic techniques are available, including laboratory tests, fine-needle aspiration, radionuclides, and ultrasound. The main objective in imaging the thyroid by techniques such as CT and MRI is to identify lesions likely to be malignant. Both modalities can contribute substantial information about the extent of a tumor or metastatic disease; however, neither able reliably to discriminate between benign and malignant tumors. Due to the relatively small number of patients and the lack of representative investigations, the debate on how best to evaluate parathyroid disease continues. At the moment it must be concluded that the routine use of imaging techniques before primary neck exploration does not improve surgical results. On the other hand, localization techniques such as MRI are considered crucial to the evaluation of persistent or recurrent hyperparathyroidism.

The recent advances in the imaging of the middle ear have resulted largely from the use of high-resolution CT, by means of which disease can be precisely localized. High-resolution CT scanning also offers higher sensitivity than plain radiography and tomographic studies in the detection of early middle ear disease.

The place of new imaging modalities of the head and neck, especially MRI and MR spectroscopy, in relation to other imaging techniques is still being defined. It is clear that MRI has become an important diagnostic tool for lesions of the skull base and the pharynx. This method has not been as useful, however, in evaluating some other diseases of the head and neck, because of low signal from the cortical bone and because of artifacts from respiratory motion. Nevertheless, MRI technology continues to evolve. Paramagnetic contrast media and faster image acquisition will improve the MRI diagnosis of some head and neck conditions.

As we look to the future, I suggest that we direct our efforts toward improving the early detection of cancer and the prediction of the biologic behavior of tumors. Achieving this goal would allow us to initiate treatment at stages when a successful outcome is far more likely and to design treatment strategies that meet, but do not exceed, the needs of the individual patient.

Since its introduction, MRI has developed into an invaluable component of clinical diagnostics. The many diagnostic applications and the
absence of harmful ionizing radiation have led to its wide spread
utilization. MRI is considerably superior to CT in the visualization of
lesions of the central nervous system and the face and neck.

Munich, April 1992                                    Thomas J. Vogl

# Acknowledgements

I would like to express my most heartfelt gratitude to my esteemed teacher Professor Dr. Dr. J. Lissner for all the guidance, support, and encouragement, both scientific and personal, that I have received from him over the years. Only at his initiative and with his understanding was I able to take a systematic approach to the analysis of the data gained in the course of a number of research projects.

It would have been impossible to carry out a braod-based study without the active support of other clinics and institutes of the Department of Medicine of the University of Munich. Special thanks are due to Dr. G. Grevers, Dr. S. Holtmann, Dr. V. Reimann, Prof. K. Schorn, Prof. K. Mees, Prof. A. Behbehani, Prof. E. Kastenbauer, and all the medical staff at the Ear, Nose, and Throat Clinic for their commitment to the clinical chapters of the book and for allowing me to use their clinical findings; and to the staff at the Neurosurgery Clinic for releasing their clinical and surgical casenotes. I am also grateful to Prof. D. Randzio and staff at the Oral Surgery Clinic for their active assistance and to Prof. S. Permanetter and staff at the Pathology Institute for their support and for making their pathology results and postmortem reports available.

The clinical studies could not have been carried out without funding for staff and materials from two research projects supported by the Deutsche Forschungsgemeinschaft and the Wilhelm-Sander-Stiftung.

I would like to extend my thanks to all the technicians and to Dr. H. Schedel and Dr. R. Brüning for their assistance with the case analysis, as well as to Mrs. D. Schulze-Ber for the excellent photographic work. Finally, I am indebted to Mrs. M. Vorbuchner for her enormous engagement and her selfless assistance in examining the patients and in collecting and collating the data.

# Contents

# 1 Introduction

## 1.1 The Problem and the Goal

The increasing expectations on radiologic diagnosis in the head and neck have clearly demonstrated the limits of the imaging techniques available to date. Refinements in microsurgical procedures and advances in radiotherapy and chemotherapy demand more accurate radiologic diagnostic procedures. Computer tomography yields good representation of osseous structures and their lesions, but its diagnostic accuracy is limited by unsatisfactory differentiation of soft tissues. Modern applications of ultrasound only partially fill this gap. All in all, the amount of topographic information that can be extracted remains insufficient.

With the progress from the first experiments with magnetic resonance to actual imaging the question must be raised of whether this technique leads to better diagnosis in the head and neck. Since inflammatory and traumatic lesions can readily be demonstrated using established modalities, we will focus on diagnosis of neoplastic lesions. Uniquely, the phenomenon of MR can be applied simultaneously for the creation of images and for investigation of the metabolism by means of in vivo spectroscopy (Table 1.1). Because of the superb differentiation of soft tissue and the multiplanar imaging possibilities, new indications emerge [28–31]. While the majority of planar imaging techniques rely on two-dimensional visualization of three-dimensional entities, the latest developments in computer technology enable threedimensional presentations. This is important for surgery and other aspects of clinical practice because of the difficulty involved in mentally translating a series of planar pictures into the three-dimensional topography. This mental transforma-

**Table 1.1.** In vivo applications of MRI: differences between techniques

| MRI | In vivo spectroscopy |
|---|---|
| Spin density | Frequency of specific atomic nucleus |
| T1 relaxation time (spin-lattice relaxation time) | Frequency of molecules with specific atomic nucleus |
| T2 relaxation time (spin-spin relaxation time) | T2 relaxation time (Spin-spin relaxation time) |
| Topographic resolution | pH value, with or without topographic resolution |

tion of the two-dimensional images is especially difficult in the head and neck as a multitude of structures are present and the lesion may present complex infiltration patterns. This book describes the diagnostic potential of specially developed three-dimensional reconstruction techniques for different types of tumors at various locations in the head and neck.

Further improvements in diagnostic information can be achieved through the use of the new paramagnetic contrast agent Gd-DTPA, which shortens the T1 and T2 relaxation times of tissues. The necessity for intravenous administration of the agent, however, means that MR tomography is no longer noninvasive. Therefore it has to be ascertained whether Gd-DTPA improves morphologic evaluation and differential diagnosis. While MRI is the most sensitive of all imaging methods by reason of its better differentiation of soft tissue, the specificity at high field strength has been unsatisfactory. The intention here is to establish, on the basis of preoperative studies and exact follow-up studies, to what extent

MRI data correlate with the information obtained from spectroscopy.

This book sets out to resolve the following problems:

*Magnetic resonance imaging*
1. Development and assessment of an optimal examination technique
2. Diagnostic value relative to other imaging methods
3. Indications for the paramagnetic contrast agent Gd-DTPA
4. Tumor specificity
5. Additional diagnostic information

*In vivo phosphorus-31 spectroscopy*
6. Metabolic information

## 1.2 Clinical Presentation

The wide spectrum of head and neck pathology can be divided for purposes of description into five topographic regions.

### 1.2.1 Temporal Bone, Skull Base, and Cerebellopontine Angle

The diagnosis and differentation of neoplasms of the base of the skull and the posterior fossa has been improved significantly by the progress in audiologic testing and by new imaging techniques. Pathology in the region of the petrous part of the temporal bone way arise from the temporal bone itself, the mastoid process, or adjacent structures such as the jugular vein, the cranial nerves, and the meninges.

The acoustic neuroma is a benign neoplasm which arises from Schwann cells of the neurilemma, usually that of the main branches of the vestibular nerve. It generally has its origin where the peripheral ganglionic neurilemma meets with the brainstem neuroglia. According to the site of origin, acoustic neuromas are divided into lateral tumors, e.g., those growing intrameatally, mediolateral tumors, and medial tumors [6].

The multitude of symptoms arise from the pressure the tumor exerts on neighboring neural structures [32]. The first functional deficits are to be expected in the vestibular and chochlear part of the vestibulocochlear nerve, because most tumors arise in the internal acoustic meatus [5, 19]. Hence, early diagnosis of acoustic neuromas and other neoplasms in the cerebellopontine angle is an important interdisciplinary task for otoneurologists and radiologists [32]. The objective clinical symptoms of these tumors are vestibular focal symptoms and retrocochlear acoustic disturbance. Besides local symptoms such as pareses of the facial and abducens nerves, symptoms of brainstem compression may also arise in advanced stages. Clinical diagnosis relies mainly on audiologic and vestibular testing methods. In spite of specific neurootologic and neuroradiologic examination procedures, before the introduction of MRI it was often impossible to diagnose small tumors reliably [43]. Preoperative confirmation of a neoplasm is, however, indispensable [1, 32].

Glomus tumors are the next most common tumors in this region. They originate from chemoreceptors (the glomera) that can be present at a great number of sites throughout the human body [9, 15]. Histologically, glomus tumors show precapillary arteriovenous shunts with a collection of nonchromaffin chemoreceptor cells. The glomera most frequently affected are those at the superior jugular bulb, the tympanic plexus, and the carotid bifurcation [39]. The glomus tumors at the base of the skull (glomus tympanicum, glomus jugulare, and glomus vagale) are located in the distribution of the glossopharyngeal nerve. In the preoperative diagnosis of these tumors, determination of the exact topographic situation and the degree of vascularization is of importance. The clinical symptoms of these tumors are diverse and depend on whether the neoplasm is located in the petrous part of the temporal bone or in the skull base [41]. Differential diagnoses in the petrous part include primary and secondary bone tumors, plasmacytoma and meningioma. Very occasionally dermoid cysts, eosinophilic granulomas, and other neoplasms arise.

## 1.2.2 Orbit

The introduction of CT represented a major advance over conventional roentgenology and tomography in the examination of the eye, but MRI has proved to be an even greater breakthrough in diagnostic imaging. Although ophthalmoscopic detection of some diseases of the orbit is often reliable, imaging procedures should nevertheless be used in all patients suspecting of having a tumor, in order to establish the presence or absence of gross retrobulbar spread, intracranial metastasis, or a second tumor. In addition, imaging may permit differentiation of retinoblastoma from lesions such as persistent hypoplastic vitreous, 'coats' disease, toxocariosis, retinal detachment, subretinal hemorrhage, or so-called pseudoglioma.

## 1.2.3 Nasopharynx and Paranasal Sinuses

Some 5% of all malignant tumors of the head and neck arise in the nasopharynx, and 90% of these histologically prove to be carcinomas [23]. The most frequent types of malignant tumors in the nasopharynx are squamous cell carcinomas and lymphoepithelial neoplasms. Lymphomas, however, are more frequent in children. A characteristic of these lymphomas is the early and extensive lymphatic metastasis. Benign tumors in the nasopharynx are rare, the most frequent being juvenile angiofibroma [2]. Although this fibroma is benign histologically, clinically its expansive growth shows features of malignancy. Mesenchymal tumors are mostly represented in the group of benign tumors of the nose and paranasal sinuses [23]. They comprise papillomas, hemangiomas, fibromas, and other rare tumors. Tumors originating in the internal nose and the paranasal sinuses make up less than 1% of all malignant neoplasms in this topographic region. Overall, the malignant tumors of the nasopharynx and paranasal sinuses can be divided into squamous cell carcinomas (60%), adenocarcinomas (20%), differentiated carcinomas (10%) and mesenchymal neoplasms (10%) [21].

Imaging procedures are usually first performed when the endoscopic findings are available.

## 1.2.4 Salivary Glands

Epithelial tumors present 90% of all neoplasms of the parotid, submandibular, and sublingual glands. The remaining 10% are comprised of tumors such as hemangiomas, lymphangiomas, periglandular tumors, and malignant lymphomas [25]. Some 85% of the benign epithelial tumors are pleomorphic or monomorphic adenomas. Cystadenolymphomas (Warthin's tumor) and other tumors are much less common. Some 25%–30% of all tumors of the salivary glands are malignant, and these malignancies typically display growth and firm infiltration and cause pain and facial paralysis. Histologically, acinus cell tumors are found in 15% of all cases and mucoepidermoid tumors in 30% [4]. Carcinomas of the salivary glands show broad histologic variation: adenoid cystic carcinomas (35%), adenocarcinomas (10%), squamous cell carcinomas (10%), and other, less frequent tumors [1].

Imaging procedures should be used to establish specifically what type of lesion is concerned, in the planning of treatment, and to follow the progress of therapy.

## 1.2.5 Oral Cavity and Oropharynx

The oral cavity and oropharynx are parts of the aerodigestive system whose patency is of vital importance [1]. Although benign tumors as a whole are uncommon in this region, all forms can be found. Common benign epithelial neoplasms are papillomas and adenomas. The most common congenital tumors are hemangioma, lymphangioma, and goiter of the base of the tongue [1, 24]. The vast majority of malignancies in the oral cavity and the oropharynx are squamous cell carcinomas; anaplastic carcinomas are less common [37]. Early carcinomas of the oral cavity and oropharynx are characterized by a lack of conspicuous symptoms. Inspection, palpation, and endoscopy are important for the diagnosis of neoplasms in this region. Imaging methods are indicated to document the exact depth of the tumors and their infiltration into neighboring structures.

### 1.2.6 Hypopharynx and Larynx

Malignant tumors of the hypopharynx most frequently originate in the piriform sinus, less frequently on the posterior wall of the pharynx [37]. In over 40% of all cases the primary symptom of these tumors is regional metastasis to lateral cervical lymph nodes.

Both benign and malignant tumors of the larynx show characteristic clinical findings, especially when they originate from the level of the glottis. Frequent benign neoplasms are polyps of the vocal cords, papillomas, and abnormalities of the laryngeal mucosa. Malignant carcinoma of the larynx is the most frequent of the head and neck carcinomas, comprising 45% of the total [1, 16]. The result of clinical laryngoscopy serves as a basis for the decision as to treatment modality: surgery, radiotherapy, or chemotherapy. In many cases imaging techniques such as CT or MRI have proved valuable in the evaluation of primary tumors and the assessment of lymph node involvement.

### 1.2.7 Neck

Most neck masses are located in the infrahyoid region. As a general rule, such masses in children are benign: most are accounted for by reactive lymphadenopathy secondary to infection or congenital lesions. The latter are mostly thyroglossal duct cysts, brachial cleft cysts, and cystic hygromas. If thyroid lesions are excluded, a unilateral neck mass in young and middle-aged adults is usually malignant. The most common disease of the neck in this age group is lymphoma. Metastatic disease accounts for most neck masses in patients over 40 years of age.

### 1.2.8 Temporomandibular Joint

The function of the temporomandibular joint (TMJ) is complex, in that the upper and lower compartments basically work as two small joints within one capsule. The purpose of any imaging of the TMJ is to depict a clinically suspected disorder. Internal derangement is a general orthopedic term referring to a mechanical fault that interferes with joint function. Internal derangement of the TMJ is thus a functional diagnosis, and for the TMJ the most common cause of internal derangement is displacement of the disk. The findings of various studies suggest that clinical examination per se is not reliable for determining the status of the joint, so it seems reasonable to assume that accurate imaging by means of MR is needed.

## 1.3 Imaging Modalities in the Head and Neck

### 1.3.1 Conventional Roentgenology

Ever since the introduction of conventional roentgenographic techniques at the turn of the century there has been rapid development in roentgenographic diagnosis of the skull and the air sinuses. Scheier and Henle [34] first reported the X-ray diagnosis of the ear and neighboring structures in 1904. In 1905 Schüller [36] published *Die Schädelbasis im Roentgenbild* ("The Skull Base in Roentgenology"). Henschen [14] described the changes of the internal acoustic meatus, acoustic neuroma and the interpretation of roentgenographic images of normal and pathological pneumatization of the mastoid. Stenvers [38] and Mayer [27] published a halfsagittal projection of the pyramid and an axial projection of the petrous part for the first time in 1917 and 1923 respectively. These projections continue to allow adequate roentgenographic diagnosis of the ear and the paranasal sinuses. For conventional tomography of the temporal bone the polydimensional technique showed the best results [7]. While conventional roentgenology has to some extent held its place, conventional tomography has disappeared from routine diagnosis.

### 1.3.2 Angiography

Diagnostic angiography is an important supplement to noninvasive imaging for the classification of intensely vascularized processes and of vascular lesions in the head and neck [3, 22, 40]. The conventional angiographic technique has been replaced almost totally by digital subtraction angiography in the past 5 years [41]. Venous DSA has not proven effective for the characterization of vascular processes in the petrous part and the facial skeleton. The reason for this lies in the simultaneous visualization of all craniocervical vessels and in the high susceptibility of this method to motion artifacts. Arterial DSA has numerous advantages over conventional angiography [41], notably higher contrast resolution, higher image frequency and the capacity for immediate reproduction of subtraction images by means of digital processing. Before a planned embolization, arterial DSA permits precise analysis of the morphology and the complex hemodynamic and angioarchitectural relations of vascular lesions and heavily vascularized tumors [40]. Despite the low complication rates of arterial DSA in the head and neck, risks remain because of the invasiveness of the method. Therefore arterial DSA should be employed only before interventional techniques, not, however, in routine diagnostic evaluation of neoplastic processes. With the establishment of arterial and venous MR angiography in clinical routine the numbers of diagnostic angiographies will continue to decrease.

### 1.3.3 Ultrasound

Ultrasound diagnosis in the head and neck has progressed in leaps and bounds since Kreidel first investigated the paranasal sinuses in the 1940s [17]. In the 1970s investigators at the University of Freiburg, FRG, analyzed A-mode and B-mode diagnosis of the paranasal sinuses in extensive clinical studies and considered the potential for general application [26]. At the moment ultrasound is utilized for various problems in the craniocervical region: A-mode imaging for the paranasal sinuses and B-mode for the facial soft tissues, the salivary glands, and the cervical soft tissues [13]. Sonographic examination of other regions, e.g., the larynx, the hypopharynx, and the pharynx [8] is in the experimental stage.

### 1.3.4 Computer-Assisted Techniques

Devices for the creation of axial tomograms with the help of computers have been constantly changed and improved, so that up to now four generations of CT scanners can be distinguished. In spite of considerable differences in the production of images and the technical execution, all CT devices rely on the same principle. A roentgen ray is rotated in a plane perpendicular to the body axis, and one or more detectors measure the attenuation of the ray in the irradiated body tissue. Different normal tissues, as well as tumors, attenuate roentgen rays proportionally to their density. The goal of CT is therefore to register the distribution of the linear attenuation coefficients [11]. Based on this principle, CT yields contrast graduation of soft tissues greatly superior to that obtained with conventional roentgenography. Also, direct portrayal of different organs in the head and neck is possible. While CT primarily produces axial images, direct coronal slices can be made with appropriate positioning of the patient [10]. Additionally, sagittal and other planes can be reconstructed from the stored data. Regarding the topographic resolution CT is superior to conventional roentgenography.

With the introduction of high-resolution CT it became possible to demonstrate the finest anatomic structures of the petrous part in detail. High-resolution CT and the special reconstruction algorithm supplement conventional roentgenography. These techniques are important in the planning of modern microsurgery of the middle ear, especially for trauma of the middle skull base or malformation of the middle ear.

Based on the discovery of magnetic resonance by Purcell [33] in 1946, the conditions for clinical MR tomography were first created by Lauterbur [20] in 1973. For diagnosis of diseases in the head and neck, modern MR tomographs have been available for some 8 years. The basic principles of image production, resolution, and special examination techniques will be elucidated in the following chapters.

## 1.4 Methods of Treatment

### 1.4.1 Surgery

In recent years otorhinolaryngology, head and neck surgery, and orofacial surgery have experienced swift and impressive progress in diagnostic and therapeutic capabilities. The introduction of the operating microscope and its application for various exploration procedures stimulated developments in ear, nose, and throat surgery as well as neurosurgery [1, 19, 32].

The choice of surgical technique for tumors of the petrous part and the cerebellopontine angle is mainly influenced by the size of the tumor. Tumors limited to the internal acoustic meatus are excised by otosurgeons via a transtemporal or a translabyrinthine approach [43]. Tumors with a diameter exceeding 25 mm and tumors which are partly intrameatal and partly extrameatal, or totally extrameatal, are excised by neurosurgeons [6]. Among the glomus tumors, tympanic neoplasms can be removed otosurgically [1]. Tumors of the glomus jugulare usually require, depending on their extension, either otosurgical or neurosurgical intervention. The facial nerve is spared if possible [9]. The first-choice therapy of neoplasms in the nose and the paranasal sinuses is radical resection; however it is not always possible to observe a margin of safety in the healthy tissue, so that additional treatment procedures must be employed [1, 12]. In the salivary glands, for both benign and malignant tumors the first operation usu-

ally determines the success of treatment and the survival chances of the patient. Only in the case of inoperable primary tumors, incomplete resections, and malignant lymphomas is therapy by other means indicated [1].

### 1.4.2 Radiotherapy

Radiotherapy is an important curative as well as palliative treatment for craniocervical tumors [35]. It may be employed primarily, or before and after operation. In a number of tumors surgery and radiotherapy are of almost equal value with regard to the success [18]. Depending on the clinical findings either surgery or primary irradiation may be employed for T1 tumors of the glottis [16, 37]. Postoperative radiotherapy with the aim of improving survival is indicated in cases where not all the tumor can be removed surgically, in extensive T3/T4 tumors, and in the case of lymph node involvement. Prerequisites for optimal radiotherapy (percutaneous or interstitial) are exact pretherapeutic diagnosis, therapy simulation and therapy planning by computer. The case for case planning of therapy by means of imaging procedures such as CT and MRI lays the best groundwork for optimal dose distribution in regions affected by tumors and for the sparing of healthy tissue.

### 1.4.3 Chemotherapy and Radiochemotherapy

Chemotherapy is indicated in primarily inoperable tumors, that are not amenable to curative radiotherapy, and in the case of distant metastasis or absolute inoperability [1]. The only patients selected for simultaneous chemotherapy and radiotherapy with curative intent are those with histologically proven squamous cell carcinomas of the oral cavity, the larynx, the oropharynx, and the hypopharynx that are limited in extent. The major applications of MRI therefore lie in pretherapeutic tumor diagnosis and in checking the results of treatment. Of great clinical interest is also the detection of recurrences after surgery or radiochemotherapy.

## References

1. Becker H, Naumann H, Pfalz C (1982) HNO-Heilkunde. Thieme, Stuttgart
2. Bloch F (1946) Nuclear induction. Phys Rev 70:460–474
3. Casjannias P, Moret J (1978) Normal and non-pathological variables in angiography aspects of the arteries of the middle ear. Neuroradiology 15:213–219
4. Casselmann JW, Mancuso AA (1987) Major salivary gland masses: comparison of MR imaging and CT. Radiology 165:183–189
5. Fisch U (1970) Transtemporal surgery of the internal auditory canal. Adv 17:203–240
6. Fisch U (1977) Die Mikrochirurgie des Felsenbeins. HNO 25:193–197
7. Frey KW, Mündnich K (1957) Schichtaufnahmen des Felsenbeins mit polyzyklischer Verwischung bei angeborenen Ohrmißbildungen. RÖFO 87:164–176
8. Frühwald F, Salomonowitz E, Neuhoff A, Pavelka R, Mailath G (1985) Tongue cancer: sonographic assessment of the tumor stage. J Ultrasound Med 6:121–137
9. Gastpar H (1961) Die Tumoren des Glomus caroticum, Glomus jugulare, tympanicum und Glomus vagale. Acta Otolaryngol (Stockh) [Suppl]167:1–23
10. Grevers G, Vogl T (1988) Die arterielle und venöse digitale Subtraktionsangiographie (DSA) – eine aktuelle Studie für die HNO-Heilkunde. Laryngol Rhinol Otol 67:221–225
11. Grevers G, Wiechell R, Vogl T, Wittmann A (1988) Der aktuelle Stellenwert multiplanarer Abbildungen für die Felsenbeindiagnostik. Arch Oto Rhino Laryngol [Suppl II]:98–100
12. Grevers G, Wilimzig C, Vogl T, Laub G (1991) Eine neue Methode zur 3D-Rekonstruktion im Kopf-Hals-Bereich. Laryngol Rhinol Otol (Stuttg) (in press)
13. Hajek PC, Salomonowitz E, Türk R, Tscholakoff D, Kumpan W, Czernbirch H (1986) Lymph nodes of the neck, evaluation with US. Radiology 158:739–742
14. Henschen A (1913) Die Akustikustumoren. RÖFO 207
15. Hildmann H, Tiedjen KV (1983) Zur Differentialdiagnose des Glomustumors. Laryngol Rhinol Otol (Stuttg) 62:502–504
16. Kleinsasser O (1987) Tumoren des Larynx und Hypopharynx. Thieme, Stuttgart
17. Kreidel W (1947) Über die Verwendung des Ultraschalls in der klinischen Diagnostik. Ärztl Forschg 2 Forschungsergeb Ges Med 1:349
18. Kurz C, Willich N, Vogl T (1987) Bestrahlung bei Chemodektomen. Laryngol Rhinol Otol 66:469–473
19. Kurze T, Doyle JB (1962) Extradural intracranial approach to the internal auditory canal. J Neurosurg 19:1033–1077
20. Lauterbur PC (1973) Image formation by induced local interactions. Examples employing NMR. Nature 242:190
21. Lloyd G, Land V, Phelps P, Howard D (1987) MRI in evaluation of nose and paranasal sinus disease. Br J Radiol 60:957–968
22. Lloyd TM, Van Aman V, Johnson JC (1979) Aberrant jugular bulb presenting as middle ear mass. Radiology 131:139–141
23. Lovrencic M, Kalousek M, Marotti M, Petric V, Virag M (1987) Tumors of nasopharynx: a CT evaluation of 52 patients. Digital radiology. Springer, Berlin Heidelberg New York, pp 265–269
24. Lufkin RB, Wortham DG, Dietrich RB, Hoover LA, Larson SG (1986) Tongue and oropharynx: findings on MR imaging. Radiology 161:69–75
25. Mandelblatt SM, Bron IF, Davis PC, Fry SM, Jacobs LH, Hoffmann (1987) Parotid masses: MR imaging. Radiology 3:411–414
26. Mann W (1975) Die Ultraschalldiagnostik der Nasennebenhöhlen. Arch Otorhinolaryngol 211:145
27. Mayer EG (1923) Otologische Röntgendiagnostik. Springer, Wien
28. Mess K, Vogl T, Seiderer M (1984) Kernspintomographie in der Hals-Nasen-Ohrenheilkunde. Fallbeispiele. Laryngol Rhinol Otol (Stuttg) 63:485–487
29. Mees K, Vogl T, Bauer M (1985) Kernspintomographie in der Hals-Nasen-Ohrenheilkunde. Diagnostische Möglichkeiten. Laryngol Rhinol Otol (Stuttg) 64:177–180
30. Mödder U, Steinbrich W, Heindel W, Lindemann J, Brusis T (1985) Indikationen zur Kernspintomographie bei Tumoren des Gesichtsschädels und Halsbereiches. Digitale Bilddiagn 5:55–60
31. Mödder U, Lenz M, Steinbrich W (1987) MRI of facial skeleton and parapharyngeal space. Eur J Radiol 7:6–10
32. Plester D, Wende S, Nakayama N (1978) Kleinhirnbrückenwinkeltumoren – Diagnostik und Therapie. Springer, Berlin Heidelberg New York
33. Purcell EM, Torry MC, Pound RV (1946) Resonance absorption by nuclear magnetic moments in a solid. Physiol Rev 69:37–38
34. Scheier H, Henle J (1904) Bericht über Versuche, den Processus mastoideus darzustellen. Versammlung Dtsch Naturforscher
35. Scherer S (1980) Strahlentherapie, 2nd edn. Springer, Berlin Heidelberg New York
36. Schüller G (1905) Die Schädelbasis im Röntgenbild. Lugas, Gräfe and Sillens, Hamburg
37. Spiessl B, Hermanek P, Scheibe O, Wagner G (1982) TNM-Atlas, UICC. Springer, Berlin Heidelberg New York

38. Stenvers HW (1917) Röntgenology of the os petrosum. Arch Radiol Electrother 14
39. Tidwell TJ, Montague ED (1975) Chemodectomas involving the temporal bone. Radiology 116:147
40. Valavanis A (1986) Preoperative embolization of the head and neck, indication, patient selection, goals and precautions. Am J Neuroradiol 7:943–952
41. Valavanis A (1986) Intraarterielle DSA in der interventionellen Neuroradiologie. In: Nadjmi M (ed) Digitale Subtrahtionsangiographie in der Neuroradiologie. Thieme, Stuttgart, pp 239–246
42. Valavanis A, Schubinger O, Naidid TP (1987) Clinical imaging of the cerebellpontine angle. Springer, Berlin Heidelberg New York
43. Young IR, Hall AS, Pallis CA, Bydder GM, Legg NJ, Steiner RE (1981) Nuclear magnetic resonance imaging of the brain in multiple sclerosis. Lancet 14:1063–1066

# 2 Basics of Magnetic Resonance Imaging

## 2.1 Principles of Magnetic Resonance

The first MR experiments were reported independently by Bloch at Stanford University and by Purcell at Harvard University in 1946. The first two-dimensional proton MR image was produced in 1972, when Lauterbur of New York State University measured a water sample [29].

These experiments were based on the principle that biologic tissue is permeable to long-wavelength radiation. MRI involves the receipt of information about the magnetic resonance of the spins in tissue exposed to a static magnetic field after induction of transitions by irradiating energy [2]. Comprehension of some basic aspects of physics is important if this phenomenon is to be understood.

### 2.1.1 Magnetism at the Atomic and Nuclear Level

The principle of magnetism is the motion of electric charges. In the atom the charges are protons and electrons. The atoms possess angular moments, the so-called spin, and the motion of the protons and electrons results in a magnetic moment (Fig. 2.1). Subnuclear charged particles of the neutron, the so-called quarks, produce a net magnetic moment about two-thirds as great as that of the proton. As the direction of the magnetic fields caused by protons and neutrons is opposite, only unpaired protons or neutrons contribute their magnetic moment to the nucleus.

When nuclei are placed in an external magnetic field, the randomly orientated dipoles line up with this field. The spin vectors experience torque when subjected to the magnetic field. As a result, the protons precess around the

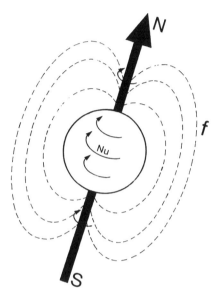

**Fig. 2.1.** Nucleus (*Nu*) with angular momentum (spin) and magnetic moment producing a magnetic field. (*f*, Field lines of magnetic field; *N*, north pole; *S*, south pole)

axis of the magnetic field at a rate given by the Larmor frequency, which varies with the field strength and the kind of nucleus.

Quantum mechanics allows the proton two energy states in the external magnetic field: the parallel and the antiparallel. The dynamic balance between these two energy states is determined by the magnetic field and the temperature. As the magnetic moments of the two energy states are opposite, the difference between the total parallel and antiparallel magnetization is the net magnetization of the volume, the so-called equilibrium (Fig. 2.2).

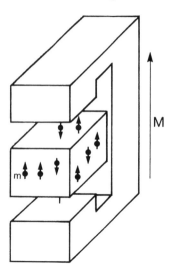

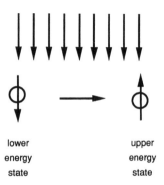

**Fig. 2.3.** The protons in the lower energy state switch direction of magnetization when transitions by radiofrequency energy applied at the Larmor frequency are induced

**Fig. 2.2.** Equilibrium direction and net magnetization (*M*) is up. The individual magnetic moments (*m*) have parallel or antiparallel direction

## 2.1.2 Resonance

Resonance occurs when transitions between low and high energy states of the nuclei present in a static magnetic field can be achieved by irradiating the nuclei with electromagnetic waves. The electromagnetic energy required for resonance has the value of the energy difference between the low and high energy states. The frequency of the electromagnetic waves has to be the same as the frequency of the nuclear spin, which depends on the static magnetic field and the kind of nucleus. When the spins are irradiated by electromagnetic waves the energy brings about a transition of the nuclei from the antiparallel to the parallel state (Fig. 2.3). This phenomenon is called "induced absorption". It can be shown that in a sample in a magnetic field there will be more transitions from the low to the high energy state, because there are more spins in the low energy state. After irradiation the spin system is no longer in thermal equilibrium. During the transition back to the lower energy state after the electromagnetic energy has been switched off, the nuclei emit electromagnetic waves which can be received by coils. This relaxation signal is called "induced emission".

The magnetization vector M has a component $M_z$ aligned with the static magnetic field and a component $M_{x,y}$ perpendicular to $M_z$. $M_z$ is called the longitudinal magnetization and $M_{x,y}$ the transverse magnetization.

At equilibrium $M_z$ is equal to M and thus equivalent to the net magnetization. $M_{x,y}$ is zero in this state. When the spin system is irradiated by an electromagnetic pulse, $M_z$ decreases and $M_{x,y}$ increases (Fig. 2.4). After the radiofrequency is switched off, $M_{x,y}$ returns to zero and $M_z$ returns to M. These processes are exponential in time and are characterized by two time constants: T1, the longitudinal relaxation time, and T2, the transverse relaxation time.

## 2.1.3 Relaxation

When the magnetization M returns to equilibrium the component $M_{x,y}$ with relaxation time T2 is lost more rapidly than the vector $M_z$ with relaxation time T1 is regained. Therefore T2 is in general shorter than T1. As the rate of return to equilibrium along the z axis depends on how fast energy can be transferred from the spinning protons to the system, T1 is called the "spin-lattice relaxation time". T1 is shorter in liquids (seconds) than in solid tissue (minutes to hours). T2 depends on the molecular structure of a sample and on the strength of the magnetic fields; these parameters affect

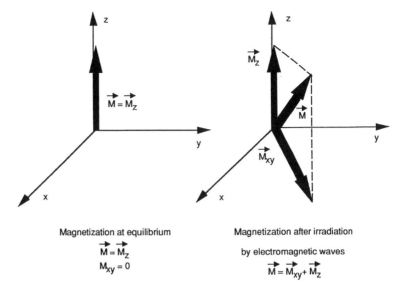

**Fig. 2.4.** Magnetization after irradiation by electromagnetic waves: $M = M_{xy} + M_z$

the rate of exchange of thermal energy by collision between the molecules. It indicates the relationship between the strength of the external field and that of the local internal field. Because T2 is determined by the exchange of energy from one nucleus to another, T2 is called the "spin-spin relaxation time".

### 2.1.4 Image Acquisition

Once the radiofrequency pulse is over, the nuclei emit energy in the form of electromagnetic waves. These waves are picked up by the receiver coils. Depending on the type of pulse, the received signal differs. The simplest MR pulse sequence is free induction decay (FID). In this sequence the magnetization vector is tilted by 90° into the x-y plane. The emission after the pulse is the FID signal. The FID for tissue is composed of sine waves of different frequencies, resulting in a short signal. The longer FID for liquids can be represented as a single sine wave, because the coherence of the precessing nuclei is much higher in liquids than in tissue. To differentiate among tissues it is necessary to use Fourier transformation

to obtain a representative frequency curve. Depending on the pulse sequence the signal varies, producing different frequency spectra for different substances.

Another response, the spin-echo, is produced by sequentially imposing two pulses of different amplitudes: first a 90° pulse, then a 180° pulse. After the 90° pulse the nuclei behave as they do after an FID pulse. The 180° pulse then reverses the direction of the net transverse magnetization. The additional 180° pulse reestablishes the phase coherence of the relaxing spins after the 90° pulse.

When resonance is produced by all nuclei in the sample, the signal emitted yields no information on the location of the nuclei; localization of the nuclei is, however, necessary for the production of images. The frequency of the received signal depends on the field strength of the static magnetic field as well as the resonance frequency. Thus, the signal from a sample in a 1.0-T field differs from the signal from the same sample in a 0.95-T field. The difference between the signals is significant and reproducible. This mechanism is used to localize the signal source. To realize this, gradients produce an increasing magnetization about the whole length of each orthogonal direction

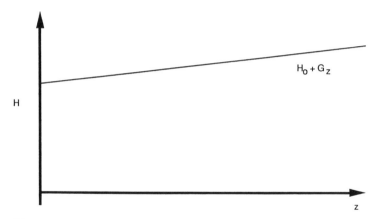

**Fig. 2.5.** Field strength $H$ of the magnetic field along the z axis. To locate the signal a gradient field $G_z$ is superimposed on the static field, producing a linear increase of the field strength

of the magnetic field. These gradients, low magnetic fields superimposed over the static magnetic field (Fig. 2.5), are available and necessary in the x-y, z-y, and z-x planes. Each point in the volume therefore has a special magnetization and the location can be calculated precisely by means of Fourier transformation.

## 2.2  Parameters of MRI

In MRI the image of the tissue displayed on the monitor depends on the RF signal that excited the protons in the static magnetic field. As the resulting images are not photographs of the tissue we have to look for criteria describing the type of tissue. The sequence can be chosen so as to yield T1-weighted or T2-weighted images; some tissues have the same signal intensity in a T1-weighted sequence but different signal intensities in a T2-weighted sequence. The choice of sequence is thus very important and depends on the region of interest and on the specific tissue concerned. There are other parameters determining the quality of the image. For instance, a number of factors associated with the imaging procedure affect the signal intensity. However, increasing signal intensity usually results in greater "noise", i.e., random RF emission from the measured tissue. Sequences and se-

quence parameters thus have to be selected with great care.

### 2.2.1  Field Strength

The field strength of any given MR device is fixed and can be modified only slightly by the user of the unit. The external magnetic field influences the contrast and the signal-to-noise ratio (S/N). The S/N tends to increase in a linear fashion with the field strength. On the other hand, RF inhomogeneities become more pronounced at higher field strengths, resulting in a decrease of S/N.

The optimal field strength does not exist; the clinical application determines the field strength needed.

### 2.2.2  Repetition Time

The repetition time (TR) has an important influence on signal intensity. The signal of the tissue is proportional to the return of longitudinal magnetization at the end of each cycle. Thus short TR reduces the signal level of the tissue with long T1 relaxation time, resulting in a T1-weighted image. Reduction of signal intensity by using short TR can be compensated by averaging. However, S/N is optimal when TR is almost T1.

### 2.2.3 Echo Time

The echo time (TE) is the time during which the magnetization received by the coils decays and is converted into a signal. For the number of the relaxing protons decreases in time the signal intensity decreases with increasing TE. Long TE values can be used to produce T2-weighted images that are generally rather noisy because of the low signal intensity.

### 2.2.4 Resolution

Each pixel of the image on the monitor corresponds to a voxel in the tissue. The volume of the tissue contained in the voxel is proportional to the signal strength. Thus, large voxels give a high S/N. However, the spatial resolution decreases when voxel size increases, impairing image quality. The choice of resolution depends on the tissue concerned.

### 2.2.5 Multiple Acquisitions

One of the factors limiting image quality is the noise that appears as a random variation in pixel intensity. In some cases the pixel intensity is increased, sometimes it is decreased. Averaging the same measurement over a series of images reduces this noise. Resolution of the noise results in a better S/N, but the acquisition time will increase proportionally with the number of measurements.

### 2.2.6 Signal-to-Noise Ratio

The S/N is a very important image parameter. The brightness of the pixels on the monitor is proportional to the intensity of the signal emitted by the tissue. In addition, random variations in signal intensity occur during measurement. This increase or decrease of the "real" signal, called noise, often impairs spatial resolution and limits long echo times. In clinical practice the S/N is often increased by increasing the number of measurements and averaging the results. The S/N can be calculated as the difference between the signal intensity (SI) of the tissue and the background signal intensity, divided by the standard deviation (SD) of the background signal intensity:

$$S/N = (SI_{\text{tissue}} - SI_{\text{background}})/SD_{\text{background}}$$

### 2.2.7 Contrast-to-Noise-Ratio

Besides the S/N, the evaluability of an MRI scan is limited by the contrast between structures. Even with excellent contrast image quality can be impaired by excessive noise. The contrast-to-noise ratio (C/N) describes the evaluability of the contrast of the image and is defined as the difference in S/N between two kinds of tissue. It can be calculated as the difference in signal intensity of two tissues divided by the square root of the sum of the squares of the standard deviation of signal intensity of both tissues.

$$C/N = \frac{(SI_{\text{tissue1}} - SI_{\text{tissue2}})}{\sqrt{SD_{\text{tissue1}}^2 + SD_{\text{tissue2}}^2}}$$

## 2.3 Equipment

Complex equipment systems are necessary for MRI. The main components are the static magnetic field, the RF unit, the computer, and the monitor. The static magnetic field can be generated by different types of magnets and is needed for the phenomenon of resonance. The RF unit consists of transmitter coils, receiver coils, and the transmitter electronics. The signals from the receiver coils are processed by the computer, which transforms the analog signals into digital image points, resulting in the MR image displayed on the monitor.

### 2.3.1 Magnets

Magnets used for whole-body imaging fall into one of three categories: resistive, superconducting, and permanent. The field strength of the system is determined by the type of magnet.

Resistive magnets generate their magnetic field by the flow of current within a wire. This wire is made of a conducting material, such as copper or aluminum, which has a specific resistance resulting in power dissipation and heating. These systems have the disadvantages of high power consumption and limited field strength (under normal conditions less than 0.5 T).

When the wire is made of superconducting material the resistance is much lower, nearly undetectable. As a result power consumption and heating are lower and therefore there is no limit on field strength. This type of magnet is used in systems with field strengths of 1.0 T and higher.

The permanent magnets are made of ferromagnetic materials in which the magnetic field has been induced at the time of manufacture. These magnets are exceeding heavy (a 0.3-T magnet weighs about 100 tons) and are used with low field strengths.

### 2.3.2 Radiofrequency Equipment

The radio waves are generated by a frequency synthesizer which produces a wide range of frequencies, amplified, and then transmitted by an RF coil. To receive the signal from the body the same coil or a separate receiver coil can be used. These coils can be divided into whole-volume coils and local surface coils. The local coils receive signal from a small region of tissue but with a high S/N. The prime consideration in choosing a coil is optimal matching of the sensitivity of the coil to the anatomic region of interest. For instance, a 5-cm coil is better than a larger coil for the imaging of the temporomandibular joint, but for the knee the coil should surround the leg in the region of the joint.

## 2.4 Pulse Sequences and Special Techniques

### 2.4.1 Spin-Echo Sequences

The distinguishing characteristic of the spin-echo (SE) sequence is the 180° RF pulse applied some time after the 90° pulse. This additional 180° pulse reestablishes the phase coherence and therefore reduces the loss in transverse magnetization. Thus the T2 component of the SE sequence is higher than in a normal FID sequence.

The SE pulse sequence was presented first by Hahn in 1950. Today it is the pulse sequence most commonly used in clinical MRI. The advantage of this sequence is the possibility of highlighting T1, T2, or spin-density effects by varying TE and TR. This is, because the three factors spin-density, T1 and T2 influence the SE signal depending on the TE and TR.

#### 2.4.1.1 T1-Weighted Sequences

If TE is set as short as possible and TR in the range of 200–700 ms, the T1 component of the signal will be high, resulting in a T1-weighted image. A typical example is the 500/20 (TR/TE) sequence.

#### 2.4.1.2 T2-Weighted and Spin-Density Sequences

Long TR (>1500 ms) provides a T2-weighted image, if additionally TE is in the range of 60–150 ms. If TE is reduced to below 40 ms and TR stays long the image will show a spin-density effect.

A frequently used T2-weighted sequence is the 3000/90 (TR/TE). Combining this sequence with the 3000/25 (TR/TE) as a double-echo sequence yields T2 and spin-density images in one scanning session. However, spin-density images do not have the same diagnostic value as T2-weighted images.

### 2.4.1.3 Clinical Applications

For head and neck lesions the SE sequence is the sequence of choice. The standard protocol comprises an axial T1-weighted sequence (500/25) and an axial T2-weighted sequence at the same slice positions. Depending on the lesion, an additional coronal or sagittal T1-weigthed scan may have to be done. The T1 SE sequence allows evaluation of tumor location, morphology, and infiltration assessment of surrounding structures and enables interpretation of changes in the CSF and the ventricular system. The SE sequence characterizes the pathology, permitting differentiation of solid and cystic tumor components and detection of regressive changes.

The administration of the contrast agent Gd-DTPA after the plain T1-sequence has proved optimal for differentiation of the tumor from the surrounding structures. The T1 of the tumor is reduced by the contrast medium.

### 2.4.2 Fast Imaging

The idea behind the gradient-echo (GE) pulse sequence introduced by Frahm and coworkers [25–27] is to shorten T2, resulting in a shorter measuring time. In the FLASH (fast low angle shot) sequence the 180° rephasing pulse used in SE sequences is eliminated and instead of the 90° pulse flip angles less than 90° are used. The signal obtained with GE imaging depends on the TR, TE, and flip angle. The T2 component of the signal is influenced by field strength and by inhomogeneities in magnetic susceptibility, because of the absence of the 180° pulse.

Thus, in most cases the T1 SE sequence can be replaced by the fast scanning technique, but a T2 SE sequence should be performed.

In the head and neck the fast scanning technique is used for imaging the enhancement provided by a contrast medium.

The most important parameter of T1 weighting is the flip angle. We use an angle of 30°–40°. TR and TE can be as short as possible and will not greatly influence the T1 component of the signal. The clinical advantage lies in better evaluation of the morphology of the lesion, especially in combination with dynamic scanning using the contrast medium Gd-DTPA.

### 2.4.3 MR Angiography: Basic Physics

The first studies of blood flow using MR were performed by Suryan in 1951 [37]. He observed that flowing liquid gave a higher signal than stationary liquid. With the development of the first imaging systems MRI soon proved superior to CT for the scanning of blood vessels. The first MR angiography (MRA) examinations employing the conventional SE sequences where flowing blood appears dark, displayed several limitations. The development of new techniques such as two-dimensional or three-dimensional flow-compensated gradient-echo sequences and RF presaturation vastly improved the visualization of the vasculature, as these techniques provide further information on velocity, volume, and direction of flow and on abnormalities or pathology of vessels. As MRA uses blood flow as a physiologic contrast medium, it therefore depends on numerous parameters which influence the appearance of flowing blood in MR images. These include tissue characteristics, imaging technique, and flow-related factors such as flow velocity, direction of flow, and flow profile (e.g., parabolic, plug).

Several magnetic effects influence the imaging of flowing blood in MR, making blood appear either bright or black. These effects are called saturation or "time-of-flight" effects and phase effects.

### 2.4.3.1 Hemodynamics

As MRA utilizes flowing blood for the visualization of the vasculature, some basic principles of flow have to be considered if MRA is to be performed with satisfactory results. Basically the signal intensity of flowing blood is influenced by a variety of parameters such as flow velocity (v), flow dynamics (d), density

($\varphi$), viscosity ($\eta$), and vessel diameter. This section briefly summarizes the influence of these parameters on the appearance of blood flow in MRI.

The most important single parameter for the visualization of the vasculature in MRI is the flow velocity, as the mode of vessel visualization depends on selection of the proper sequences, which in turn are predefined for imaging of either fast or slow blood. The consideration of flow velocity is especially important when flow-compensated GE sequences are being used.

The simplest model of a blood vessel is a cylindrical straight tube of length l and diameter d with constant flow. According to the principles of Bernoulli, flow velocity in a tube is at any two points of the tube the same, which is expressed by the formula

$$v_1 \times A_1 = v_2 \times A_2 \quad \text{or} \quad v_1 = v_2 \times (r_2/r_1)^2$$

where $v$ = velocity, $A$ = area and $r$ = tube radius. This formula also expresses the fact that, when vessel diameter is reduced by a factor of 2, e.g., due to a stenosis, flow velocity is increased by a factor of 4 within the stenosis [21].

In supraaortic vessels which are not pathologically altered the flow velocity is highest in the center of the vessel. With SE sequences, the more slowly flowing blood adjacent to the vessel wall is enhanced, whereas the faster flow in the center is imaged as flow void. This boundary layer effect is physically the result of frictional forces among blood particles and between vessel wall and flowing blood [17, 21, 30, 36].

### Laminar and Turbulent Flow

Laminar flow prevails when the layers of blood within the vessel glide along each other without actually mixing. An alteration of any of the parameters of blood flow leads to changes from laminar to turbulent flow, causing signal loss in flow-compensated GE imaging. The conditions for changes from laminar to turbulent flow are determined by the Reynolds number (Re):

$$Re = d \times v/\eta \text{ [21]}$$

The critical value above which laminar flow changes to turbulent flow is Re = 2320; however, much higher values for Re can be observed under physiologic conditions due to vessel curvature and oscillatory blood flow. For laminar flow the velocity profile, that is the distribution of velocities across the vessel lumen, is parabolic, whereas the velocity profile of turbulent flow is plug-like. Due to an increasing intravascular velocity, which predicts that flow layers no longer glide past each other, vortices are formed along the course of flow with little velocity variation across the vessel lumen.

### 2.4.3.2 Time-of-Flight Effects

Time-of-flight (TOF) effects are created by changes in longitudinal magnetization which are a function of the RF pulses employed and the T1 relaxation time [17, 36]. Basically, TOF effects can be explained by the motion of spins through an imaging slice. Depending on the type of pulse sequence used (SE or GE), one can distinguish between "wash-out effects" and inflow enhancement. A number of parameters influence the signal intensity of flowing blood, causing either high or low signal intensity.

*Wash-out effects* result in total signal void of flowing blood on SE sequences. In order to create a measurable signal, tissue must be exposed to both the 90° (labeling) and 180° (detecting) RF pulses, which are separated in time by TE/2. In conventional SE imaging blood flowing rapidly through the imaging slice is labeled by the first 90° RF pulse but has left the slice by the time of the 180° RF pulse, and is not visualized. In order for flowing blood, to return a high signal, the blood bolus has to remain within the imaging slice for at least TE/2 and thus be exposed to both RF pulses. These effects can be reduced by employment of GE sequences. A GE sequence is, expressed simply, an SE sequence which lacks the second RF pulse.

*Inflow enhancement* (paradoxical enhancement) can be observed with GE sequences and is caused by unsaturated spins of flowing

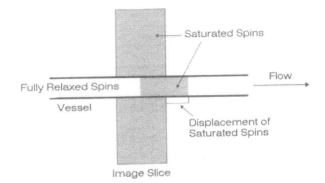

**Fig. 2.6.** Time-of-flight effect. Spins of stationary soft tissue are saturated after continuous RF pulses. Blood flowing into the imaging slice replaces saturated with unsaturated spins, causing high signal intensity compared with the adjacent soft tissue. (With courtesy to Dr. R. Hansmann, Siemens, FRG [36])

blood entering the imaging slice and replacing saturated spins (Fig. 2.6). Note that unsaturated blood flowing into an imaging slice produces a higher signal than stationary saturated tissue within the slice. During image acquisition the protons of stationary tissue are progressively saturated by continuous RF pulses. The signal intensity is proportional to the degree of saturation, flow velocity, and slice thickness. As flowing blood within an imaging slice is continuously provided with unsaturated spins, its signal intensity remains high, and flowing blood is therefore visualized with high signal intensity although its T1 relaxation time is long (1.2 s at 1.5 T) [36].

*Influence of TR*

The degree of saturation also depends on an equilibrium of TR and T1 (Fig. 2.7). The spins of stationary tissue are increasingly saturated if TR is shortened, with a resulting attenuation of signal intensity in GE sequences. Simultaneously, blood is also saturated, but is visualized with high signal intensity due to the fact that fresh unsaturated spins replace the saturated spins. Prolonged passage through an imaging slice, large imaging volumes, multislice imaging, and shortened TR raise the probability that flowing blood will become saturated.

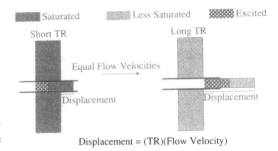

Displacement = (TR)(Flow Velocity)

**Fig. 2.7.** Influence of TR in SE sequences: With short TR (*left*), stationary tissue is partially saturated since the longitudinal magnetization can not fully recover between excitations. Saturated blood is replaced by unsaturated, providing high signal intensity in blood relative to the surrounding soft tissue. When TR is long (*right*), stationary tissue can recover between excitations, providing high signal intensity. Blood flows out of the imaging slice before refocusing, causing signal void [36]

### 2.4.3.3 Phase Effects

Phase effects are created by an alteration in transverse magnetization of spins moving through an applied gradient field, relative to stationary spins. These effects have different impacts on MR images, depending on intravascular flow behavior, and can be employed for the acquisition of flow images and for quantitative statements about flow velocity.

Basically, phase effects result from frequency encoding methods, which are used for spatial localization of a signal in the imaging plane [21, 35, 36]. Under the influence of an external magnetic field, spins defocus due to differences in their precessional frequency. This can be avoided by application of a second gradient in the opposite direction, which refocuses all spins at the echo time TE, enabling the recording of a measurable signal at the even echoes.

Flowing spins are also dephased by the external gradient, but, as they have changed location by the time of the second rephasing gradient, cannot be exactly refocused. The result is a net velocity-dependent flow phase producing a measurable signal. Spins moving in-plane along the frequency encoding gradient with the same velocity distribution across the vessel lumen all have the same phase shifts, resulting in a high signal intensity. With laminar velocity profiles, the faster-flowing spins in the center of a vessel accumulate a larger phase shift than the slower-flowing spins at the vessel boundary.

These intravoxel velocity differences, also referred to as velocity dephasing, produce a decrease in signal intensity and even may result in total signal loss (signal void). Note that any alteration of constant flow velocity (e.g., turbulent or pulsatile flow) results in additional phase shifts and a corresponding increase in velocity dephasing and leads to flow voids.

Any reduction of pixel size reduces these effects by decreasing the amount of spins included and therefore lowers phase dispersion and increases S/N.

### 2.4.3.4 Flow Compensation Technique

As described before, spins flowing through an imaging slice experience velocity dephasing with resulting signal reduction. These flow-induced phase shifts can be diminished with employment of additional gradient fields, which rephase stationary spins and spins flowing at constant velocity in even echoes. This technique is referred to as gradient motion rephasing (GMR; Fig. 2.8). The number of gradient fields applied depends on the type of motion within the imaging volume. "Higher order" motion, such as turbulent flow or acceleration, can be compensated by using more than three additional gradient fields, which, however, increases TE and makes the sequence more susceptible to artifacts.

Note that this technique does not increase the signal intensity of flowing blood, but merely restores it to a level comparable to that which could be achieved without velocity dephasing, e.g., to that of stationary blood.

### Magnitude Contrast MRA

In magnitude contrast angiography two sets of data are obtained, one with high signal intensity of vascular structures, acquired using the GMR technique, and a second, flow dephasing data set with low signal intensity. In order to reduce acquisition time and dis-

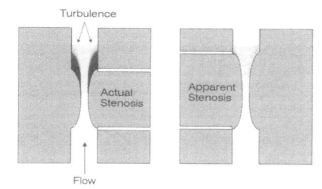

**Fig. 2.8.** Limitations of GMR. Turbulent flow, acceleration, other high-order motion proximal to the stenosis can not be compensated by constant velocity GMR, leading to signal voids proximal to the stenosis, This can lead to the stenosis being overestimated [36]

**Table 2.1.** Flow effects in MRA

*SE sequences*

Time-of-flight effects:
- Signal loss due to wash-out effects
- Signal loss due to RF presaturation
- High signal intensity due to slow blood flow, short TR, large imaging volumes

Phase effects:
- Boundary layer effect (donut sign)

*GE sequences*

Time-of-flight effects:
- Inflow enhancement
- Flow voids due to large imaging volumes

Phase effects:
- Flow enhancement due to GMR
- Flow enhancement due to small pixel size

**Table 2.2.** Performance of flow-imaging techniques in MRI

|  | 2D TOF | 3D TOF | Magnitude contrast | Phase contrast |
|---|---|---|---|---|
| Acquisition time | 3 | 3 | 2 | 1 |
| Spin saturation | 2 | 1 | 3 | 3 |
| Turbulence sensitivity | 2 | 3 | 1 | 1 |
| Pulsatile sensitivity | 2 | 3 | 1 | 1 |
| Spatial resolution | 3 | 3 | 2 | 3 |
| Direction sensitivity | 3 | 3 | 1 | 3 |
| T1 sensitivity | 3 | 1 | 3 | 3 |
| Background suppression | 2 | 1 | 3 | 3 |

1, average; 2, good; 3, excellent.

placement artifacts due to gross motion on the part of the patient, these two data sets are obtained in interleaved mode. An internal subtraction step totally eliminates soft tissue, which has the same signal intensity in both data sets, and leaves only vascular structures. A requirement for this technique is laminar blood flow, providing velocity dephasing, otherwise the dephasing sequence is not effective (Tables 2.1, 2.2).

The advantages of this technique are high sensitivity for slow blood flow, high spatial resolution, and total elimination of soft tissue. Disadvantages are higher sensitivity for turbulent flow artifacts, long acquisition time, and the lack of directional sensitivity [36].

*Inflow Angiography*

Inflow enhancement and GMR are powerful tools for producing flow images. An excited volume is partitioned into several contiguous thin slices using a second phase-encoding gradient, providing partial saturation of stationary soft tissue. Flowing blood replaces the saturated spins with unsaturated spins, causing the vessel to be visualized with bright signal intensity. Several factors influence the appearance of flowing blood on 3D or 2D inflow angiography. Depending on TR, the flip angle

$\alpha$, flow velocity, and slice thickness, blood will also become saturated after a certain distance. Slow-flowing spins are saturated shortly after entering a 3D volume, whereas fast-flowing spins can travel deeper into the volume before being saturated. The choice of sequence (3D FISP or 2D FLASH) therefore depends on the flow velocity. In addition, slice thickness must be kept to a minimum in order to obtain high-quality angiograms, avoid flow saturation, and increase spatial resolution (Fig. 2.9). Since constant velocity GMR is used, inflow angiography is rather sensitive to higher order motion such as acceleration or turbulence, resulting in velocity dephasing and signal loss. 3D FISP sequences, however, allow small pixel sizes which reduce phase dispersion effects. One of the major drawbacks of 3D inflow MRA is the fact that slow-flowing spins are saturated shortly after entering the imaging volume. This problem can be overcome with the employment of 2D multislice GE sequences (2D FLASH) with a slice thickness of 2–3 mm. Advantages of this technique are the ability to visualize slow-flowing blood over the entire 2D volume and the sensitivity for unidirectional flow. A major disadvantage is the fact that the slices do not have ideally rectangular slice profiles and that the thinnest slices are still thicker than those of 3D sequences. This leads to a diminishing of spatial

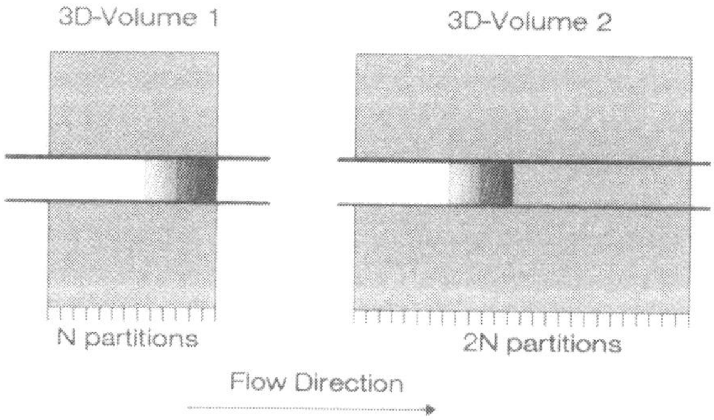

3D-Volume 1          3D-Volume 2

N partitions          2N partitions

Flow Direction

Fig. 2.9. Influence of slice thickness on signal intensity of flowing blood. Inflow is only effective to a limited slice thickness. Blood penetrating through large imaging volumes is continuously saturated, leading to progressive loss of signal intensity [36]

resolution and an increase in phase dispersion [30, 35, 36].

### 2.4.3.5 Flow Separation

Due to the multitude of vascular structures in the head and neck it is necessary to perform selective arterial or venous MRA, using one of several subtraction or presaturation techniques. The most common method for selective MRA is the application of a presaturation RF pulse close to the imaging volume, which suppresses flow-related enhancement. Blood flowing through the saturation slice appears dark in the imaging volume. This technique allows selective arterial MRA through the elimination of venous flow and vice versa (Fig. 2.10).

Another method for selective MRA is the subtraction technique, which requires the acquisition of two sets of data. This is usually achieved by means of a rephasing/dephasing FISP 3D sequence, followed by internal subtraction. A major disadvantage of this technique is the doubling of acquisition time with a resulting increase of artifacts due to gross motion or pulsation [30, 33, 35].

### 2.4.3.6 Postprocessing of MRA Images

The Maximum-intensity projection (MIP) technique is used to process a series of slices acquired by 2D or 3D methods. Several parallel rays, each representing one pixel, are projected through the original data set. With the ray-tracing method only pixels with the brightest voxel are projected on the final image. Since the brightest voxel usually represents only vascular structures, soft tissue is eliminated (Fig. 2.11). MIP allows reconstruction in multiple projections or fully rotatable 3D images. In some cases, e.g., after Gd-DTPA injection, soft tissue also contains bright voxels and can not be subtracted with the MIP algorithm.

*Cine Mode.* MIP provides the possibility to perform repeated projections with an increase of the rotation angle after each projection. Displaying these projections in a cine loop provides the impression that the vessels are rotating in space. This technique is especially useful for evaluating of vessels that normally obscure each other.

*Targeted MIP.* The reduction of the region of interest for MIP processing in the original MRA data set not only reduces computing time, but also increases spatial resolution and image quality. This is because fewer random pixels and less soft tissue with high signal intensity (e.g., fatty tissue) are included in the projection [1, 36].

### 2.4.4 3D Imaging

New techniques in CT and MR enable 3D-reconstruction of lesions. This increases the value of these imaging modalities for diagnosis and especially for the planning of surgery and radiotherapy. The idea of 3D imaging is not

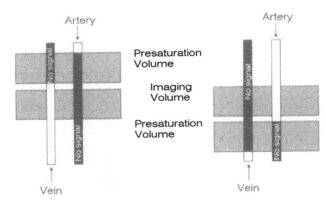

**Fig. 2.10.** Flow separation. Localization of additional RF pulses above (*left*) or below (*right*) the imaging volume eliminates either arterial (*left*) or venous (*right*) blood flow [36]

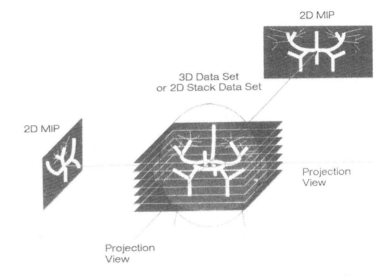

**Fig. 2.11.** Maximum-intensity projection (*MIP*): The 3D or 2D data set is computed with ray-tracing algorithm, projecting only voxels with maximum intensity onto a 2D plane [36]

new; it was originally presented in 1975 for use in the reconstruction of fractures. The technique of 3D CT has become more widespread over the past 10 years and is now frequently used in clinical practice.

3D MRI, however, is a very young discipline and much less experience has been accumulated and reported. Especially in the head and neck, 3D visualization of the structures is difficult due to topographical complexity. Nevertheless, this new technique demonstrates head and neck lesions excellently. Special hardware and software are required, either in the form of a separate workstation or built into the standard tomograph. 3D MRI is most often performed using a 3D FLASH sequence with and without the contrast medium Gd-DTPA. For 3D reconstruction, contiguous MR slices define a 3D lattice of data that is then analyzed by a succession of rays descending through the data cube from a point of view outside the original data set. This ray-tracing mode (Fig. 2.12) reconstructs the surface of the patient's head, resulting in an ex-

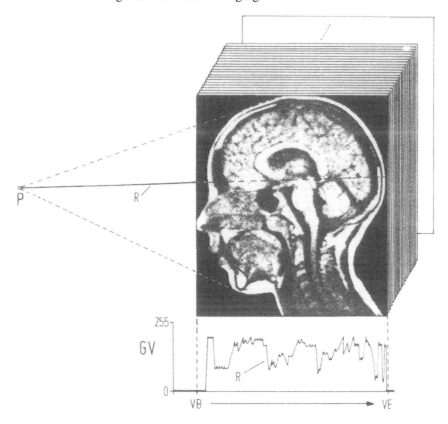

**Fig. 2.12.** Ray-tracing method. Contiguous MR slices define a lattice of data that is detected by a succession of rays descending through the data cube from a point of view outside the original data set. The gray values of one of the rays which traces each of the slices are demonstrated in the curve under the image. *GV*, gray value; *R*, ray; *VB*, volume beginning; *VE*, volume end; *P*, point of view

cellent 3D simulation (Fig. 2.13 a). The progress in the quality of computer reconstruction becomes apparent by comparing the reconstruction with a photograph of the patient (Fig. 2.13 b).

To display the lesion inside the reconstructed head a section has to be "cut off", exposing the relevant structures (Fig. 2.14). In order to cut off part of the data cube of this selected region of interest within a chosen slice, it has to be marked by overlaying a window. This window is displayed within the 3D-reconstructed head projecting the relevant parts of the original slice. The most important step is the determination of the location and size of the window.

These parameters are determined in cooperation with the clinicians and vary depending on the kind of lesion. In all cases the results of the 3D FLASH technique are compared with those of an SE examination regarding the characteristics of the lesion and its demarcation from the surrounding tissue. It is assumed that 3D FLASH imaging has a higher S/N than 2D imaging. The reason for this is that each section in a 3D acquisition of 128 sections contributes signals 128 times more often than with 2D FLASH. The result is a better S/N, if all parameters of the sequences are identical. But this is not realistic because the total imaging time of the 3D acquisition would be 128 times greater. Thus, TR has to be decreased to 40 ms. Comparison of the S/N and C/N of 2D FLASH, T1-weighted SE, T2-weighted SE, and 3D FLASH reveals that the SE technique is superior in this respect. For

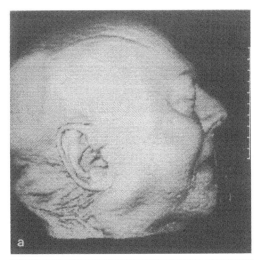

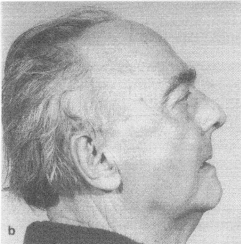

**Fig. 2.13a, b.** Comparison of 3D reconstruction and photograph of patient
**a** 3D reconstruction by the technique
**b** Photograph of the patient

the moment, then, the SE technique has a higher diagnostic value than the 3D technique [3–8].

The 3D examination, however, enables simultaneous viewing of multiple slices in different orientations relative to the surface of the head. Therefore, although this method has no additional diagnostic value, it is useful in evaluating the lesions with respect to the planning of surgery or radiotherapy. Using a separate workstation with a high-speed image processor for planning, all slices acquired by the 3D examination can be interactively demonstrated and the primarily sagittal slices transformed into each required orientation. These 3D reconstructions can be used to visualize the anatomic relationships and pathologic structures encountered during surgery. A series of 3D reconstructions should be calculated following the path that will be taken by the surgeons.

In tumors affecting the neck, glomus tumors, adenomas, hemangiomas, and metastases of other tumors, 3D images can be obtained from any angle visualizing the tumor and its relation to the surrounding structures. The tumor's relation to the carotid artery and the jugular vein is of particular diagnostic significance [9, 10, 12, 13]. The topography of the nasopharynx and the muscles is also important and can be depicted in good detail with the 3D technique owing to the slice thickness of 1–2 mm. Vascularization of lesions has been studied with and without Gd-DTPA. In 80% of tumors there is a significant increase in signal intensity with the contrast medium. The current most widespread method of analyzing MR images is sequential observation of individual 2D slices and subsequent "mental reconstruction" of the topography. However, the important aspects of lesions are much easier to evaluate on 3D-reconstructed images. The technical progress to reach the current 3D techniques has been impressive indeed. In some disciplines, such as orthopedics, neurosurgery, and angiography, 3D reconstructions have already proved their clinical worth. The clinical promise of 3D MRI is just as great as that of 3D CT, but several limitations have emerged [24]. The extent of the lesion and the pattern of infiltration can be demonstrated in a series of 3D reconstructions with varying window depth. It has been shown that width and orientation of the window are decisive parameters of the value of the 3D image. The wider the window, the better the evaluability of the structures of interest and the surrounding tissues. However, topographic landmarks such as nose, cheek, and eye are lost when a wide window is selected. For this reason the width of the window should be chosen for each patient individually, depending on the

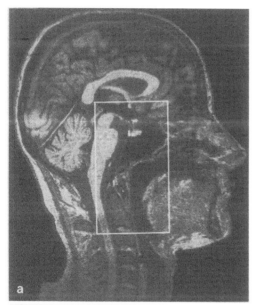

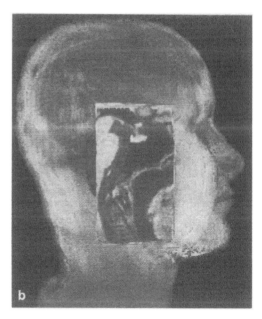

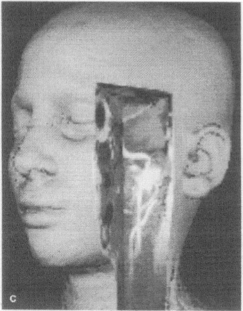

**Fig. 2.14a–c.** 3D reconstruction of the head of a volunteer
**a** Image in sagittal plane
**b** 3D reconstruction with adapted window
**c** 3D reconstruction on a 1.5-T machine, ray-tracing technique

location and extent of the lesion, to optimize the diagnostic value of the 3D reconstruction technique. A further step in investigation will be T2-weighted FLASH sequences to improve the sensitivity and specificity of this fast imaging procedure.

## 2.5 Biologic Effects and Safety Considerations

The diagnostic advantages of MR tomography and spectroscopy have led to widespread use of this new imaging method. The safety regulations that govern the use of medical equipment demand extensive knowledge of the effects of magnetic and electromagnetic fields on the human body. This is of particular concern regarding the exposure of the whole body or part of the body to static and dynamic magnetic fields. Apart from the known effects on ferromagnetic objects such as prostheses, surgical clips, and pacemakers, no adverse effect on health has yet been established [38]. Nevertheless, the various fields do induce reversible biologic effects [39].

In 1981 the British National Radiological Protection Board established guidelines for the operation of MR units, and similar guide-

**Table 2.3.** Limits of exposure to MR laid down by national bodies in the UK, USA, and FRG

| | NRPB (1981, 1983) | BRH (1981) | BGA (1983) |
|---|---|---|---|
| Static magnetic field | 2.5 T (whole and partial body) | 2 T (whole and partial body) | 2 T (whole and partial body) |
| Changing magnetic fields | 20 T/s for SP 10 ms and longer; $\left(\dfrac{a\beta}{at}\right)^2 t < 4$ for SP shorter than 10 ms | 3 T/s (whole and partial body) | Max. 3 μA/cm$^3$ or 3 mV/cm for SP 10 ms and longer; 30/τ μA/cm$^2$ or 30/τ μV/cm for Sp shorter than 10 ms (τ in ms) |
| Radio-frequency fields | 1 °C increase of body temperature SAR = 0.4 W/kg (whole body), SAR = 4 W/kg (av$^1$) | SAR = 0.4 W/kg (whole body); SAR = 2 W/kg (av$^1$) | SAR = 1 W/kg (whole body); SAR = 5 W/kg (partial body for every 1 kg of tissue excl. eye) |

*SP*, switching period; *SAR*, specific absorption rate; av$^1$, averaged over any 1 g of tissue.
NRPB, British National Radiological Protection Board; BRH, US Bureau of Radiological Health; BGA, German Federal Board of Health.

lines were adopted 1 year later by the US Bureau of Radiological Health (Table 2.3). However, these guidelines are only temporary recommendations and are somewhat arbitrary. Similar recommendations have been issued by agencies in other countries, such as the Federal Board of Health in the Federal Republic of Germany.

The constant technological improvement and the continuing increase in magnetic field strengths are leading to increasingly better images and to shorter examination times. Commercial MR units with static magnetic fields between 0.5 T and 2 T are now being used. There is a tendency in the areas of research and spectroscopy toward higher field strengths of up to 4 T. Side effects from these strong magnetic fields can in all probability be expected.

## 2.5.1 Biologic Effects

### 2.5.1.1 Static Magnetic Fields

It has been shown that static magnetic fields can influence electromagnetic processes in organisms. These effects include impulse conduction in the heart (ECG), the velocity of nerve conduction, and membrane potentials (Fig. 2.15). The extent of the effects depends on the strength of the field. At a strength of above 2 T a decrease in nerve conduction velocity and effects on enzyme reaction have been found, while between 0.35 T and 1 T orientation effects on DNA and on retina cells are seen.

Static magnetic fields of strengths greater than 0.3 T are associated with abnormalities clearly visible on the ECG. The changes in the T wave are related to induced potentials, resulting from the flow of blood through the field. This flow in turn is dependent on field strength, flow velocity, and the diameter of the vessel in question.

Our own studies on 20 volunteers using field strengths of 0.35 T and 1 T showed that the static magnetic field induces no arrhythmia and no change in the heart rate. However, it does produce a slight increase in the T-wave amplitude and artificial waves following the QRS complex.

Studies have demonstrated no reproducible mutagenic effects or effects on hematopoietic and other fast-growing tissues [40]. Static magnetic fields could conceivably affect different molecules whose magnetic properties vary with direction. The field reorients these molecules and changes their position in larger molecular aggregates. This could lead to changes in enzyme kinetics. Thus, it is recommended that checks on the circulatory system

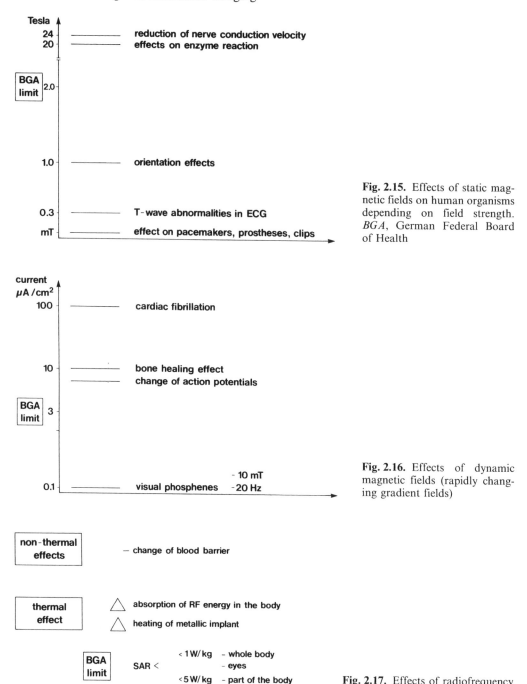

Fig. 2.15. Effects of static magnetic fields on human organisms depending on field strength. *BGA*, German Federal Board of Health

Fig. 2.16. Effects of dynamic magnetic fields (rapidly changing gradient fields)

Fig. 2.17. Effects of radiofrequency

should be performed if a static magnetic field strength higher than 2 T is used.

### 2.5.1.2 Rapidly Changing Gradient Fields

Rapidly changing magnetic fields are superimposed on the main static field to obtain spatial information in MR imaging. These gradient fields, changing at up to 3 T/s, generate interval electric currents of 3 μAs by means of induction (Fig. 2.16). The best-documented effect of these fields is the induction of visual light flashes known as magnetic phosphenes. These have a threshold field change of 2–5 T/s. Stimulation of the action potential in nerves and muscles is found at currents greater than 0.9 μA. The most important potential hazard is cardiac fibrillation; this effect is dangerous only at currents of 80 μA or more.

### 2.5.1.3 Radiofrequency Pulses

Radiofrequency pulses do have nonthermal effects, but the main concern relates to possible thermal reactions. Specific absorption rate (SAR) is used to measure these effects and serves as a parameter for RF radiation. The limit fixed for exposure of the whole body is 1 W/kg and for part of the body 5 W/kg (Fig. 2.17). Theoretical estimates of the RF radiation absorbed during MRI vary between 1 and 100 mW/kg body weight. Our experiments have shown that neither the central body temperature nor the peripheral temperature in humans undergoes any significant change during MRI for clinical purposes with magnetic field strengths of up to 1.5 T.

The use of some special coils in MRI might harbor some risk. Usually, surface coils are constructed strictly for receiving, however, unfavorable coupling of the transmitting and receiving coils due to switching errors or to incorrect positioning might amplify the RF field in the area of the coil, causing the release of higher energy to adjacent tissues.

## 2.5.2 Safety Considerations

The MR imaging environment has well-documented effects upon hardware such as ferromagnetic instruments, prostheses and implants.

### 2.5.2.1 Loose and Removable Metallic Objects

Loose ferromagnetic objects may become projectiles, moving into the magnetic field and causing serious injury. The force of attraction depends on the size and shape of the ferromagnetic object, its distance from the magnet, and its susceptibility to magnetization. This serious danger can be avoided by having all staff and patients pass through a metal detector gate before entering the magnet room. Removable metallic objects such as hairclips and earrings should be taken off and stored safely during the examination.

### 2.5.2.2 Implanted Metallic Objects

Exposure to MR of a patient with a metallic implant can have grave consequences. Serious harm may be done by heating, torque, and electrical interaction.

#### Cardiac Pacemakers

Cardiac pacemakers are an absolute contraindication to MR imaging. Persons with pacemakers should remain outside the 5 G ($5 \times 10^{-4}$ T) line of the field around the magnet, which should be specially marked around all MR units.

The static magnetic field exerts a twisting force on the pacemaker, potentially damaging or dislocating the leads. Static magnetic fields and RF energy may interfere with the demand function of the pacemakers, and varying fields and RF energy can induce electric potentials. These effects could simulate normal heart activity, causing the pacemaker to cease cardiac excitation.

### Heart Valve Prostheses

Artificial valves manufactured before 1984 can contain ferromagnetic materials and thus contraindicate MRI. All modern valves are nonferromagnetic and hence safe.

### Surgical Clips

Hemostatic or aneurysm clips have a high nickel content and so can experience torque when the patient is moved into the MR scanner. Intracranial aneurysm clips are recognized as a contraindication for most MR examinations; any significant torque may cause damage to a vessel. The nonferromagnetic aneurysm clips available today do not preclude MRI. Patients with surgical clips in other areas of the body can be examined without any danger, provided more than 2 weeks have elapsed since the operation and the clip is fixed within connective tissue.

### Orthopedic Implants

Most stainless steel orthopedic implants and prostheses are not ferromagnetic and so no harm is caused by MRI. Due to the high conductivity of metal, artificial hips or dentures may absorb considerable RF energy during long imaging sequences and can undergo significant heating. Numerous patients with prosthetic implants have undergone MRI, and no side effects have yet been reported.

#### 2.5.2.3 Metallic Foreign Bodies

Routine practice in an MR department must exclude the presence of a metallic foreign bodies in patients and members of staff. Slivers of metal in the eye are a known danger, and in the case of doubt lateral skull radiography has to be performed. Metal workers are especially at risk.

### 2.5.3 Summary

The hazards presented by hardware such as metallic implants and ferromagnetic hospital devices are of critical importance in the operation of clinical MR systems.
Strict criteria should be applied to the selection of women during the early weeks of pregnancy.
For MR units of up to 1.5 T, there is no indication of any significant influence on living organisms.
The current tendency in MR technology however, is towards higher strengths of magnetic field and RF energy. This calls for extensive investigation of possible effects on the human cardiovascular system and thermoregulation.

*The absolute contraindications to MRI are*:

- Cardiac pacemaker
- Other electromechanical implants
- Intracranial aneurysm clips (ferromagnetic)
- Heart valve prostheses (ferromagnetic)
- Metallic splinters in the brain or near a blood vessel

## References

1. Anderson C, Saloner D, Tsuruda J et al. (1990) Artefacts in maximum-intensity-projection display of MR angiograms. AJR 154:623–629
2. Aue WP (1983) Topische Kernspin-Resonanz – eine nichtinvasive Sonde für biochemische Messungen in Lebewesen. Radiologie 23:357–360
3. Bauer M, Obermüller H, Vogl T, Lissner J (1984) MR bei zerebraler alveolärer Echinokokkose. Digitale Bilddiagn 4:S 129–131
4. Bauer M, Baierl P, Vogl T, Wendt T, Lissner J (1986) Efficacy and secondary intracranial tumors before and after radiotherapy. Society of Magnetic Resonance in Medicine, 5th annual meeting, Montreal, Canada. Book of abstracts vol 3, pp 590–591
5. Bauer M, Baierl P, Fink U, Vogl T, Rohloff R (1986) Verlaufskontrolle von primären und sekundären Hirntumoren nach Strahlentherapie mittels Kernspintomographie im Vergleich zur Computertomographie. In: Vogler E, Schneider GH (eds) Digitale bildgebende Verfahren – Integrierte digitale Radiologie. 84th Radiological Symposium, Graz, 3–5 at 1985. Schering, Berlin, pp 151–155
6. Bauer M, Fenzl G, Vogl T, Fink U, Lissner J (1986) Indications for the use of Gd-DTPA in MR of the CNS. Invest Radiol 5:12
7. Bauer WM, Baierl P, Obermüller H, Bise K, Valenti M (1985) Comparison of plain and contrast-enhanced MR in intracranial tumors – report on 37 cases confirmed by histology. In: Society of Magnetic resonance, 4th annual meeting, London. Book of abstracts, pp 310–311
8. Bauer WM, Baierl P, Vogl T, Obermüller H (1985) Contrast-enhancement in intercranial tumors – a comparison of CT and MR. Radiology 157 (P):126
9. Becker H, Vogelsang H, Schwarzrock R (1985) Vergleichende MR- und CT-Untersuchungen bei ausgewählten neuroradiologischen Fragestellungen. RÖFO 142:23–30
10. Becker H, Naumann H, Pfalz C (1982) HNO-Heilkunde. Thieme, Stuttgart
11. Beimert U, Grevers G, Vogl T (1988) Zum Stellenwert der digitalen Subtraktionsangiographie bei der Diagnostik von Glomustumoren. Arch Otorhinolaryngol [Suppl II]:100–101
12. Bender A, Bradac GB (1986) Erfahrungen in der radiologischen Diagnostik kleiner Akustikusneurinome. Rontgengenblätter 39:36–39
13. Bentson J (1980) Combined gascisternography and edge enhanced computed tomography of the internal auditory canal. Radiology 136:777–779
14. Bottomley PA, Foster TH, Aegersinger RE, Pfeiffer LM (1984) A review of normal tissue hydrogen NMR relaxation times and relaxation mechanism from 1–1000 MHz: dependence on tissue type, NMR frequency, temperature, species, excision and age. Med Phys 11:112
15. Bongartz G, Vestring T, Fahrendorf G, Peters PE (1990) Einsatz schneller Sequenzen bei der kraniozerebralen MR-Diagnostik. Fortschr Geb Rontgenstr 153(6):669–677
16. Brindle KM, Campbell ID (1984) Hydrogen nuclear magnetic resonance studies of cells and tissues. In: James TL (ed) Biomedical magnetic resonance. Radiol Research and Education Foundation, San Francisco, pp 243–255
17. Brown DG, Riederer SJ, Jack CR et al. (1990) MR-angiography with oblique gradient-recalled echo technique. Radiology 176:461–466
18. Carpinelli G, Podo F, Di Vito M, Gresser I, Proietti E, Belardelli F (1985) 31P-NMR study on metabolic modulations of phosphomonoesters and phosphodiesters in experimental tumors during regression in vivo. Society of Magnetic Resonance in Medicine, 4th annual meeting, London. Book of abstracts, p 454
19. Creasy JL, Price RR, Presbrey T et al. (1990) Gadolinium-enhanced MR-angiography. Radiology 175:280–283
20. Dumoulin CL, Souza SP, Walker MF, Wagle W (1989) Three dimensional phase contrast angiography. Magn Reson Med 9:139–149
21. Edelman RR, Hesselink JR (1990) Clinical magnetic resonance imaging. Saunders, Philadelphia, pp 110–182
22. Edelman RR, Mattle HP, Atkinson DJ, Hoogewoud HM (1990) Magnetic resonance angiography. In: Cardiovascular imaging. American Roentgen Ray Society, Categorial Course Syllabus, pp 51–60
23. Edelman RR, Wentz KU, Mattle HP et al. (1989) Intracerebral arteriovenous malformations: evaluation with selective MR-angiography and venography. Radiology 173:831–837
24. Ehricke H-H, Laub G (1990) Integrated 3D display of brain anatomy and intracranial vasculature in MR imaging. J Comput Assist Tomogr 14 (6):846–852
25. Frahm J, Haase A, Mathai D et al. (1985) FLASH MR imaging: from images to movies. Radiology 157:156 (Abstract)
26. Frahm J, Merbold KD, Hänike W, Haase A (1985) Stimulated echo imaging. J Magn Reson 64:81–93
27. Frahm J, Haase A, Matthaei D (1986) Rapid three-dimensional MR imaging using the FLASH-technique. J Comput Assist Tomogr 10:363–368
28. Krayenbühl H, Yaşargil MG (1979) Zerebrale Angiographie für Klinik und Praxis, 3rd edn. Thieme, Stuttgart, pp 38–241
29. Lauterbur PC (1973) Image formation by induced local interactions. Examples employing NMR. Nature 242:190

30. Lissner J, Seiderer M (1990) Klinische Kern-spintomographie, 2nd fully revised edn. Encke, Stuttgart, pp 59–83, 570–607
31. Marchal G, Bosmans H, van Fraeyenhoven L et al. (1990) Intracranial vascular lesions: optimization and clinical evaluation of three dimensional time of flight MR-angiography. Radiology 175:443–448
32. Masaryk TJ, Modic MT, Ruggieri PM et al. (1989) Three-dimensional (volume) gradient-echo imaging of the carotid bifurcation preliminary clinical experience. Radiology 171:801–806
33. Nadel L, Braun IF, Kraft KA, Fatouros PP, Laine FJ (1990) Intracranial vascular abnormalities: values of MR phase imaging to distinguish thrombus from flowing blood. AJNR 11:1133–1140
34. Peters PE, Bongartz G, Drews C (1990) Magnetresonanzangiographie der hirnversorgenden Arterien. Fortschr Rontgenstr 152(5):528–533

35. Sevick RJ, Tsuruda JS, Schmalbrock P (1990) Three-dimensional time-of-flight MR angiography in the evaluation of cerebral aneurysms. J Comput Assist Tomogr 14(6):874–881
36. Siemens (1990) Angiography Numaris II/Version A 2.1, Edition 05/1990: Magnetom SP User Guide. Siemens AG, Erlangen, FRG
37. Suryan G (1951) Nuclear resonance in flowing liquids. Proc Indian Acad Sci Sect A 33:107
38. Vogl T (1988) Influence of MR imaging on the human organism. Enke, Stuttgart
39. Vogl T, Paulus W, Fuchs A, Krafczyk S, Lissner J (1991) Influence of magnetic resonance imaging on evoked potentials and nerve conduction velocities in humans. Invest Radiol 26:432–437
40. Vogl T, Krimmel K, Fuchs A, Lissner J (1988) Influence of magnetic resonance imaging on human body core and intravascular temperature. Medical Physics 15:4:562–566

# 3 Examination Technique

All of the MRI examinations presented in this book were carried out on superconducting MRI devices (Siemens Magnetom). In the period from 1 July 1984 to 31 December 1985 the studies were conducted at a field strength of 0.35 T. After upgrading to 1.0 T (gradient field 6 mT) in January of 1986 special sequences, software and surface coils for studies in the head and neck region were developed. Single measurements were carried out on prototypes devices in the Siemens research center in Erlangen, Germany. Since spring 1990 numerous studies have been performed on a 1.5-T machine of the newest generation (Magnetom 63 SP). All examinations are conducted only after intensive investigation and questioning of the patient about possible risks. Every subject has to give written consent for the procedure to be carried out; an additional briefing is given during the clinical examination if administration of the contrast agent Gd-DTPA is planned (phase III trials). Depending on the protocol the examination lasts between 30 and 60 min. About 1% of examinations have to be aborted because of claustrophobic reactions on the part of the patient.

## 3.1 Coil Technology

The complexity of the topographic relations in the head and neck requires adaptation of the examination technique to meet the needs of each individual patient [1]. The three-dimensional resolution and S/N achieved using the body coil are totally unsatisfactory for this area. Most examinations of the petrous part of the temporal bone, the middle skull base and the salivary glands are carried out using the standard headcoil supplied by the manufacturer. The field of this coil is 30 cm in diameter. With a matrix of $256 \times 256$ pixels the spatial resolution is 1 mm³. In the case of lesions of the middle ear and the internal auditory canal selected patients are additionally examined using a round surface coil developed in cooperation with Siemens, Erlangen. This supplementary hardware yields a further improvement in spatial resolution. For the oropharynx and neck region we use the Helmholtz coil of our own design. The S/N with this coil is 4.3 times better than with the head coil, and the spatial resolution is 1 mm³. With this arrangement the primary tumor and the cervical lymph node masses can be staged in one procedure without having to reposition the patient.

## 3.2 Sequences and Specific Examination Protocols

A variety of MR examination sequences and parameters are available for the head and neck. After extensive preliminary studies emphasis is now placed on SE sequences and fast imaging techniques. Two types of examinations can be distinguished: rapid sequences for morphologic image interpretation, and dynamic investigation of contrast enhancement.

### 3.2.1 Petrous Part, Middle Skull Base, and Face

For general clinical purposes axial images using long and short TR (2000–3000/25,90 and 500/25) are performed after a sagittal scout sequence (Table 3.1). The slice thickness should not exceed 4 mm, and in no case are gaps between slices permitted. This protocol is concluded with a short coronal sequence; if

**Table 3.1.** Examination protocol for MRI of the temporal bone and middle skull base

| Sequence number | Plane | Mode | TR (ms) | TE (ms) | Slice thickness (mm) |
|---|---|---|---|---|---|
| 1 | Sagittal | SE | 200 | 30 | 10 |
| 2 | Axial | SE | 2000 | 25/90 | 4 |
| 3 | Axial | SE | 500 | 25 | 4 |
| | Dynamic MRI (FLASH) with Gd-DTPA (0.1 mmol/kg BW), GE mode, time 8 min | | | | |
| 4 | Axial | SE | 500 | 25 | 4 |
| 5 | Coronal | SE | 500 | 25 | 4 |

necessary, a paraaxial plane along the vestibulocochlear nerve can be imaged.

In more than 70% of examinations Gd-DTPA is injected, at a dose of 0.1 mmol/kg body weight. Axial and coronal sequences are then performed with short TR. The dynamics of contrast agent uptake is analyzed and evaluated regarding differential diagnosis (Chap. 4). In most cases the time-consuming T2-weighted sequence is dropped if an acoustic neuroma is suspected.

### 3.2.2 Oropharynx and Neck

In the oropharynx and neck examinations are performed solely with the Helmholtz neck coil. As in the other regions of the head and neck, T1- and T2-weighted sequences are the gold standard. Swallowing motions impair image quality in 18% of examinations. In some patients dynamic MRI is used to determine tumor vascularization. Depending on the clinical and endoscopic localization of a process images are obtained in the coronal or sagittal plane.

## 3.3 Fast Sequences and Dynamic MRI

When Gd-DTPA is used to assist diagnosis, T1-weighted sequences are routinely performed before and after administration of the paramagnetic contrast agent. The good S/N results in superb topographic resolution. The velocity of contrast agent uptake can not be measured effectively because the characteristic differences in signal intensity appear during the first few minutes after administration. Such measurement demands a shorter sequence in order to register the variations in signal intensity as exactly as possible. The more times this sequence is started consecutively, the more precisely the storage of contrast enhancement can be documented.

In dynamic MRI, carried out in slices that show the lesion optimally, GE sequences are performed before and after administration of Gd-DTPA. With this technique the ordinary SE experiment is modified by elimination of the 180° high-frequency pulse. The refocusing of the spin is achieved by inversion of the gradient direction. In this way TR is shortened. Provided the excitation angle is smaller than 90° and TR is significantly shorter than T1, a balance between excitation and longitudinal relaxation is achieved.

In rapid imaging, contrast is achieved not by modification of TR, but by variation of the excitation angle. In order to get GE images with high signal intensity as well as the best possible contrast we utilize an excitation angle of 30°. TE is fixed at 12 ms for technical reasons. With a matrix of $256 \times 256$ pixels and optimal acquisition of data, imaging times shorter than 5 s are possible. Several technical modifications are possible, under the condition of a short acquisition time, that offer a good S/N and satisfactory resolution.

The GE sequence we use is started every 30s during the phase of rapid contrast agent uptake by the tumor. After 120 s the rhythm is changed to 60 s. After 360 s the examination is completed, and the T1-weighted sequence presented above is performed to record the details. This procedure is useful for simultaneous evaluation of morphology and dynamic contrast enhancement.

## Reference

1. Requard H, Sauter R, Bayerl J, Weber H (1987) Helmholtzspulen in der Kernspintomographie. Electromedia 55 (2):61–67

# 4 Contrast Media

Magnetic resonance imaging is being used with increasing frequency for the evaluation of diseases in the head and neck. MRI, with its superior soft tissue contrast, depicts tumor margins more clearly than CT and differentiates inflammatory changes more accurately from solid space-occupying lesions. Knowledge of not only the exact topographic relations, but also the vascular supply and the degree of vascularization, is essential for preoperative diagnosis. With the introduction of the paramagnetic contrast medium Gd-DTPA, which helps provide this information, the superiority of MRI over other imaging modalities in the assessment of lesions in the neck is increasing even further [4, 5].

Initially it seemed that the excellent soft tissue contrast obtained with plain MRI would obviate the need for contrast media, retaining the advantage of a completely noninvasive procedure. However, in view of the improved diagnostic accuracy achieved with iodinated contrast media in general radiology and CT, contrast agents for MRI were developed. This chapter will provide the reader with an understanding of the physical principles of contrast enhancement in MRI and describe specific pharmacologic paramagnetic contrast agents and their applications in various areas of the head and neck.

The following advantages are expected from the use of contrast media in MRI:

1. *Increased sensitivity* via contrast enhancement of small tumors
2. *Increased specificity* via characteristic enhancement patterns of different lesions
3. *Information on tissue perfusion* via dynamic scanning before and after administration of the contrast agent
4. *Reduction of examination time*
5. *Information on motion disorders of the pharynx and esophagus* via oral administration

## 4.1 Basic Principles

In 1946 Bloch [2] found that the T1 nuclear relaxation rate of water protons could be enhanced by the addition of paramagnetic agents such as nitrate. In 1973 Lauterbur [6] described the use of paramagnetic contrast agents in experimental animals. The "ideal" contrast-enhancing agent should be nontoxic and highly effective with its effect confined to specific areas. Additionally the substance should have good water solubility and should be rapidly excreted. Parenteral paramagnetic contrast agents were first used in man in the early 1980s and clinical trials have shown the contrast medium Gd-DTPA to be beneficial and safe for use in MRI. Experimental and clinical studies on other paramagnetic materials such as Fe, nitroxide, and various chelates are currently under way.

The production of contrast by the increased absorption of X-rays, as with conventional contrast media, is not applicable to MRI, because the source of the signal lies within the body itself. It is not reasonable to introduce extra protons to enhance contrast because of the extremely high proton concentration in the body. The effects of contrast media in MRI can, therefore, only be due to changes in parameters such as T1, T2, and proton density.

### 4.1.1 The Theory of Proton Relaxation

Some knowledge of the theory of proton relaxation is helpful in understanding how paramagnetic contrast media exert their effect. Unenhanced MRI provides its contrast by the difference in relaxation times of protons in various tissues.

In conventional SE imaging the T1 (spin-lattice or longitudinal) relaxation time, the T2 (spin-spin or transverse) relaxation time, proton density and signal void caused by flowing blood are responsible for providing contrast.

Proton relaxation theory can perhaps best be understood through basis quantum mechanics. Protons in nature possess angular momentum or spin, which leads to a magnetic moment associated with the proton. This magnetic moment $\mu$ is an expression of the direction and strength of the magnetic field around the proton and can be represented as a vector quantity. Until placed in a static magnetic field ($B_0$), protons normally exist in a random array. Under the influence of the static magnetic field, hydrogen protons exist in one of two states, aligned either parallel (spin up), which means a low energy level, or antiparallel (spin down) with the magnetic field. The basis for the generation of the MR signal is the so-called net magnetic moment, which arises because slightly more of the protons are in the low energy level or parallel state when placed in the magnetic field.

When an RF pulse is introduced at the frequency of the nuclear precession of the protons, magnetic resonance is induced, converting some of the protons from their low-energy state to their high-energy state. By means of transverse magnetization perpendicular to the static magnetic field (created by a 90° RF pulse) magnetic resonance absorption of the RF pulse can be detected. In SE imaging a second 180° RF refocusing pulse is applied and after a period of time an RF signal is detected. By Fourier transformation the intensity of this signal is converted to an intensity of gray on the final MR image. Two relaxation processes, which can be examined individually, are induced by the loss of energy on the part of the excited protons after the end of the RF pulse:

*T1 relaxation time*
- *Longitudinal relaxation:* the time taken for the net proton magnetic moment to return to its original orientation
- *Spin-lattice relaxation:* the time taken for the protons to release their excess energy to their surroundings

*T2 relaxation time*
- *Spin-spin relaxation:* the process whereby the excited proton exchanges excess energy with other protons

The signal intensity of tissues in conventional SE images is therefore, a function of both T1 and T2 relaxation times. Overall, proton relaxation enhancement produces shortening of both T1 and T2, which are, however, competing effects. On the other hand, MR signal intensity can be increased by shortening T1 or prolonging T2. The predominant effect of paramagnetic agents in conventional doses is shortening of T1.

### 4.1.2 Contrast Enhancement

#### 4.1.2.1 General

The deposition of a material in a magnetic field causes magnetization of the material. The ratio of induced magnetism to that of the magnetic field is defined as magnetic susceptibility. There exist four classes of magnetic behavior: diamagnetic, paramagnetic, superparamagnetic, and ferromagnetic. Nearly all organic compounds are diamagnetic and have paired electrons in the outer orbital shells. These materials are not susceptible to magnetization (Table 4.1).

Paramagnetic, superparamagnetic, and ferromagnetic materials are all characterized by unpaired electrons in their outer orbital shells. They all possess magnetic susceptibility, magnetism is induced if they are placed in an external magnetic field. Due to the crystalline matrix, superparamagnetic and ferromagnetic materials acquire large magnetic moments.

**Table 4.1.** Classes of magnetic behavior

| | |
|---|---|
| 1. Diamagnetic: | – organic compounds<br>– paired electrons in outer<br>  orbital shells<br>– no magnetic susceptibility |
| 2. Paramagnetic: | – unpaired electrons<br>– magnetic susceptibility<br>  (medium)<br>– no retention of magnetization |
| 3. Superpara-<br>   magnetic: | – unpaired electrons<br>– magnetic susceptibility<br>  (strong)<br>– no retention of magnetization |
| 4. Ferromagnetic: | – unpaired electrons<br>– magnetic susceptibility<br>  (strong)<br>– permanent magnetization |

**Table 4.2.** Paramagnetic substances (unbalanced electron spins)

1. Ions containing unpaired electrons

   Lanthanide series
   $Gd^{3+}$
   $Eu^{2+}$

   Transition metal series
   $Mn^{2+}$, $Mn^{3+}$
   $Fe^{2+}$, $Fe^{3+}$
   $Ni^{2+}$
   $Cr^{2+}$
   $Cn^{2+}$

2. Unpaired electrons
   Nitric oxide
   Nitrogen dioxide

3. Paired electrons with parallel spins
   Molecular oxygen

4. Stable free radicals

**Table 4.3.** Paramagnetic contrast agents

| Paramagnetic materials: shortening of T1 | |
|---|---|
| *Chelates of lanthanide series* | Gd-DTPA<br>Gd-DOTA |
| *Transitional metal* | Fe |
| Superparamagnetic materials: shortening of T2 | |

No magnetization is retained by paramagnetic and superparamagnetic materials when the magnetic field is removed (Table 4.1). Ferromagnetic particles, however, remain partially magnetized and show properties of a permanent magnet.

### 4.1.2.2 Paramagnetic Contrast Agents

Paramagnetic substances are characterized by having at least one unpaired electron, which has a magnetic moment at least 1000 times stronger than that of a proton (Tables 4.2, 4.3). As a result of motion (rotation, diffusion, etc.) the paramagnetic compound produces rapid fluctuation in the local magnetic field. This facilitates energy transfer among the excited protons and also from the protons to their lattice. The relaxation times of the protons are influenced via a magnetic dipole-dipole interaction with the paramagnetic center of the contrast agent. At the molecular level, many complex factors determine to what degree the relaxation times change. The effect of a paramagnetic compound is, for example, influenced by the correlation time and the distance between the water molecule and the paramagnetic center. Other factors include frequency, magnetic field strength, and the number of binding sites of the water molecules. Paramagnetic compounds always shorten, never prolong, the relaxation times. All paramagnetic compounds generally affect both T1 and T2 relaxation times (Fig. 4.1). In rare cases, using superparamagnetic materials, T2 is shortened to a much greater degree than T1. Bloembergen [3] has calculated the degree of shortening the relaxation times using a model. A change in the relaxation rate $1:T_1$ can be mathematically expressed as

$$\Delta \frac{1}{T_1} = \frac{K + p^2 \times \mu^2 \times N}{r^6}$$

where $r$ is the distance between the paramagnetic material and the water molecules, $p$ is the gyromagnetic contrast, $N$ is the concentration and $\mu$ is the effective magnetic moment of the paramagnetic substance (Fig.

4.2). An increase in the relaxation rate $1 : T_1$ is proportional to the concentration of the paramagnetic material and the square of its magnetic moment. The effectiveness of a paramagnetic contrast medium, which is independent of the concentration, is called relaxivity. This value is calculated by the following mathematical expression:

$$\text{relaxivity} = \frac{1}{N} \times \left( \frac{1}{T_a} - \frac{1}{T_b} \right)$$

where $N$ is the concentration, $T_a$ is relaxation time after administration of the paramagnetic substance and $T_b$ is the relaxation time before administration of the paramagnetic substance.

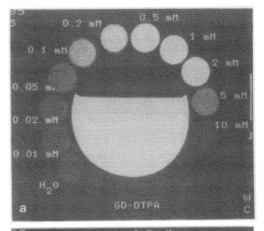

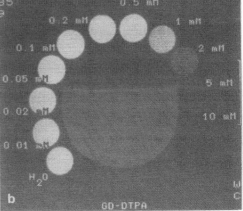

▷

Fig. 4.1 a, b. Spin-echo images from probes with different concentrations of Gd-DTPA in a NaCl solution
a T1 weighted
b T2 weighted, 2500/80
Using a low contrast medium concentration, T1 reduction causes an increase in signal intensity in comparison with the plain NaCl solution. With T1 weighting, a significant increase in signal intensity is achieved via the use of Gd-DTPA. No significant effect is seen with T2 weighting. (With courtesy to Dr. H. Schmid, FRG)

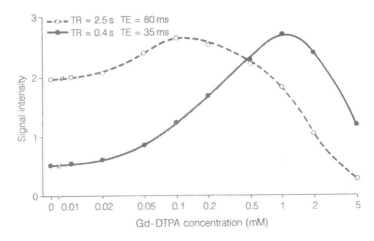

Fig. 4.2. The relative increase in signal intensity with T1 and T2 weighting at various concentrations of Gd-DTPA

Relatively low concentrations of paramagnetic contrast medium (0.1–1 mmol/kg body weight) are necessary in order to obtain significant enhancement of different human tissues. For applications in the head and neck the main interest is focused on parenteral contrast agents. There are few indications for oral administration.

### Parenteral Contrast Agents

Many of the metal ions composing the lanthanide and transition metal series in the periodic table show paramagnetism due to the unpaired electrons in their outer orbital shells. $Gd^{3+}$, with seven unpaired electrons in the 4f electron orbits, is the most efficient in enhancing relaxation of the hydrogen protons of the water molecule (Fig. 4.3). In its ionic form $Gd^{3+}$ is toxic, the $LD_{50}$ in animal studies being 0.1 mmol/kg. This toxicity was the reason for the development of a carrier ligand to prevent dissociation and to allow rapid excretion.

Two types of carrier ligands have already demonstrated clinical use. The multidentate chelate form of DTPA (diethylenetriamine pentaacetic acid) has received the most attention in regard to $Gd^{3+}$. The gadolinium ions form an extremely stable complex with the DTPA ligand (stability constant 10–22). The strongly hydrophilic Gd-DTPA cannot permeate intact plasma membranes and cannot cross the blood-brain barrier, and is excreted from the body within a few hours in the administered form. Thus, its pharmacokinetic behavior essentially resembles that of urographic contrast media. EDTA (ethylenediamine tetraacetic acid) has also been examined as a potential ligand, but has been rejected because of its higher toxicity. Other gadolinium compounds are currently being investigated as potential MR contrast agents, among them the gadolinium cryptelates. Of these Gd-DOTA appears to be a potential alternative MR contrast agent (Table 4.4); studies in vitro and in vivo have demonstrated that its stability in vivo is higher than that of Gd-DTPA. The first clinical trials of Gd-DTPA have just started in Germany. Enormous efforts are also being expended on researching a large number of other potential MR contrast media such as metalloporphyrines, nonionic agents, and special agents for the liver and spleen.

The use of radiolabeled antibodies as tumor-specific agents for immunoscintigraphy has sparked off experimental efforts to adapt this technique for paramagnetic labeling of monoclonal antibodies. Preliminary results have also been obtained for a blood pool contrast medium, with gadolinium-labeled albumin as a nondiffusible agent.

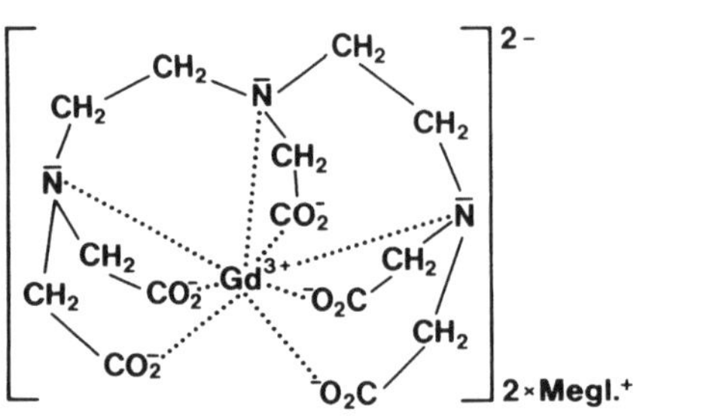

**Table 4.4.** List of paramagnetic contrast agents

1. Nonspecific
   Metallic ion complexes (parenteral, oral)
      chelates:    – Gd-DTPA
                   – Gd-EDTA
      cryptelates: – Gd-DOTA
   Nitroxide stable free radicals

2. Specific
   Metalloporphyrins?
   Nonionic agents
   Hepatobiliary agents
   Monoclonal antibodies
   Gadolinium-labeled albumin

**Fig. 4.3.** Chemical structure of Gadolinium diethylentriamine pentaacetic acid/Di-N-methylglucamine (Gd-DTPA)

## 4.2 Pharmacology of Gd-DTPA

To date the clinical experience of contrast-enhanced MRI has mainly been with parenteral Gd-DTPA though there are some preliminary data on the possible use of oral Gd-DTPA. In contrast to the free, nonchelated gadolinium ion, intravenously administered Gd-DTPA is excreted from the body within a few hours. Its pharmacokinetic behavior is identical to that of established angiographic and urographic contrast media. The agent Gd-DTPA shows nonspecific biodistribution with rapid intravascular distribution and diffusion into the extracellular space (Table 4.5). After intravenous administration the complexes are mainly eliminated via the kidneys; the portion excreted extrarenally is extremely small. The half-life of the agent is determined by two factors, the biodistribution volume of the substance in the body and the GFR. The half-life of Gd-DTPA in the human body is approximately 90 min. Within 24 h after intravenous administration 90% of the dose given is eliminated via the urine. Within the first hour after injection the plasma and interstitial concentrations are sufficient to have a significant effect on MR relaxation times. West German health authorities (Bundesgesundheitsamt, BGA) were the first to approve Gd-DTPA dimeglumine as a contrast agent for MRI, and late in 1983, in the Department of Radiology of the Klinikum Charlottenburg, Berlin, the first clinical trials were carried out in volunteers and patients with cerebral tumors [8, 9]. Table 4.6 shows the recommended dosage and administration protocol for the parenteral use of Gd-DTPA. At the moment the recommended dosage is 0.2 ml/kg with a maximum total dose of 20 ml. The rate of injection should not exceed 10 ml/min.

## 4.3 Safety Profile of Gd-DTPA

The paramagnetic contrast medium Gd-DTPA has already been used in clinical trials on over 10 000 patients in Europe, the United States, and Japan. So far the agent has been well tolerated at dosages up to 0.2 mmol/kg

**Table 4.5.** Biodistribution of intravenous Gd-DTPA

Nonspecific biodistribution:
– Vascular perfusion of tissue
– Capillary permeability
– Diffusion into extracellular space

Time course:
– Initially within intravascular compartment
– Diffuses throughout extravascular space

T1 agent, similar to radiographic contrast agents

**Table 4.6.** Dosage and administration of Gd-DTPA

1. Recommended dosage: 0.2 ml/kg i.v.
   Maximum total dose: 20 ml
2. Rate of injection: not to exceed 10 ml/min
3. Injection followed by a 5-ml flush of normal saline
4. Imaging to be completed within 1 h after injection

**Table 4.7.** Safety profile of intravenous Gd-DTPA

Well tolerated in clinical trials

Asymptomatic transient rise in serum iron in 15%–30% of cases

Adverse reactions among 410 patients:

| | |
|---|---|
| Headache | 4.9% |
| Nausea | 3.4% |
| Vomiting | 1.5% |
| Other | <1.0% |

(Table 4.7). In 15%–30% of patients a transient rise in serum iron is found. To date there have been no reports of severe side effects such as circulatory changes or significant allergic reactions. A study published by the manufacturer of Gd-DTPA reported that headache and nausea occurred in about 4% of 410 patients. Our own experience in more than 2000 patients confirms these results; so far no significant adverse reactions have been encountered.

## 4.4 Examination Protocols

Paramagnetic metal ion chelates and conventional iodinated contrast media show some similarities. Because their molecular weights are comparable, their patterns of biodistribution are also analogous. However, contrast enhancement is better on MRI than on CT. Detection and depiction of lesions is also better by virtue of the multiplanar imaging capacity of MRI. Another important advantage of paramagnetic over conventional radiographic contrast agents appears to be the low

incidence of side effects. While iodinated contrast media act directly by attenuating the X-ray beam, paramagnetic contrast agents act indirectly through alteration of the local magnetic susceptibility.

### 4.4.1 Sequences

Prior to the parenteral administration of Gd-DTPA, images have to be obtained using T1-weighted sequences. In the case of a variety of clinical findings precontrast T2-weighted se-

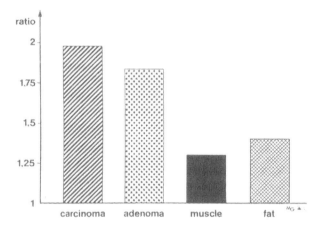

**Fig. 4.4** (*left*). Mean relative signal enhancement in neck tumors and normal tissues

**Fig. 4.5** (*below*). Contrast enhancement before and at various times after injection of contrast medium

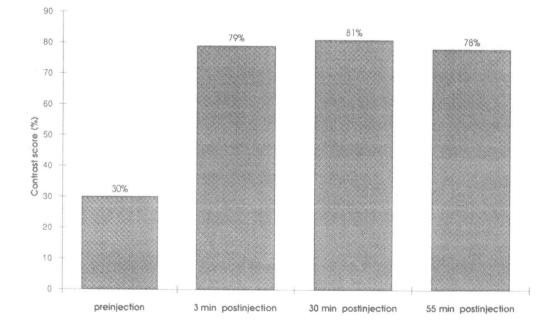

quences are also obtained. While for skull base lesions images only have to be obtained in one plane before administration of the contrast agent, for all other areas images in a second plane are recommended. Gd-DTPA is then administered intravenously at a dose of 0.1 mmol/kg body weight and a rate of 1 ml/ 6 s, followed by a 5-ml saline flush. Following the administration of Gd-DTPA only T1-weighted images are obtained, usually in two different planes. All tissues that accumulate gadolinium show an increase in signal intensity in T1-weighted sequences due to shortening of T1 relaxation times (Fig. 4.4). The greatest enhancement by Gd-DTPA is found in images acquired 3 min after injection, however, there is a comfortable 20- to 30-min window of time following injection of Gd-DTPA during which imaging can be performed (Fig. 4.5). The sequence protocol has to be changed for additional dynamic studies of a lesion. In this case fast imaging sequences have to be carried out before, during, and after injection of the contrast medium.

### 4.4.2 Subtraction Technique

In head and neck tumors, vascularized malignant tissue, fat, and hemorrhage show similar intensities on Gd-DTPA-enhanced T1-weighted MR sequences, so it is often difficult to distinguish vascularized portions of a lesion from the high-intensity fat in adjacent bone marrow and soft tissue. We have thus developed a special subtraction technique for contrast-enhanced MR images, the advantages and disadvantages of which are listed in Table 4.8.

#### 4.4.2.1 Method of Subtraction

In all patients T1-weighted images (500/ 15 ms) are obtained before the paramagnetic contrast agent Gd-DTPA is given. Gd-DTPA is then administered slowly via a previously installed vascular access device or via a peripheral intravenous catheter without movement of the patient. The T1-weighted se-

**Table 4.8.** MR subtraction technique

*Advantages:*
1. Better delineating of:
– tumor margins
– areas with mild enhancement

2. Increased contrast between tumor and:
  – adjacent fatty tissue
  – bone marrow

3. Differentiation of tumor recurrence and fibrosis

*Disadvantages:*
1. No subtraction with complex motion of patient
2. Misregistration artifacts appear as bright lines

quences are then repeated with the same slice selection criteria and imaging parameters as before the administration of the contrast medium. Images before and after contrast enhancement are then chosen for subtraction. The images are compared on the monitor to determine whether motion has occurred between the sequences. The standard software on our system enables us to display the contrast-enhanced image and electronically subtract the nonenhanced image on a pixel by pixel basis.

#### 4.4.2.2 Clinical Results

This subtraction technique is found to be useful in about 10% of MR examinations in the head and neck. In the majority of cases increased contrast between the tumor and adjacent fatty tissues is achieved. Subtracted images also improve contrast between the enhanced tumor and adjacent bone marrow of the mandible, maxilla, or spinal column. In some cases subtraction can improve discrimination of an enhancing tumor and hemorrhage or scar tissue, thus enabling, for example, the differentiation of a highly vascularized recurrent tumor from nonenhancing fibrosis. The subtraction technique is especially advantageous for lesions adjacent to the orbital fat and the skull base. A major disadvantage of the technique is that it cannot be used if the patient moves between acquisition of the enhanced and unenhanced sequences. If movement does occur, image degradation is caused by misregistration artifacts appearing as bright lines according to the type of motion.

In summary, this technique is already of significant use for some head and neck studies. Technical advances in pixelshifting could further improve its diagnostic capabilities.

### 4.4.3 Dynamic MRI

The dynamic MRI technique is based on the use of fast imaging sequences. The time dependence of the Gd-DTPA enhancement is recorded by imaging the same slice 8–12 times, once every 30 s. A 40° flip angle FLASH sequence (30/12) is used in our protocol with an acquisition time of 2 s beginning at the time of the bolus injection of Gd-DTPA.

The short exposure GE sequences repeated in a standardized pattern allow measurement of the degree of enhancement as well as its time dependence. Similar to the profile of density

over time in dynamic CT, the dynamic enhancement is analyzed and used for differential diagnosis (Fig. 4.7). Paragangliomas, for example, typically show uptake of the paramagnetic contrast agent immediately after injection and then a gradual decrease toward the end of the examination. This enhancement/time pattern with the washout effect helps to differentiate paragangliomas from tonsil tumors and neck cysts.

### 4.4.4 Oral Administration of Contrast Medium

In 1985, Runge et al. [7] suggested that the development of an oral contrast medium for MRI could follow the barium sulfate model, and his group suggested gadolinium oxalate as a potential agent. Other nonabsorbable paramagnetic iron preparations such as ferric hydroxide dextran have also been investigated as potential oral contrast agents. Recently, Gd-DTPA has successfully been used in human studies. This oral contrast agent could have some indications for examinations of the

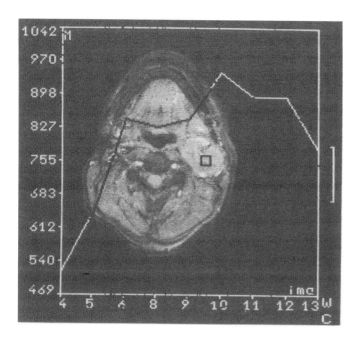

**Fig. 4.6.** Example of fast imaging technique in a glomus caroticum tumor. After administration of Gd-DTPA dynamic scanning allows the evaluation of the increase and decrease in signal intensity versus time. Characteristically the washout effect causes a loss in signal intensity after 8–10 min

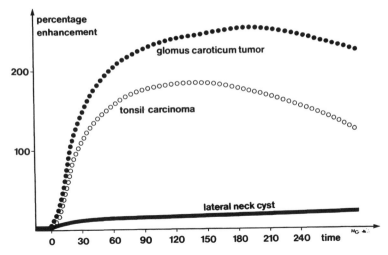

**Fig. 4.7.** Signal enhancement in different tissues after Gd-DTPA administration using the dynamic MRI technique

oro- und hypopharynx and cervical esophagus, since in combination with fast MRI techniques the movement of different muscle structures can be observed (Fig. 4.8). Fast MRI combined with oral paramagnetic contrast medium is still in its infancy, but rapid progress is to be expected.

## 4.5 Clinical Indications

Gd-DTPA and similar paramagnetic agents enhance contrast differences between normal and pathologic tissue while keeping examination times short. The clinical applications will be extensively demonstrated in the following chapters, but some basics have to be stated here.

### 4.5.1 Normal Topography

The MRI signal of all richly vascularized structures, such as the mucosa of the pharynx and the nasal turbinates, is enhanced by Gd-DTPA. Muscles, fascial planes, and vessels, on the other hand, typically present no significant enhancement. In the nasopharynx and tongue base, submucosal lymphoid tissue is characterized by a low increase in signal intensity after administration of the contrast medium (Table 4.9).

### 4.5.2 Benign Tumors

Because of the lack of enhancement of muscles and the enhancement of tumors, T1-weighted sequences after administration of Gd-DTPA provide improved tumor-muscle contrast. In the majority of cases anatomic details such as the preservation of tissue planes are better appreciated and so a benign tumor can often be diagnosed more confidently than without Gd-DTPA.

### 4.5.3 Malignant Tumors

In malignant neoplasms of the head and neck the role of MRI with Gd-DTPA is to define the extent of disease, differentiate malignant from benign tumors, and identify deep soft tissue extension and invasion of cartilage and bone. T2-weighted sequences provide higher tumormuscle contrast but lower spatial resolution and are more susceptible to motion artifacts, T1-weighted sequences yield better de-

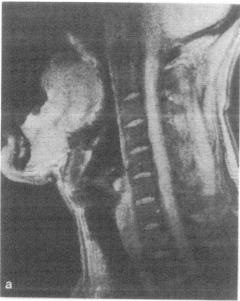

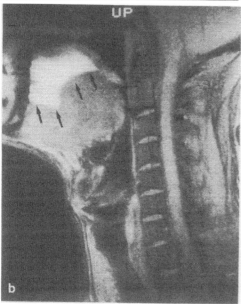

**Fig. 4.8 a, b.** Examination of the swallowing process with fast GE sequences
**a** Plain T1-weighted FLASH with mouth open as wide as possible
**b** T1-weighted FLASH after oral administration of Gd-DTPA. Due to the long examination time with the sequences used, exact recording of the movements that occur is not possible. Delineation of the superficial structures after oral administration of contrast medium

**Table 4.9.** Signal characteristics and Gd-GTPA enhancement of tissues in the head and neck

|  | T1 | T2 | Gd-DTPA enhancement |
|---|---|---|---|
| 1. Cartilage, surface | Low | Low | None |
| 2. Cartilage, interior | High | High | None |
| 3. Cavernous sinus | Low | Variable | High |
| 4. False vocal cords | High | High | None |
| 5. Fat | High | High | None |
| 6. Mucosa | Low-medium | High | High |
| 7. Muscle | Low | Low | None |
| 8. Parotid | High | Medium | Low |
| 9. Thyroid | Medium | High | High |
| 10. Tonsils | Low-medium | Medium | High |
| 11. True vocal cords | Medium | Medium | None |
| 12. Turbinates | Variable | High | Variable |

tection of invasion of bone and bone marrow and higher S/N.

In extracranial malignancies Gd-DTPA proves most helpful in demonstrating the tumor invasion to surrounding tissues.

### 4.5.4 Posttreatment Control

Tumors of the head and neck may be managed by surgery, irradiation, chemotherapy, or a combination of these strategies. The high risk factors for tumor recurrence are advanced disease, narrow surgical margins, extranodular spread, persistent pain or other symptoms, and persistent post-irradiation edema.

Patients who have been treated by surgery, radiotherapy, or chemotherapy are difficult to examine due to scarring or induration especially in relatively unaccessible areas. The following tissues and lesions have to be taken into account for the interpretation of MR images: recurrent tumor, residual tumor cells within fibrotic tissue, myocutaneous flaps, inflammation, and chondronecrosis or perichondritis. High signal intensity on T2-weighted images after treatment may represent a variety of tissue changes such as recurrent tumor, inflammation, or edema. Early after surgery, T1-weighted sequences with contrast medium are not helpful for differentiating tumor from edema. After a period of at least 3 months, however, fibrosis and tumor recurrence can be differentiated on the basis of their different uptake of contrast agent.

## 4.5.5 Inflammatory Disease

On T2-weighted sequences inflamed mucosa has a high signal intensity with no clear demarcation from the retained secretion. Patients with sinusitis display marked enhancement of inflamed mucosa and mucoperiosteal thickening. While retained secretions enhance in normal or partially obstructed sinuses, they never enhance in completely obstructed sinuses. Retention cysts are characterized by low signal intensity in T1-weighted images, high signal intensity in T2-weighted images, and no significant enhancement after administration of contrast medium.

In summary, T2-weighted sequences do not differentiate clearly between inflamed mucosa and secretions, while T1-weighted sequences with contrast medium differentiate inflamed mucosa, mucoperiosteal thickening, and mucosal secretions in partially obstructed sinuses.

## 4.6 Summary

The paramagnetic contrast agent Gd-DTPA has the following general indications in the head and neck:

- Clear delineation of tumor margins using T1-weighted sequences
- Identification of intracranial and skull base lesions with pathologic blood-brain barrier
- Improved localization of small submucosal tumors
- Differentiation of tumor recurrence and fibrosis

The following limitations exist in routine clinical practice:

- no differentiation of benign and malignant lymphadenopathy
- no discrimination between edema and tumor in extracranial lesions.

Plain MRI of the head and neck is a safe and efficacious imaging modality. Diagnostic sensitivity and specificity is further improved, however, by the use of paramagnetic contrast agents. Further improvement may come with the development of other contrast agents allowing specific distribution to organs and tumors. Using these new compounds, the radiologist may not only highlight specific structures but also demonstrate physiologic processes not accessible to other imaging modalities.

## References

1. Aue WP (1983) Topische Kernspin-Resonanz – eine nichtinvasive Sonde für biochemische Messungen in Lebewesen. Radiologie 23:357–360
2. Bloch F (1946) Nuclear induction. Phys Rev 70:460–474
3. Bloembergen N (1957) Proton relaxation times in paramagnetic solutions. J Chem Phys 27:572–573
4. Frahm J, Haase A, Matthaei D (1986) Rapid three-dimensional MR imaging using the FLASH-technique. J Comput Assist Tomogr 10 (2):363–368
5. Friedburg H, Bockenheimer S (1983) Klinische NMR-Tomographie mit sequentiellen T2-Bildern (Carr-Purcell-Spin-Echosequenzen). Radiologe 23:353–356
6. Lauterbur PC (1973) Image formation by induced local interactions. Examples employing NMR. Nature 242:190
7. Runge VM, Clanton JA, Price AC, Wehr CJ, Herzer WA, Partain CL, James AE (1985) The use of Gd-DTPA as a perfusion agent and marker of blood-brain barrier disruption. Magn Reson Imaging 3:43–55
8. Schoerner W, Semmler W, Felix R, Laniado M, Speck U, Niendorf HP (1984) Zur Wahl der Aufnahmesequenzen in der Kontrastmittel-Kernspintomographie: Kontrastverhalten von Hirntumoren nach Gd-DTPA-Anwendung bei unterschiedlichen Spin-Echo-Verfahren. Röntgenpraxis 37:323–326
9. Schörner W, Felix R, Claussen C et al. (1984) Kernspintomographische Diagnostik von Hirntumoren mit dem Kontrastmittel Gd-DTPA. ROFO 141:511–516

# 5 Signal Intensity and Relaxation

The basis for the interpretation of MRI measurements is the knowledge of signal intensity and relaxation times of normal and pathologic structures in the head and neck region. For the determination of T1, double SE images with equal TE and differing TR are important. T2 is calculated from double SE images with equal TR and differing TE. In addition, the signal intensities of various tissues are determined on T1-weighted images before and after administration of the paramagnetic contrast agent Gd-DTPA.

Comparative evaluation is done by using histologically verified diagnoses to establish a score for reliability of MRI findings. The score ranges from 0 for diagnostically insufficient to 3 for optimal image information (Table 5.1).

The *sensitivity* refers to the group in which the disease sought is present, and is an index for the capability to recognize an illness. The *specificity* relates to the group without the disease. The *accuracy* refers to the proportion of the total number of diagnoses that are correct, and thus defines the efficiency of the method. Other measures used are positive predictive value, negative predictive value, and prevalence.

## 5.1 In Vivo Results

If plain T1-weighted images are used, the statistical evaluation of signal intensities in MRI shows significant differences for muscle, fat, and white matter (Table 5.2). The most significant difference ($p < 0.0001$) is that between muscle and fatty tissue. The tumors (in this example, tumors of the temporal bone), with a mean signal intensity of 144, differ very significantly ($p < 0.0001$) from fatty tissue and white matter. The difference between tumor tissue and muscle is of borderline significance ($p = 0.087$).

**Table 5.1.** Diagnostic reliability and statistical evaluation of MR images

| Score: diagnostic value | | |
|---|---|---|
| 0 | Insufficient | Anatomic detail insufficient |
| 1 | Satisfactory | Distinct anatomic detail, recognition of tumors larger than 2 cm |
| 2 | Good | Clear delineation of smaller tumors |
| 3 | Optimal | In addition to tumor delineation: visualization of tumor necrosis, vascularization |

Statistical evaluation

$$\text{Sensitivity (\%)} = \frac{\text{true positive}}{\text{true positive} + \text{false negative}} \times 100$$

$$\text{Specificity (4)} = \frac{\text{true negative}}{\text{true negative} + \text{false positive}} \times 100$$

$$\text{Accuracy (\%)} = \frac{\text{true positive} + \text{true negative}}{\text{total number of examinations}} \times 100$$

The lowest values for T1 are found in fatty tissue (Table 5.2). Fat differs very significantly ($p<0.001$) from muscle and white matter. The T1 relaxation times of muscle and white matter do not differ significantly ($p=0.33$). The tumors differ from all three reference tissues at a high level of significance.

The T2 values for the different tissues show great variation with high standard deviation (Table 5.2). The lowest T2 is displayed by muscle. White matter and muscle can be precisely differentiated on T2-weighted images ($p<0.0001$). Because tumor tissue on average shows a prolonged T2 relaxation time, T2-weighted sequences have diagnostic capabilities. A limitation, however, is the very high standard deviation, which makes differentiation more difficult in the individual case.

Overall, the diagnostic differentiation of tumors from other tissues by MRI is severely restricted in spite of the great differences in signal intensity and relaxation times. New possibilities are opened up by the specific pharmacodynamic reactions that occur as a result of the administration of paramagnetic contrast media such as Gd-DTPA. Differences in signal intensity are observed in T1-weighted sequences before and after Gd-DTPA. Comparison of the different tissues shows that reference and tumor structures differ significantly in contrast agent uptake (Table 5.2). The signal intensity of fatty tissue increases significantly ($p<0.0001$). The increase in white matter is also significant, though less so ($p<0.01$). In contrast, no sig-

**Table 5.2.** Signal intensity and relaxation times on T1-weighted MRI (in patients with tumors of the temporal bone)

| Signal intensity | | |
|---|---:|---:|
| TU | 145± | 72 |
| MU | 173± | 68 |
| FA | 621± | 192 |
| WM | 258± | 76 |
| **T1 (ms)** | | |
| TU | 2249± | 1031 |
| MU | 1529± | 722 |
| FA | 539± | 325 |
| WM | 1515± | 628 |
| **T2 (ms)** | | |
| TU | 137± | 107 |
| MU | 37± | 19 |
| FA | 51± | 18 |
| WM | 75± | 22 |
| **Signal intensity with Gd-DTPA** | | |
| TU | 217± | 65 |
| MU | 180± | 60 |
| FA | 701± | 215 |
| WM | 328± | 84 |

TU, tumor; MU, muscle; FA, fat; WM, white matter.

nificant change in signal intensity on administration of Gd-DTPA is found in muscle ($p=0.99$). The tumors show highly significant increase in signal intensity after Gd-DTPA injection ($p<0.0001$). The accumulation of Gd-DTPA is greater than for the three reference tissues. This characteristic is of utmost importance in the evaluation of MRI findings in the head and neck.

# 6 Temporal Bone, Middle Skull Base, and Cerebellopontine Angle

## 6.1 Clinical Findings

Many different diseases affect the temporal bone and the middle skull base. The clinician encounters mainly diseases of the middle and inner ear. Common examples of middle ear disorders are acute and chronic otitis media, cholesteatoma, otosclerosis, congenital abnormalities, and fractures of the temporal bone. Disorders of the inner ear include congenital and acquired sensorineural hearing loss, sudden deafness, presbyacusis, noise-induced hearing impairment, ototoxicity of various causes, metabolic hearing loss, Menière's disease, and labyrinthitis. Tumors are relatively rare but may involve the middle ear, mastoid, and temporal bone primarily, metastatically, or by extension from a contiguous area. Acoustic neuroma is important in the differential diagnosis of sudden hearing loss, vertigo, and tinnitus. Many inner ear diseases show one or more of these symptoms, and if the origin of such a disease is unclear an acoustic neuroma must be excluded. The most common benign neoplasms of the middle ear are glomus tumors, which, though histologically benign, usually tend to grow aggressively. Patients suffering from a glomus tumor may present with a variety of different signs and symptoms depending on the vascularity of the lesion and its propensity to erode surrounding structures. The most common symptoms, in order of frequency, are hearing loss, tinnitus, discharge, otalgia, vertigo, bleeding, cranial nerve palsies, a mass in the external canal and a mass visible behind the tympanic membrane.

In middle ear diseases, the use of a binocular microscope is obligatory to obtain adequate information. If there is a defect in the tympanic membrane the situation inside the middle ear can be evaluated, depending on the size of the defect. Besides this physical examination of the middle ear, several hearing tests such as impedance, pure-tone audiometry, and speech audiometry have to be undertaken in most cases.

Inner ear diseases can not be diagnosed by otoscopy. Audiometric evaluation is absolutely mandatory to distinguish between cochlear and retrocochlear lesions of the auditory system. If conventional audiometry arouses suspicion of a retrocochlear origin of the lesion, other, more complicated audiologic tests such as the tone decay test, the short-increment sensitivity index (SISI), and Békésy audiometry have to be carried out. Auditory brainstem response (ABR) audiometry has become an important diagnostic tool in the evaluation of inner ear diseases. Additionally, a lesion of the inner ear usually requires examination of the peripheral vestibular organ. In acoustic neuroma, for instance, the alternate bithermal caloric test shows a reduced caloric response on the side of the lesion in almost 80% of patients.

**Demands on the Radiologist.** Tumors of the temporal bone usually require further diagnostic evaluation by the radiologist. The surgeon needs an exact assessment of the lesion's topography, vascularization, extent, and infiltration of surrounding tissues. The definitive histologic diagnosis is also essential for the decision on the therapy of choice (surgery, radiotherapy, chemotherapy). In glomus jugulare tumors there is no consensus on the therapy of choice. While surgery is generally favored as a standard treatment of glomus tumors, some authors prefer radiotherapy, at least if incomplete resection or neurologic sequelae of surgery seem inevitable.

**Table 6.1.** General diagnostic protocol for MRI of the temporal bone and middle skull base

| Sequence number | Plane | Mode | TR (ms) | TE (ms) | Slice thickness (mm) |
|---|---|---|---|---|---|
| 1 | Sagittal | SE | 200 | 30 | 10 |
| 2 | Axial | SE | 2000 | 25, 90 | 4 |
| 3 | Axial | SE | 500 | 25 | 4 |
| | Dynamic MRI (FLASH) employing GE technique with Gd-DTPA (0.1 mmol/kg b.w.), acquisition time 8 min | | | | |
| 4 | Axial | SE | 500 | 25 | 4 |
| 5 | Coronal | SE | 500 | 25 | 4 |

In the case of a vascularized tumor, the vessels supplying the lesion have to be identified to optimize therapeutic planning.

## 6.2 Examination Technique

The general diagnostic protocol for MRI of the temporal bone and middle skull base features axial sequences with long and short TR after a short sagittal localizer (Table 6.1). Using the head coil, the region of interest is imaged in contiguous 4-mm-thick slices. If required, a paraaxial T1-weighted sequence in the plane of the vestibulocochlear nerve can be obtained. Prior to the advent of paramagnetic contrast medium (Gd-DTPA) into clinical routine an additional multiecho sequence was used for plain MRI. Nowadays axial and coronal sequences with short TR are carried out after administration of Gd-DTPA.

The time course of contrast agent uptake is analyzed for the diagnosis of specific lesions via dynamic MRI. If there is clinical suspicion of an acoustic neuroma the T2-weighted sequence is usually omitted because of the high acquisition time. If a vascular lesion is suspected in the region of the middle skull base, temporal bone, or jugular bulb, arterial or venous MR angiography should be performed. For the planning of surgery or radiotherapy, 3D MRI offers new diagnostic possibilities.

## 6.3 The Topographic Basis for the Evaluation of MR Images

The temporal bone, the bony basis of the middle skull base (Fig. 6.1), is made up of four osseous segments: the tympanic, mastoid, petrous, and squamous parts. The tympanic cavity and the bony parts of the eustachian tube constitute the middle ear, which is bounded medially by the basal narrowing of the cochlea and laterally by the tympanic membrane (Fig. 6.2a). Dorsally, the tympanic part of the temporal bone joins with the mastoid part. The petrous portion contains the labyrinth, the internal carotid artery, and the facial and vestibulocochlear nerves. With the promontory of the cochlea the petrous part bounds laterally on the tympanic part. The area of the temporal bone adjacent to the cerebrum forms a part of the middle cranial fossa and constitutes the anterolateral boundary with the posterior cranial fossa. The upper parts of the posterior boundary of the temporal bone are formed by the squamous portion, which is thus in close vicinity to the facial canal and the mastoid part.

Within the internal auditory canal and the cerebellomedullar cistern the *facial nerve* accompanies the superior and inferior vestibular parts and the cochlear part of the vestibulocochlear nerve (Fig. 6.2d, e). In the region of the so-called Bill's bar the facial nerve leaves the internal auditory canal to anterior [35]. This segment, termed the labyrinthine part, extends between the vestibule and the basal turn of the cochlea. At the genicular ganglion the nerve turns at right angles, giving off the major petrous nerve. The subsequent horizontal segment of the facial nerve (Fig. 6.3 a, b) extends within the tympanic cavity to the external genu, from where it runs inside the vertical oriented mastoid canal (Figs. 6.2 c, 6.3 c).

Because of the lack of compact bone signal the temporal bone only shows up indirectly, but can be identified well by means of the adjacent structures. The hypointense bone structure cannot be differentiated from the pneumatized portions. The nerve bundle of the facial and vestibulocochlear nerves, with medium signal intensity, serves as a reference structure inside temporal bone. Both nerves come from the brainstem, cross the cerebel-

lopontine cistern, and run into the internal auditory canal (Fig. 6.2 a). At the fundus of the internal auditory canal the nerve bundle divides in a superior compartment comprising the facial nerve and the utricular nerve (superior vestibular nerve) and an inferior compartment comprising the saccular nerve (inferior vestibular nerve) and the cochlear nerve. The superior and inferior parts are subdivided in anterior and posterior compartments by the vertical crest (Bill's bar) (Fig. 6.2 e):

– Anterosuperior: facial nerve
– Anteroinferior: cochlear nerve
– Posterosuperior: utricular nerve
– Posteroinferior: saccular nerve

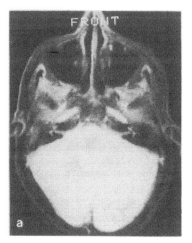

◁
**Fig. 6.1 a, b.** Normal topography at the level of the middle of the pyramid in a postmortem specimen **a** Plain axial MRI (SE, 2000/9) at the level of the internal auditory canal: high signal intensity of all liquid-containing structures **b** Diagram

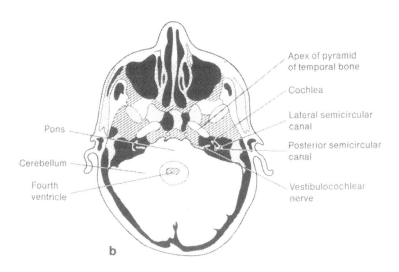

Apex of pyramid of temporal bone

Cochlea

Lateral semicircular canal

Posterior semicircular canal

Pons

Cerebellum

Fourth ventricle

Vestibulocochlear nerve

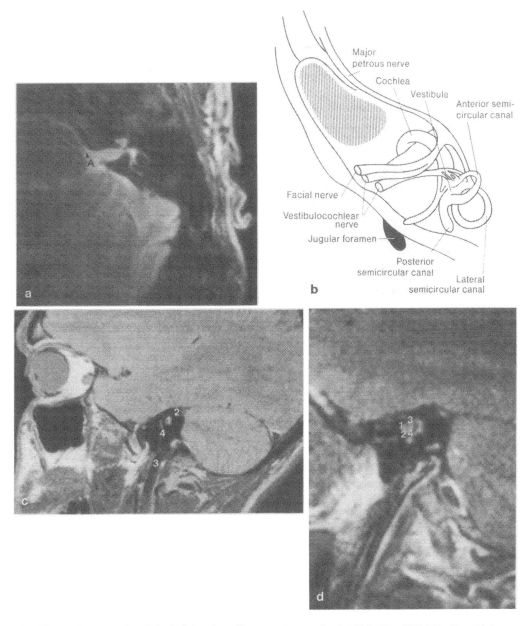

Fig. 6.2a–e. Topography of the facial and vestibulocochlear nerves and structures of the tympanic cavity using T2-weighted sequences and a surface coil

Plain axial MRI (SE, 2000/90). Axial sequences reliably delineate the CSF-containing structures of the cerebellomedullar cistern, the internal auditory canal, and the cochlea and vestibular system. *A*, anterior inferior cerebellar artery

Schematic demonstration of internal structures of the temporal bone in the axial plane

c Parasagittal MRI (SE, 2000/22) slice thickness 3 mm. Visualization of the soft tissues of the internal auditory canal as central area of high signal in the pyramid. *1*, Soft tissue of nerve bundle; *2*, apex of pyramid; *3*, internal carotid artery; *4*, facial nerve (vertical segment)

d Parasagittal MRI (SE, 2000/60) slice thickness 3 mm. *1*, facial nerve; *2*, cochlear nerve; *3*, superior vestibular nerve; *4*, inferior vestibular nerve

e see p. 52

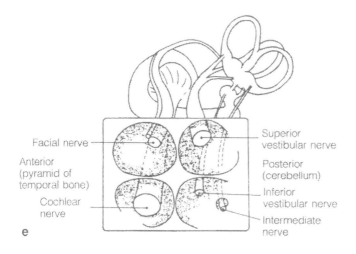

Facial nerve

Anterior
(pyramid of
temporal bone)

Cochlear
nerve

e

Superior
vestibular nerve

Posterior
(cerebellum)

Inferior
vestibular nerve

Intermediate
nerve

**Fig. 6.2. e** Schematic demonstration of neural internal structures in the sagittal plane

The facial nerve continues within the facial canal, which now runs steeply caudal and dorsal into the region of the posterior wall of the tympanic cavity. The course of the nerves can be followed reliably, especially in sagittal slices (Fig. 6.3).

With appropriate T2-weighting the cerebrospinal fluid (CSF) surrounding the facial and vestibulocochlear nerves has a higher signal intensity than the nerve structures. Moreover, the distal course of the nerves can be evaluated best on a T2-weighted image (Fig. 6.3 b, c). However, the proximal branches of the vestibulocochlear nerve are imaged to best advantage with spin density weighting, because this shows tumors more clearly against the CSF. Administration of the paramagnetic contrast medium Gd-DTPA leads to no significant change of signal in the area of the cerebellomedullary cistern and the facial and vestibulocochlear nerves if the blood-brain barrier is intact. A significant increase of signal is always found in the transverse and sigmoid sinuses and in the superior bulb of the jugular vein (Fig. 6.4 a – c).

In diagnostic MRI of the *cerebellopontine angle* two important vessels must always be identified: the loop of the anterior inferior cerebellar artery and the petrosal vein (Fig. 6.2 a,b). According to Valavanis [47, 48] the loop of the anterior inferior cerebellar artery is outside the internal auditory pore in 53% of cases, at the pore in 52%, and in-

trameatal in 22% (Fig. 6.2 a). In T2-weigthed sequences this vessel stands out as an arched linear structure of lower signal intensity within the high-intensity CSF. The labyrinthine artery, originating from the internal auditory pore, is not detected by MRI. The petrosal vein is seen to best advantage in coronal and axial images and often exhibits zones of increased signal intensity because of the slow blood flow (Fig. 6.3 a). Comparison of T1-weighted sequences with and without contrast medium, and in individual cases the evaluation of subtraction images are thus a prerequisit for exact classification of tumors in this area.

The *jugular foramen* can be described in terms of two topographically important parts, the vascular part and the nervous part:

| Vascular part: | superior jugular bulb vagus nerve accessory nerve |
| Nervous part: | glossopharyngeal nerve inferior petrosal sinus |

The jugular vein shows up on MRI with variable signal intensity depending on blood flow (Fig. 6.4 a – c). Using a surface coil, in some individual cases the band-shaped vagus nerve can be demonstrated within the jugular foramen and the hypoglossal nerve can be visualized in the medial segment of the hypoglossal canal.

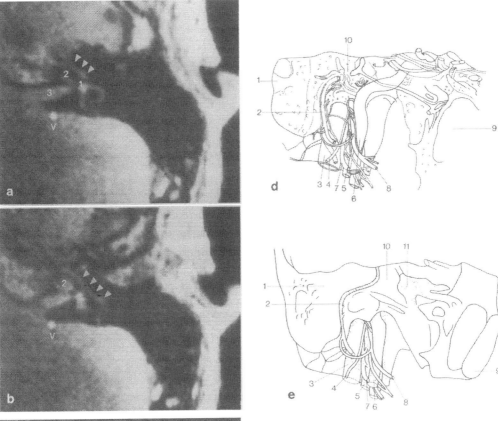

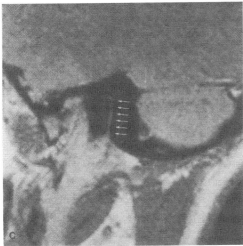

**Fig. 6.3 a–e.** Demonstration of the tympanic and mastoid course of the facial nerve on MRI of the temporal bone

**a, b** Axial MRI (SE, 2000/60). Demonstration of the first part of the tympanic segment of the facial nerve shortly after the first genu. *Arrowheads,* horizontal part of facial nerve; *1,* vestibule; *2,* cochlea; *3,* internal auditory canal; *V,* petrosal vein

**c** Parasagittal MR (SE, 2000/60) Demonstration of the vertical segment of the facial nerve (*arrowheads*) as a linear area of signal in the mastoid and the proximal segments of the parotid gland

**d, e** Diagram showing topographic relations of internal carotid artery, facial nerve and various skull base structures. *1,* mastoid bone; *2,* facial nerve; *3,* internal jugular vein; *4,* accessory nerve; *5,* vagus nerve; *6,* internal carotid artery; *7,* hypoglossal nerve; *8,* glossopharyngeal nerve; *9,* maxillary sinus; *10,* petrous bone; *11,* trigeminal nerve

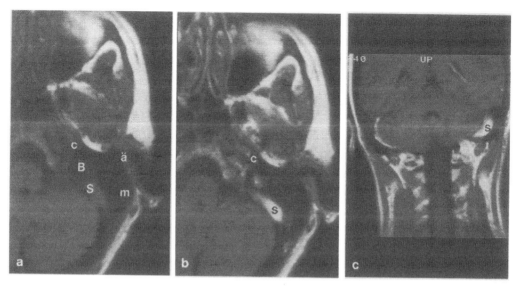

**Fig. 6.4a–c.** Normal topography of the superior jugular bulb and the sigmoid sinus before and after administration of Gd-DTPA in T1-weighted sequences. *S*, sigmoid sinus; *B*, jugular bulb; *C*, Internal carotid artery; *m*, mastoid; *ä*, external auditory canal
**a** Plain axial MRI (SE, 500/17). Low signal intensity of the basal segments of the temporal bone. The jugular bulb and the sigmoid sinus show medium signal intensity

**b** Axial MRI (SE, 500/17) with Gd-DTPA. Exact demarcation of the transverse and the sigmoid sinus as well as the ventrally located jugular bulb due to the high signal intensity after administration of Gd-DTPA
**c** Coronal MRI (SE, 500/17) with GD-DTPA. Demonstration of the sigmoid sinus

The course of the *trigeminal nerve* is characterized by a linear zone of medium signal intensity on T1-weighted sequences in the area of the middle skull base.

The checklist in Table 6.2 shows what structures of the temporal bone, middle skull base, and cerebellopontine angle should be investigated.

## 6.4 Sensitivity and Specificity of MRI in Relation to Other Imaging Modalities

A prospective study was carried out to ascertain the diagnostic efficacy of MRI. The subjects were patients who, on the grounds of subjective and objective manifestations, were suspected to have lesions of the temporal bone and the cerebellopontine angle. Beside the classical focal symptoms there were clinical symptoms of brainstem compression.

All patients underwent audiologic tests, a check of the vestibular nerve, and electric response audiometry (ERA). For conventional X-ray diagnosis, films were taken in Schüller's and Stenvers' projection. All patients underwent contrast-enhanced CT, and in a few cases CT combined with air cisternography was also carried out.

Table 6.3 shows that for acoustic neuroma, the sensitivity, specificity, and accuracy of MRI were near 100%. In the whole series of 290 patients there were no false negatives and only six false positives (Table 6.4). Overall, the sensitivity of MRI was 100% and the specificity was 96% for tumors of the temporal bone. The low prevalence of 43% is explained by the large number of true negative. With overall accuracy of 98% MRI was far superior to the other imaging techniques (Table 6.5). Contrast-enhanced CT, analyzed by three independent examiners, showed a sensitivity of

**Table 6.2.** Checklist for temporal bone, middle skull base, and cerebellopontine angle

1. Temporal bone

| Normal | Abnormal | |
|---|---|---|
| | | tympanic cavity |
| | | mastoid |
| | | internal auditory canal |
| | | jugular foramen |
| | | eustachian tube |
| | | vestibule |
| | | cochlea |
| | | semicircular canals – superior |
| | |             – horizontal |
| | |             – posterior |
| | | internal carotid artery |
| | | facial nerve |

2. Cerebellopontine angle

| Normal | Abnormal | |
|---|---|---|
| | | cerebellomedullar cistern |
| | | superior vestibular nerve |
| | | facial nerve |
| | | inferior vestibular nerve |
| | | cochlear nerve |
| | | internal auditory artery |

3. Adjacent structures

| Normal | Abnormal | |
|---|---|---|
| | | sphenoid sinus |
| | | great wing of sphenoid bone |
| | | small wing of sphenoid bone |
| | | sigmoid sinus |
| | | basilar artery |
| | | posterior cerebral artery |

| Normal | Abnormal | |
|---|---|---|
| | | fourth ventricle |
| | | vermis |
| | | flocculus |
| | | clivus |
| | | pituitary gland |
| | | prepontine cistern |

**Table 6.3.** MRI prediction vs postoperative histology: acoustic neuroma

| | | Postoperative histology | |
|---|---|---|---|
| | | Yes | No |
| MRI | Yes | 72 tp | 0 fp |
| | No | 0 fn | 149 tn |

tp, true positive; tn, true negative; fp, false positive; fn, false negative.

**Table 6.4.** MRI prediction vs postoperative histology: all tumors ($n=290$)

| | | Postoperative histology | |
|---|---|---|---|
| | | Yes | No |
| MRI | Yes | 125 tp | 6 fp |
| | No | 0 fn | 159 tn |

**Table 6.5.** Comparison of the results of MRI, CT and conventional roentgenology in the area of the temporal bone and the cerebellopontine angle

| | MRI | CT, enhanced | CT, air cisternography | Conventional roentgenology |
|---|---|---|---|---|
| $n$ | 290 | 115 | 12 | 171 |
| Sensitivity (%) | 100 | 76 | 83 | 58 |
| Specificity (%) | 96 | 80 | 83 | 45 |
| Overall accuracy (%) | 98 | 77 | 80 | 50 |
| PPV (%) | 95 | 83 | 83 | 43 |
| NPV (%) | – | 29 | 16 | 38 |
| Prevalence (%) | 43 | 57 | 50 | 41 |

PPV/NPV, positive/negative predictive value.

**Table 6.6.** MRI prediction vs postoperative histology for five groups of tumors

| | | Postoperative histology | | | | |
|---|---|---|---|---|---|---|
| | | Acoustic neuroma n | Glomus tumor n | Meningioma n | Cholesteatoma n | Other tumors n |
| MRI | Acoustic neuroma | 72 | | | | |
| | Glomus tumor | | 28 | | | |
| | Meningioma | | | 9 | | 1 |
| | Cholesteatoma | | | | 8 | 2 |
| | Other tumors | | | 1 | 1 | 9 |

Overall accuracy 96%.

76% and a specificity of 80%. The results of CT with air cisternography proved slightly better but should be interpreted with caution in view of the small number of patients.

The lowest sensitivity, specificity, and overall accuracy were found for conventional roentgenography.

In Table 6.6 the MRI findings are correlated with the postoperative tumor histology for five groups of tumors. For acoustic neuroma and glomus tumor the MRI diagnosis was true positive in all cases. One meningioma was falsely assigned to the rare tumors, and one cholesteatoma was wrongly classified as a meningioma. Among the rare tumors, one metastasis and one plasmacytoma were diagnosed as cholesteatomas, and a sarcoma infiltrating the temporal bone showed the typical morphologic criteria of a meningioma. The overall accuracy of diagnostic MRI for the patients with tumors involving the temporal bone was 96%.

### 6.4.1 Value of the Various MRI Sequences

The superiority of diagnostic MRI in the region of the temporal bone is seen in improved soft tissue contrast and the multiplanar imaging.

*T1-weighted sequences* allow evaluation of tumor localization, morphology, internal structures, and the displacement of adjacent structures, including the interpretation of slight structural changes in the hypointense CSF and cerebroventricular system.

*T2-weighted sequences* allow especially the characterization of pathological tissue structures and favor the differentiation of solid and cystic tumor components as well as the diagnosis of regressive changes of extraaxial tumors. With heavily T2-weighted sequences, differentiation of tumor and surrounding edema is possible in more than 70% of cases.

*In T1-weighted sequences with contrast medium* differentiation of the surrounding structures is significantly improved by the administration of Gd-DTPA. This agent is able to permeate a pathologically changed blood-brain barrier, resulting in a reduction of tumor T1. All extraaxial and axial lesions of the skull base can be identified precisely via this technique.

## 6.5 Acoustic Neuroma

The development of MRI to a routine procedure necessitates an urgent change in diagnostic practice regarding acoustic neuromas [19]. The initial clinical examination and neurootological investigations (audiology, ERA, vestibular tests) will retain their primary role [10, 17]. Conventional x-ray techniques (Schüller's and Stenvers' projections), though providing information of low specificity often indicate the presence of processes, especially

**Table 6.7.** Growth patterns of acoustic neuroma

| Type | Expansion | Diameter (mm) | Clinical findings |
|------|-----------|---------------|-------------------|
| Lateral | Intrameatal | 1–8 | Focal symptoms |
| Mediolateral | Intra- and extrameatal | <25 | Focal symptoms, local signs |
| Medial | Extrameatal, cerebellopontine angle | >25 | Focal symptoms, local signs, brainstem compression |

in the middle ear, and hence remain useful [24].

Hitherto more specific examination of the temporal bone has been obtained mostly using CT, in some cases combined with air cisternography for intrameatal tumors. This technique, however, is hampered by a high proportion of false positives, ranging between 5% and 12% [14, 15]. The reasons for this misinterpretation are soft tissue adhesions, arachnoid cysts, and abnormalities of the arachnoid vessels such as aneurysms or ectatic loops of the inferior anterior cerebellar artery [18].

The primary use of MRI for tumors within the internal auditory canal, the vessel-nerve bundle and the cerebellopontine angle, is recommended because of the lack of invasiveness and the low costs in comparison with CT with air cisternography [23, 34]. On MRI the demarcation of tumor expansion is better due to the superior soft tissue contrast and the lack of signal from surrounding osseous structures. For optimal results an appropriate head coil or a small-diameter surface coil using a variable slice thickness have to be available. Additionally it is advantageous to image slices parallel to the course of the vestibulocochlear nerve. Interestingly enough, some authors report a very high sensitivity of nonenhanced MRI for primary diagnosis of acoustic neuromas but the results of several recent studies show that the sensitivity of MRI, especially for intrameatal acoustic neuroma, can be clearly increased by the administration of Gd-DTPA.

In our own series on plain MRI the T1 and T2 relaxation times of the tumor versus white matter had limited diagnostic potential in the individual case due to the wide standard deviation of these parameters [57]. Only inflammatory processes such as primary or secondary cholesteatomas can be detected on the basis of their extremely prolonged T1 and T2 relaxation times.

Diagnostic results with the fast imaging technique and a dynamic series over a period of 7 min after administration of Gd-DTPA hint at specific behavior of acoustic neuromas. Overall accuracy of nearly 100% can be achieved using MRI for the diagnosis of these lesions.

### 6.5.1 Classification

On clinical and MRI criteria three types of acoustic neuromas can be differentiated (Table 6.7) [57, 59]:

– Lateral (intrameatal) tumors. This type originates in the area between the glial cells and Schwann cells of the superior vestibular nerve.
– Mediolateral (intra- and extrameatal) tumors. This was the most frequent type in our own series.
– Medial (extrameatal) tumors. These arise primarily from the nerve bundle in the cerebellopontine angle and do not expand within the internal auditory canal.

The different signal characteristics of the three types of acoustic neuromas and their location with reference to the pyramid apex and the internal auditory canal allow exact classification and differential diagnosis by means of MRI.

### 6.5.2 MRI Characteristics

Reproducible MRI diagnosis of acoustic neuroma is based on the following characteristics of the tumor: location and size, homogeneity, T1 (T2) relaxation time, and increase in signal intensity after administration of paramagnetic contrast medium.

Acoustic neuromas regularly show signal intensity comparable to that of brain parenchyma in T1-weighted sequences (see Fig. 6.8 a). Regressive changes such as necrosis show up as intratumoral areas of lower signal intensity. Recent or older hemorrhages are visualized as hyperintense areas. The demarcation of CSF, the pons, and the cerebellum is achieved via T2-weighted sequences (see Fig. 6.8 c).

Comparative analysis of T2 reveals small differences between acoustic neuromas and other tumors of this area. Cholesteatomas and other inflammatory tumorous lesions, however, can reliably be differentiated from the remaining classes of tumors on the basis of their longer T2 times (Fig. 6.5). The highest overall accuracy in the diagnosis of acoustic neuroma is achieved after administration of Gd-DTPA, which causes a signal increase of the tumor due to a disturbance of the blood-brain barrier (see Fig. 6.8 a, b, d, e). With this contrast agent neuromas down to a few millimeters in diameter can be detected. The percent increase in signal intensity is calculated from enhanced and nonenhanced T1-weighted sequences. At a Gd-DTPA dose of 0.1 mmol/kg bodyweight, the highest increase is shown by meningioma (215%), followed by acoustic neuroma (180%) and glomus tumor (140%). Due to the intact blood-brain barrier only a nonspecific increase in signal intensity is found in the white matter (Fig. 6.6).

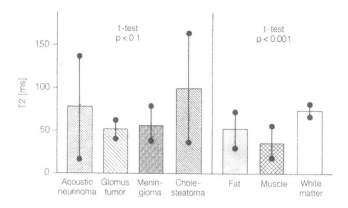

**Fig. 6.5.** T2 relaxation times (mean ± SD) for tumors of the temporal bone

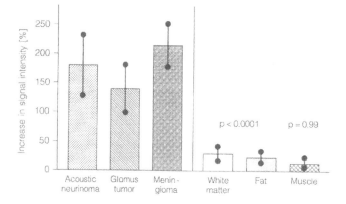

**Fig. 6.6.** Percent increase in signal intensity of temporal bone tumors after administration of Gd-DTPA

The possibilities of the tumor differentiation by using fast imaging sequences and the dynamic analysis of the contrast enhancement will be presented in the section concerning glomus tumors (Sect 6.7).

### 6.5.2.1 Extrameatal Acoustic Neuroma

The mean MRI tissue parameters exhibited by extrameatal acoustic neuromas correspond to the overall average for other acoustic neuromas. While plain MRI seems comparable to enhanced CT, the administration of Gd-DTPA allows optimal evaluation of all structures as well as the edematous and necrotic components of a tumor (Fig. 6.7a, b).

In T1-weighted as well as T2-weighted sequences delineation of the tumor from the surrounding brain parenchyma is possible. The surrounding edema and the necrotic areas are also differentiated clearly.

For exact delineation between tumorous tissue and the vessel-nerve bundle it is important to evaluate coronal slices parallel to the course of the vestibulocochlear nerve.

### 6.5.2.2 Intra-Extrameatal Acoustic Neuroma

The intrameatal part of the tumor and the part located free in the cerebellopontine angle must always be differentiated (Fig. 6.8a–e). The extrameatal component can be demonstrated by CT, but the intrameatal component cannot be reliably detected by CT without air cisternography.

In 80% of patients the involvement of the cranial nerves is reliably demonstrated on plain MRI, in the remaining 20% only after administration of GD-DTPA. The facial nerve is often displaced against the anterosuperior pole of the tumor, whereas the vestibulocochlear nerve rarely shows displacement, usually disappears in the medial contour of the tumor. Figure 6.8b clearly shows a characteristic growth pattern of this form on MRI which we have called the "whistle sign".

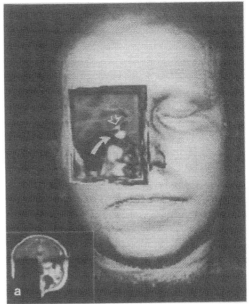

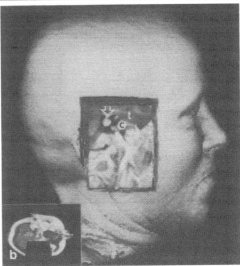

**Fig. 6.7a, b.** Extrameatal acoustic neuroma in a preoperative 3D sequence
**a** Coronal MRI (turbo-FLASH, ray tracing) with Gd-DTPA. Demonstration of an extrameatal acoustic neuroma in the cerebellopontine angle (*white arrow*). Additional demonstration of an enhanced venous part of the dura directly adjacent to the apical portion of the tumor (*open arrow*)
**b** Parasagittal MRI (turbo-FLASH, ray tracing reconstruction) with Gd-DTPA. Verification of the position of the tumor within the cerebellopontine angle. *c*, Hyperintense internal carotid artery; *t*, temporal lobe

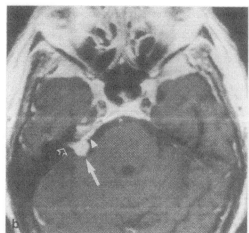

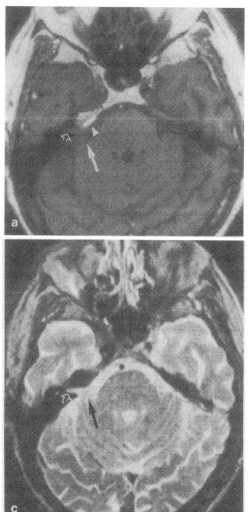

**Fig. 6.8 a–e.** Intra-extrameatal acoustic neuroma on the right side: comparison of various MRI sequences and planes
**a** Plain axial MRI (SE, 500/17). Demonstration of a tumor within the internal auditory canal and the cerebellopontine cistern. The lesion is isointense to brain parenchyma. *Open arrow,* intrameatal segment; *white arrow,* extrameatal segment; *arrowhead,* dura and clivus
**b** Axial MRI (SE, 500/17) with Gd-DTPA. Significant increase in signal intensity in the area of the

intra- and extrameatal segments of the tumor after administration of Gd-DTPA. Medially, the tumor is adjacent to the pons and the cerebral peduncles. The primarily hyperintense fatty tissue in the area of the dura and the clivus can reliably be demarcated from tumorous involvement due to the low increase in signal intensity after injection of Gd-DTPA (*arrowhead*)
**c** Plain axial MRI (SE, 2000/90). Low contrast between the lesion (*arrow*) and the CSF within the cerebellomedullar cistern
**d, e** see p. 61

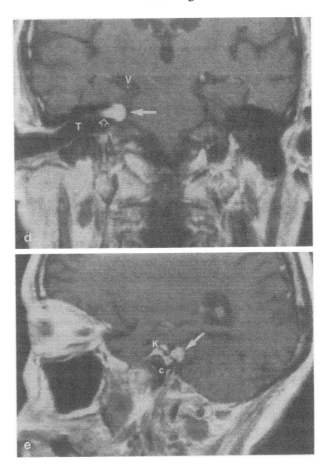

**Fig. 6.8. d** MRI (SE, 500/17) with Gd-DTPA. Verification of the intra-extrameatal localization (arrows). In particular compression of the pons can be excluded via this slice orientation. *T,* tympanic cavity; *V,* petrosal vein

**e** Sagittal MRI (Se, 500/17) with Gd-DTPA. Demonstration of the close relationship of the hyperintense tumor (*white arrow*) to the clivus and the cerebral peduncles. *c,* internal carotid artery; *k,* clivus

### 6.5.2.3 Intrameatal Acoustic Neuroma

In intrameatal acoustic neuromas MRI allows direct differentiation of the tumor from the nerve bundle (Figs. 6.9, 6.10). Inflammatory cohesions of the meninges are also found within the internal auditory canal and can be misinterpreted as intrameatal acoustic neuromas.

### 6.5.2.4 Recklinghausen's Disease

In MRI of patients with neurofibromatosis (Recklinghausen's disease) the simultaneous involvement of several cranial nerves in different stages of growth can be demonstrated (Fig. 6.11). Diagnosis of postoperative changes and the demonstration of recurrence also fall within the domain of MRI. Due to its sensitivity for small lesions in the cerebellopontine angle and the internal auditory canal, MRI is the technique of choice for the verification of all pathologic lesions in this area [48].

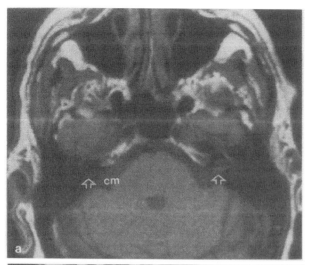

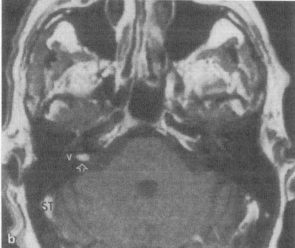

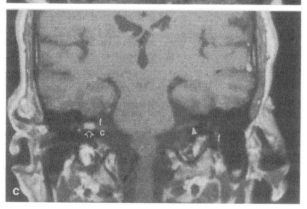

**Fig. 6.9 a–c.** Right intrameatal acoustic neuroma: evaluation via T1-weighted sequences in two planes
**a** Plain axial MRI (Se, 500/17). Wide cerebellomedullar cistern, symmetric internal auditory canals, no reliable demonstration of a tumor. *Arrows,* internal auditory canal; *cm,* cerebellomedullary cistern
**b** Axial MRI (SE, 500/17) with Gd-DTPA. Significant increase in signal intensity of soft tissue ($5 \times 3 \times 3$ mm) within the right internal auditory canal after administration of Gd-DTPA. Lateral expansion of the tumor to the vestibule (*V*). No contact with the cerebellomedullary cistern. *Arrow,* right intrameatal acoustic neuroma. No significant contrast agent uptake on the left side. Clear enhancement in the transverse sinus (*ST*)
**c** Coronal MRI (SE, 500/17) with Gd-DTPA. Verification of the intrameatal localization of the tumor. Medially, the bundles of the facial nerve (*f*) and the cochlear nerve (*c*) can be differentiated. No lesion is visible on the left side (*arrowhead*). Within the left facial canal the facial nerve (*f*) shows enhancement

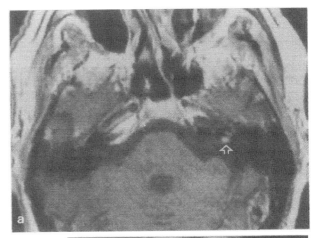

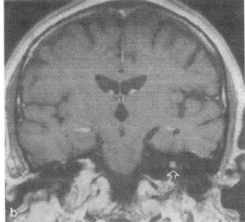

**Fig. 6.10a, b.** Left intrameatal acoustic neuroma (3 × 4 mm) originating from the area between glial cells and Schwann's cells of the superior vestibular nerve
**a** Axial MRI (SE, 500/17) with Gd-DTPA
**b** Images in two planes localize the small tumor precisely to the vestibule and parts of the labyrinth. The whole tumor could be exstirpated via the translabyrinthine approach, preserving all functions of the cranial nerves (*arrow*)

**Fig. 6.11.** Recklinghausen's disease with bilateral intra-extrameatal acoustic neuromas. Coronal MRI (SE, 500/17) with Gd-DTPA. Demonstration of an intra-extrameatal acoustic neuroma on the right side. The extrameatal component shows wide expansions within the cerebellomedullary cistern and displaces parts of the medial temporal lobe cranially. Small inhomogeneous internal structures are seen within the strongly enhancing tumor. Verification of an intra-extrameatal acoustic neuroma on the left side involving the complete intrameatal nerve bundle and a small meningioma in the apical area of the left parietal lobe (*arrow*), extrameatal tumor component; *i*, intrameatal tumor component

## 6.6 Other Neuromas

In the differential diagnosis of acoustic neuroma several other neuromas originating from neighboring cranial nerves have to be taken into consideration, i.e. facial neuromas, trigeminal neuromas, and neuromas of the inferior cranial nerves (Fig. 6.12) [21, 27, 53]. The majority of facial neuromas originate

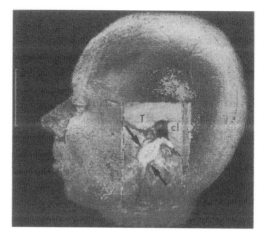

**Fig. 6.13.** Right hypoglossal neuroma. Sagittal MRI (3D FLASH, ray tracing) with Gd-DTPA. Demonstration of the intracanicular tumor component (*open arrow*) within the hypoglossal canal. Large, central, inhomogeneous neuroma located anteriorly in the paravertebral space (*black arrows*). *cl,* Cerebellum; *T,* temporal lobe

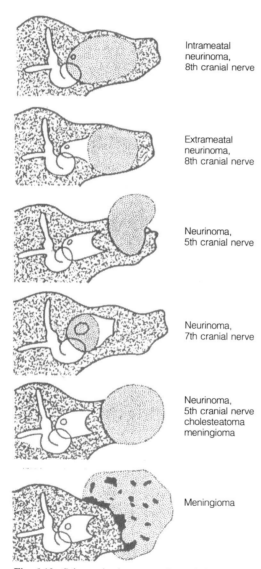

Intrameatal neurinoma, 8th cranial nerve

Extrameatal neurinoma, 8th cranial nerve

Neurinoma, 5th cranial nerve

Neurinoma, 7th cranial nerve

Neurinoma, 5th cranial nerve cholesteatoma meningioma

Meningioma

**Fig. 6.12.** Schematic demonstration of the growth patterns of various tumors infiltrating the internal auditory canal and the pyramid apex

from the genicular ganglion and expand into the labyrinthine as well as the tympanic segment of the facial nerve. Facial neuromas are characterized by a circular or oval cross section, a close topographic relationship to the facial canal, and a clear signal increase after administration of Gd-DTPA. Contrast-enhanced MRI is the optimal diagnostic technique because all growth patterns can be documented precisely. Circumscribed meningioma and hemangioma also have to be taken into account in differential diagnosis. These tumors can also affect the tympanic cavity and the internal auditory canal. Neuromas of the inferior cranial nerves represent the second most frequent tumor type in the jugular foramen. Hypoglossal neuromas (Fig. 6.13) show up as circular or oval homogeneous masses of soft tissue with an intense uptake of contrast agent.

An important diagnostic criterion is the ipsilateral hemiatrophy of the tongue muscles caused by paresis, with clearly increased T2. In contrast to glomus jugulare tumors, neuromas grow only expansively, often with involvement of the parapharyngeal area. This growth pattern tends to show up as an hourglass configuration on coronal and sagittal slices.

In contrast to the masses described above, the trigeminal neuroma is located in the ventral part of the cerebellopontine angle. Advanced tumors destroy the pyramid apex, infiltrate Meckel's cave, and show an hourglass configuration.

## 6.7 Glomus Tumors

The various glomus bodies of the human organism display anatomic and functional similarities (Fig. 6.14). The terms paraganglioma, glomerocytoma, and chemodectoma have been used as synonyms for glomus tumors [25, 33, 45, 56].

Extremely rich vascularization is characteristic for this group of tumors [33, 46]. Generally the whole glomus is interlaced with a dense network of arterioles that join with wider veins located especially on the surface of the tumor. The varying origin of tumors of the glomus jugulare and glomus tympanicum explains the extraordinary variability of the clinical findings and demands painstaking diagnosis. Besides clinical investigation, which especially has to embrace symptoms like tinnitus and conductive hearing loss, audiometry and neurootological examination have to be carried out.

Prior to the advent of CT, selective angiography of the external carotid artery and the vertebral artery was used for diagnosis. In the early stages of skull base glomus tumors, blood is supplied via branches of the external carotid artery (see Fig. 6.19h), while larger processes are supplied via the vertebral and basilar artery [5]. Angiography is especially helpful in identifying surgically relevant variants of vessels such as lateral displacement of the internal carotid artery in the petrosal segment or an unusually cranial location of the superior jugular bulb (Fig. 6.15).

Hitherto diagnostic CT was performed in order to determine the category and the expansion of glomus tumors. High-resolution CT can demonstrate the relationship to the cervical soft tissue as well as the intratympanic and

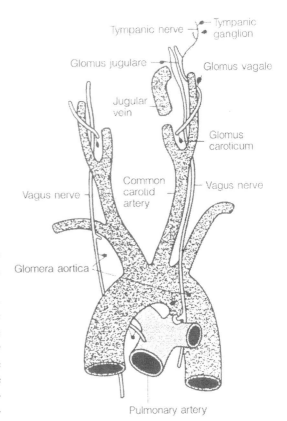

**Fig. 6.14.** Typical localization of the glomera in the human organism

intracranial expansion. In the majority of cases glomus tumors can be differentiated from other skull base diseases by dynamic CT and the time-density profile [11, 38].

The CT findings, however, include a relatively high proportion of false negatives and false positives, especially if CT is primarily carried out after intravenous administration of contrast agent [37]. Small tumors, especially those originating from the glomus tympanicum, render diagnosis more difficult because they only show up as hypointense areas without osseous destruction. MRI, with its superior soft tissue contrast, is proving to be the modality of choice for the diagnostic imaging of these tumors.

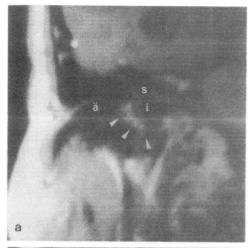

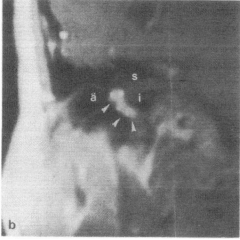

**Fig. 6.15a, b.** Glomus hypotympanicum tumor (type B): evaluation using surface coil
**a** Plain MRI (SE, 500/17). Demonstration of soft tissue in the area of the caudal segments of the tympanic cavity and hypotympanic cavity. Exact delineation of the relations of the tumor to the segments of the cochlea as well as the superior vestibular nerve (*s*) and the inferior vestibular nerve (*i*) ä, external auditory canal
**b** Coronal MRI (SE, 500/17) with Gd-DTPA. Homogeneous enhancement of the glomus hypotympanicum tumor on the right side. The neural structures show no enhancement

### 6.7.1 Classification

Glomus tympanicum and glomus jugulare tumors can be differentiated according to origin and site. Several different classifications exist, for the glomus tumors of the temporal bone and skull base, but the classification by Valavanis and Fisch has proved valuable for diagnosis and for planning of surgery [20, 21]:

Type A   Glomus tympanicum tumor
Type B   Glomus hypotympanicum tumor: intact cortical border of bulb, erosion of hypotympanic osseous structures
Type C   Glomus jugulare tumor without intracranial expansion
        C1   Minimal erosion: vertical segment of carotid canal
        C2   Complete erosion: vertical segment of carotid canal
        C3   Erosion: horizontal segment of carotid canal
        C4   foramen lacerum, cavernous sinus
Type D   Glomus jugulare tumor with intracranial expansion
        De   Extradural (De 1–3)
        Di   Intradural (Di 1–3)

### 6.7.2 MRI Characteristics

Several factors favor primary evaluation of glomus jugular tumors by MRI. First, MRI shows better soft tissue contrast than CT by virtue of the lack of signal from the surrounding bone [2, 22, 33]. However, the use of a head coil is obligatory, because the superior jugular bulb is located centrally in the skull base. The main reason for the superiority of MRI is the imaging of flowing blood due to the flow phenomenon. The topographic relations of the carotid siphon and the superior jugular bulb can reliably be distinguished on plain MRI [4, 22, 25]. MRI is able to differentiate optimally between a glomus tumor and a high-sited jugular bulb. The tumor and its extension into the jugular vein can be diagnosed on coronal slices. Retrograde phlebography

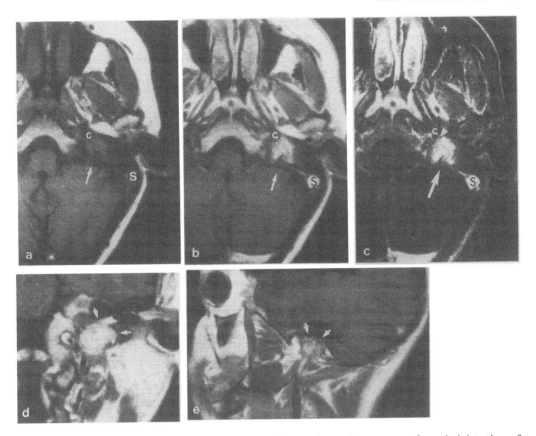

**Fig. 6.16a–e.** Left glomus jugulare tumor (type C1). Involvement of the superior jugular bulb with erosion of the vertical segment of the carotid canal
**a** Plain MRI (SE, 500/28). Tumor (10 × 12 mm) within the left jugular bulb (*c*, internal carotid artery; *S*, sigmoid sinus
**b** Axial MRI (SE, 500/28) with Gd-DTPA. Increase in signal intensity of the indistinctly demarcated tumor with central inhomogeneities and hypo-intense internal structures after administration of Gd-DTPA. The dorsal segments of the carotid canal are eroded
**c** Subtraction image (**a** – **b**). Exact demarcation of areas of strong enhancement and the erosion of the carotid canal (type C1) (*arrowhead*)
**d, e** Coronal and parasagittal MRI (SE, 500/28) with Gd-DTPA. Preoperative evaluation of the craniocaudal expansion (*arrows*)

of the jugular vein has thus become completely obsolete.

Type C tumors more than 1.5 mm in diameter can be characterized exactly as to location and size. These tumors show a typically lobular outline and rich vascularization (Figs. 6.16, 6.17).

In some patients with small glomus tumors plain MRI is of limited diagnostic value (Figs. 6.16a, 6.17a). The use of the fast imaging technique and the administration of Gd-DTPA optimizes the diagnostic potential. Similar to the time-density profile in dynamic CT, the time course of the signal intensity of the glomus tumor can be calculated by analyzing eight GE sequences with a total acquisition time of 7 min (see Fig. 6.11). In all untreated glomus tumors a rapid and high increase in signal intensity, with an average factor of 2.5, is found in the first 60 s after administration of Gd-DTPA. The maximal enhancement is reached after 120–160 s. In all cases the signal intensity decreases about 300–350 s after administration of Gd-DTPA (Fig. 6.18). This course of signal intensity after injection, due to the high degree of vascularization of the tumor, correlates with the findings of dynamic CT.

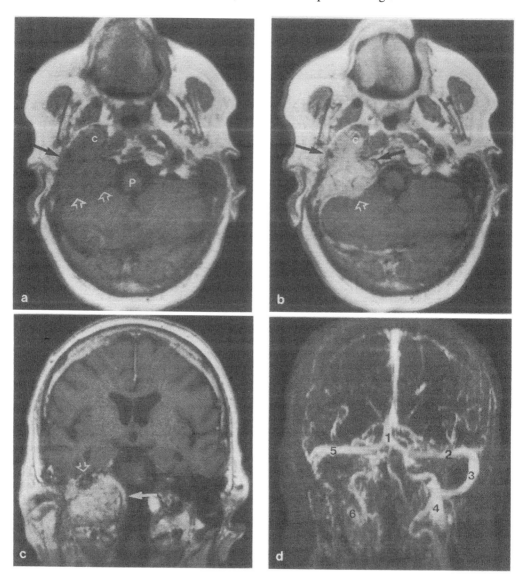

**Fig. 6.17a–d.** Glomus jugulare tumor with intracranial expansion (type D). Value of the administration of contrast agent as well as venous MR angiography (MRA).

**a** Plain axial MRI (SE, 500/17). Hypointense tumor with central zones of lower signal in the area of the jugular fossa. Involvement of the infratemporal fossa and the retromaxillary space. Suspicion of intradural expansion (*arrows*). Anteriorly displaced internal carotid artery (*c*). On the right side the sinus system and jugular vein are not visualized. *P,* pons

**b** Axial MRI (SE, 500/17) with Gd-DTPA. After administration of Gd-DTPA the whole tumor shows inhomogeneous enhancement. Centrally low-signal internal structures due to tumor vessels. Clear enhancement in the area of the dura and in the direction of the cerebellum. Suspicion of intradural infiltration (*open arrow*). Exact demarcation of the tumor in relation to the parapharyngeal space and to dorsal after Gd-DTPA

**c** Coronal MRI (SE, 500/17) with Gd-DTPA. Verification of the topographic relations of the tumor in the area of the infratemporal fossa. The characteristic linear internal structures are vessels. Additional demonstration of the convex outline of the tumor with displacement of the CSF system (*white arrow*). Compact bone is visible only at the apical parts of the pyramid (*open arrow*)

**d** Legend see p. 69

The signal intensities of nonenhanced and en-hanced sequences (field strength 1.0 T) are compared. On average, the Gd-DTPA uptake increases the signal intensity by 205% in tumor tissue, 23% in muscle, and 51% in fatty tissue.

In the majority of cases, optimal imaging with exact delineation of the vascularized parts of the tumor (Figs. 6.16b, 6.17b) is achieved with administration of Gd-DTPA. In some patients with large tumors no additional information is obtained via contrast enhancement.

A study was carried out to compare the diagnostic accuracy, the topographic orientation, and the demarcation of glomus jugulare and glomus tympanicum tumors on MRI and CT. Judged by these criteria, MRI was superior to CT in 13 cases and of equal value in three cases. Especially in processes with infiltration of the middle cranial fossa (Fig. 6.17c), coherent mastoiditis, and small glomus tympanicum tumors (Fig. 6.19) enhanced MRI

shows its superior diagnostic potential. The CT findings in patients with glomus jugulare were false positive in three cases and false negative in four cases. All patients with glomus tumors of the skull base or the temporal bone undergo a supplementary angiographic study, either digital subtraction angiography or, more recently, MR angiography (Fig. 6.17d). This yields important additional information on the exact vascularization of the tumor and on the hemodynamic situation in the circle of Willis. Vascular supply via branches of the posterior auricular artery is the most frequent type. Other glomus tumors are supplied via the ascending pharyngeal artery.

The high overall accuracy of MRI is based especially on the reliable demonstration of other tumors of the temporal bone and the cerebellopontine angle.

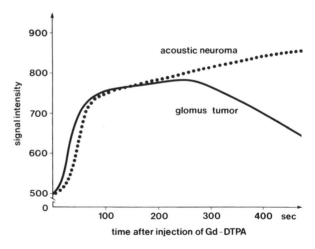

**Fig. 6.18.** Course of signal intensity of glomus jugular tumors in comparison to acoustic neuromas. Analysis with gradient echo sequences over 7 min after administration of Gd-DTPA

◁

**Fig. 6.17. d** MRA after arterial saturation with demonstration of the venous system: 2D FLASH sequence in AP projection. Normal demonstration of confluence of sinuses (*1*). Left transverse sinus (*2*), sigmoid sinus (*3*), jugular vein (*4*). Still normal perfusion of the involved right transverse sinus (*5*). Obstruction of sigmoid sinus with demonstration of multiple collaterals. Obstruction of the collateralized jugular vein with a small aperture remaining (*6*). Complete obstruction of the jugular bulb and the sigmoid sinus is demonstrated by MRA

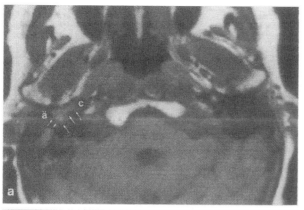

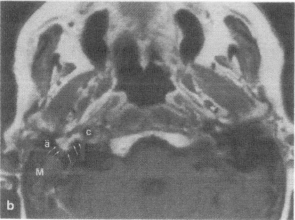

**Fig. 6.19 a–h.** Left glomus tympanicum tumor (type A): value of spin echo sequences, administration of contrast agent, dynamic series, and 3D techniques

**a** Plain axial MRI (SE, 500/17). Demonstration of a tumor in the area of the tympanic cavity in a T1-weighted sequence. Expansion within the complete middle ear. *c*, internal carotid artery, *ä*, external auditory canal

**b** Axial MRI (SE, 500/17) with Gd-DTPA. Homogeneous enhancement of the clearly demarcated tumor in the area of the tympanic cavity after administration of Gd-DTPA. No proof of other infiltration in the surrounding tissue. The tumor is in contact with the internal carotid artery (*c*). Inflammatory changes in the area of the mastoid show up as hyperintense structures, with no significant enhancement. *M*, mastoiditis

**c** Plain axial MRI (SE, 2000/90). In T2-weighted sequences the tumor shows low and slightly inhomogeneous signal intensity (*arrows*); inflammatory changes in the mastoid show up with a clearly increased signal intensity. *M*, mastoiditis

**d, e** Axial MRI (FLASH), plain (**d**) and with Gd-DTPA (**e**). Dynamic MRI sequences are carried out before and after administration of contrast agent. In the plain image, tumor (*T*) and mastoiditis (*M*) show equal signal intensity. In the area of the parapharyngeal space there is hyperintense fatty tissue (*F*). After injection of contrast medium there is significantly increased signal intensity in the area of the jugular bulb (*B*) and the tumor (*T*); regular flow within the sinus system. These sequences allow exact analysis of the dynamic enhancement, but show lower topographic resolution

**f** Coronal MRI (SE, 500/17) with Gd-DTPA. Exact demonstration of the relationship of the tumor and the external auditory canal (*ä*), the temporal lobe (*T*) and the pyramid apex (*P*). Normal findings on the left, with hypointense signal within the temporal bone. *M*, mastoid

**c–f** see p. 71
**g, h** see p. 72

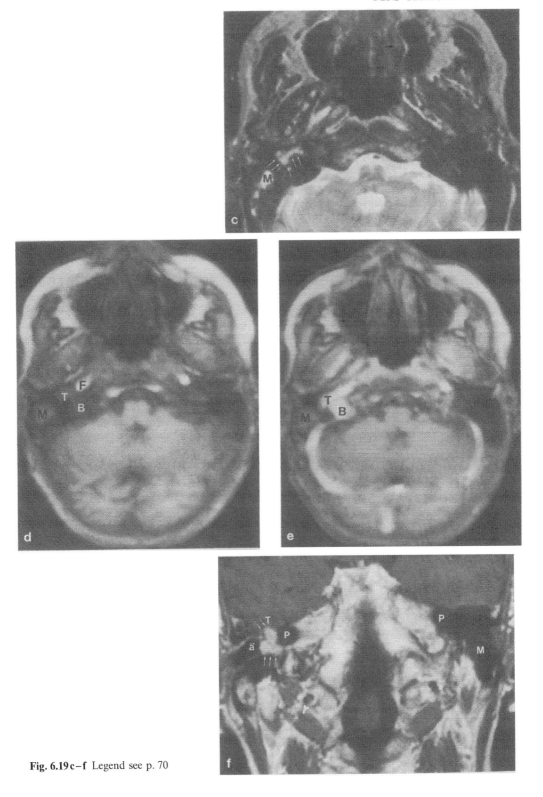

**Fig. 6.19 c–f** Legend see p. 70

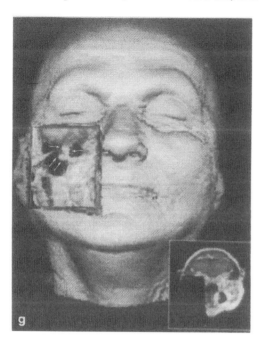

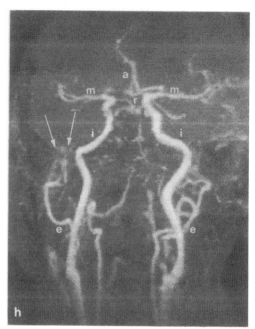

**Fig. 6.19. g** Coronal MRI (3D turbo-FLASH, ray tracing) with Gd-DTPA. Demonstration of the tumor in a 3D sequence (lower spatial resolution compared to a T1-weighted sequence, (*f*) with exact topographic relations to the external auditory canal, the pyramid apex, and the temporal lobe **h** MR angiography, arterial after venous saturation 3D FISP. Demonstration of normal course of internal carotid artery (*i*), medial (*m*) and anterior (*a*) cerebral artery system, and anterior communicating artery (*r*). Slightly hyperintense segment in the course of the terminal branches of the ascending pharyngeal artery (branch of the external carotid artery) after administration of Gd-DTPA of Gd-DTPA. Based on this localization the glomus tympanicum tumor is not shown and only the supplying vessel can be differentiated (*arrows*)

Acoustic neuroma, the most frequent tumor of this region, is identified and delineated by the typical topographic relations and by the characteristic course of signal intensity after administration of Gd-DTPA. In contrast to glomus tumors, acoustic neuromas show a slow rise in signal intensity early after injection and a constant increase up to 7 min after injection (Fig. 6.18).

The following features of glomus tumors are characteristic:

- Location in the middle skull base and the cerebellopontine angle without involvement of the vestibulocochlear nerve
- Lobular outline
- Rich vascularization
- Prolonged T2 in relation to white matter
- Rapid increase in signal intensity after administration of contrast agent and decrease after 300 s (wash-out effect)

### 6.7.2.1 Glomus Tympanicum Tumor

The most frequent benign tumors of the middle ear are the glomus tympanicum tumors. Originating from the medial osseous border of the middle ear, these tumors are located in the territory of the tympanic branch of the glossopharyngeal nerve (Jacobson's nerve) and the auricular branch of the vagus nerve (Amald's nerve). These tumors are always clearly delineated on MRI (Fig. 6.19) and adapt to the shape of the tympanic cavity with a rectilinear outline. These homogeneous soft tissue masses are in extensive apposition to the cochlear promontory and the carotid canal (6.19 a, b). The erosion of the promontory, visualized on high-resolution CT, cannot be seen on MRI.

The MR characteristics of glomus tympanicum tumors are as follows:

1. Localization: tympanic cavity, adjacent to cochlear promontory and carotid canal
2. Clear delineation
3. Homogeneous signal intensity
4. High contrast agent uptake (Fig. 6.19)

As differential diagnoses, hemangiomas of the middle ear and various vessel abnormalities must be considered. Hemangioma of the middle ear originates from the perineurium of the facial nerve and shows a clear morphology like facial neuroma. After administration of contrast medium the characteristic signal intensity profile of hemangioma is found with a slow increase and a long plateau.

Two vascular abnormalities are more frequent than others: (1) There is sometimes atresia of internal carotid artery from the carotid bifurcation to the petrous segment. Collateralization and the caroticotympanic artery compensates for the missing segment. (2) The cranial jugular bulb is caused by diverticular bulging of the superolateral part of the superior jugular bulb into the hypotympanic cavity. These vessel variants can clearly be differentiated after administration of Gd-DTPA or on MR angiography (Fig. 6.19h).

## 6.8 Meningioma

Meningioma is regarded as the third most frequent tumor of the middle skull base and the temporal bone. These clearly demarcated extraaxial tumors are located in the convexity and also in the area of the sphenoid bone, the olfactory canal, the posterior cranial fossa, and along cranial nerves [39]. Meningioma of the temporal bone and the pyramid apex was found less frequently in our patient material than in other studies [26]. The MRI criteria for the exact evaluation of meningiomas are above all the topographic features (Fig. 6.20b). In contrast to other tumors of the cerebellopontine angle, meningiomas always show extensive contact with the pyramid (Fig. 6.20b) and form a wide angle with the posterior border of the temporal bone. This is the most important criterion for differentiating between meningeomas and acoustic neuromas in the majority of patients, as acoustic neuromas have a small area of contact and a narrow angle with the posterior border of the temporal bone. In T1-weighted sequences meningiomas show a signal intensity similar to that of brain parenchyma (Fig. 6.20a). Accordingly, small meningiomas originating from arachnoid cell aggregations at the posterior border of the temporal bone cannot be diagnosed on plain MRI. Administration of the paramagnetic contrast agent Gd-DTPA always causes a homogeneous and intensive increase in signal intensity due to the reduction of T1 [48, 49] (Fig. 6.20b). In the case of a meningioma expanding within the internal auditory canal the infiltration can be detected by means of the increase in signal intensity after injection of Gd-DTPA. In specific cases the diagnosis should be verified by high-resolution CT [48]. The majority of meningiomas cause a circumscribed exostosis of bone in the area of their origin. Large and medium-sized exostoses are visualized by MRI, but small exostoses generally escape detection. The following MRI characteristics are regarded as typical for meningiomas:

1. Topography
   - extensive apposition (Fig. 6.20)
   - extraaxial location
   - invasion of the venous sinus system, in rare case apically along the pyramid apex (Fig. 6.21)
2. Plain MRI
   - T1 weighted: hypointense to white matter
   - T2 weighted: hyperintense to white matter (Fig. 6.20c), heterogeneous appearance, cystic, calcification, hypointense margin
3. Gd-DTPA
   - high uptake, homogeneous, dynamic, rapid in first 3 min, T1 + Gd-DTPA

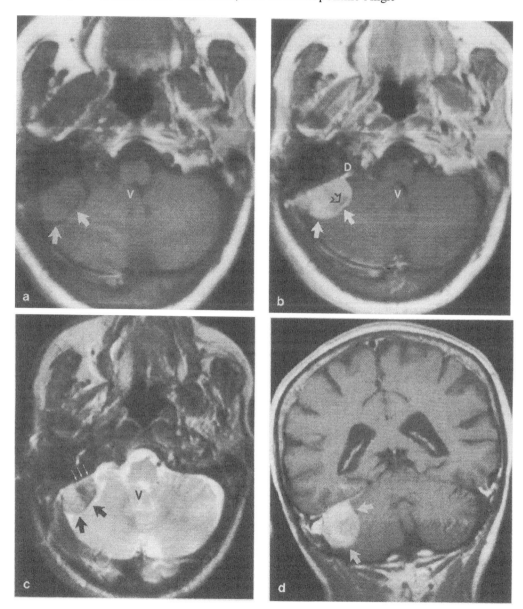

**Fig. 6.20a–d.** Meningioma along the pyramid with compression of the right hemisphere of the cerebellum
**a** Plain axial MRI (SE, 500/17). Tumor (*arrows*) along the pyramid in T1-weighted sequences, isointense to the normal cerebellar parenchyma. The fourth ventricle (*V*) is displaced to the left. Regular osseous structures of the temporal bone
**b** Axial MRI (SE, 500/17) with Gd-DTPA. Slightly inhomogeneous enhancement of the large tumor along the pyramid, central zone of calcification (*open arrow*), additional enhancement in the area of medial dural parts (*D*)

**c** Plain axial MRI (SE, 2000/90). In T2-weighted sequences the meningioma shows up as a hypointense structure in comparison to the hyperintense CSF and the white and gray matter. Internal central structures of lower signal are equivalent to calcification zones. Regular demonstration of the temporal bone
**d** Coronal MRI (SE, 500/17) with Gd-DTPA. Verification of the topographic relations of the inhomogeneously enhancing meningeoma to the cerebral falx and the cerebellar lobes

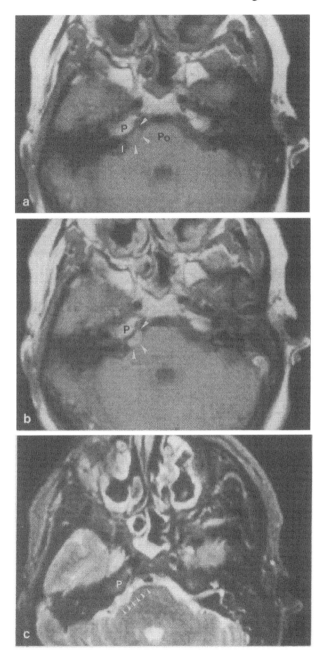

**Fig. 6.21 a–e.** Meningioma along the apical and anterior apex of the pyramid and the cerebellomedullary cistern. Demonstration of the tumor in different planes and sequences
**a** Plain axial MRI (SE, 500/17). Demonstration of an elliptic tumorous lesion (*arrowheads,* 10 × 6 mm) in the area of the cerebellomedullary cistern, contact with the pyramid apex (*P*). Clear demarcation of the tumor from CSF (*l*); medially the tumor borders on the segments of the pons (*Po*). Regular imaging of the soft tissue within the internal auditory canal

**b** Axial MRI (SE, 500/17) with Gd-DTPA. Homogeneous increase in signal intensity in the area of the elliptic tumor after administration of Gd-DTPA. Clear demarcation from the pyramid and the pons (*arrowheads*)
**c** Plain axial MRI (SE, 2000/90). Isointense demonstration of the complete cerebellomedullary cistern (*arrowheads*). The presence of the tumor cannot be proved in T2-weighted sequences
**d, e** see p. 76

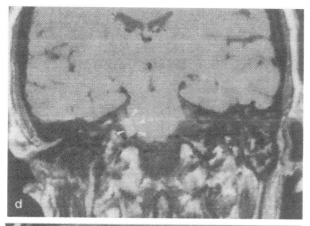

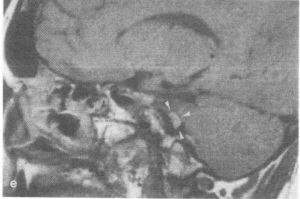

**Fig. 6.21. d, e** Coronal (*d*) and parasagittal (**e**) MRI (SE, 500/17) with Gd-DTPA. Verification of the topographic relations of the tumor in two planes. Slight compression of the pons and contact, with the pyramid (*arrowheads*)

It seems almost paradoxical that MRI has been become the diagnostic modality of choice for meningiomas although they can escape detection by plain MRI. However, using the paramagnetic contrast agent Gd-DTPA and fast sequences in multiple planes, the preoperative planning for these tumors has been decisively improved.

## 6.9 Epidermoid

In the literature the epidermoid is reported as one of the most frequent tumors of the cerebellopontine angle (3%–6% of the tumors) [48]. This lesion's low signal intensity in T1-weighted sequences (Fig. 6.22 a) and the significantly prolonged T2 time are important in diagnosis. This signal behavior is also found in arachnoid cysts of this region, but in contrast to such cysts epidermoids show cisternal expansion within the preformed subarachnoid spaces (Fig. 6.22 c) and enclose larger vessels without displacing them. An intratumorally extending anterior cerebellar artery or basilar artery is thus characteristic for epidermoids. Similar to arachnoid cysts, epider-

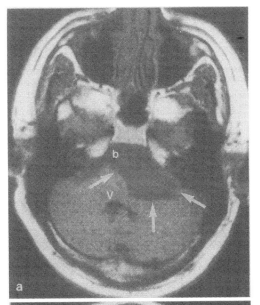

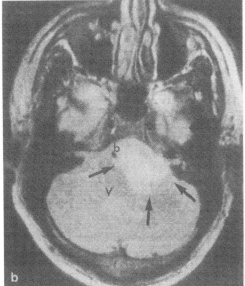

**Fig. 6.22 a–c.** Epidermoid in the cerebellopontine angle and the left hemisphere of the cerebellum; comparative analysis of different sequences
**a** Plain axial MRI (SE, 500/28). The tumor is isointense to the CSF (*arrows*) and shows slight displacement of the basilar artery to medial (*b*) and compression of the 4th ventricle (*v*). Regular structures of the internal auditory canal
**b** Plain axial MRI (SE, 2000/90). Increased signal intensity of the tumor in T2-weighted sequences. Displacement of the basilar artery, no demonstration of other internal structures
**c** Coronal MRI (Se, 500/17) with Gd-DTPA. Verification of the cisternal expansion of the tumor after administration of Gd-DTPA. Little increase in signal intensity after injection in comparison with the CSF system. *i*, internal auditory canal; *P*, pons

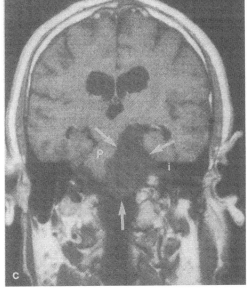

moids can cause pressure erosion of the posterior surface of the temporal bone. In contrast to epidermoids, lipomas show high signal intensities in T1-weighted and T2-weighted sequences. Lipomas are often spherical and smaller than epidermoids [48]. An important diagnostic criterion for epidermoids is the lack of contrast agent uptake due to the minimal vascularization of their keratin and cholesterol content.

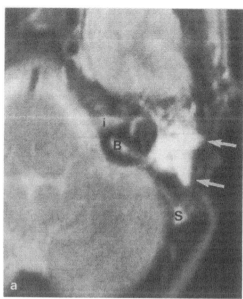

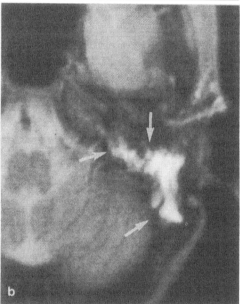

**Fig. 6.23a, b.** Left cholesteatoma in the tympanic cavity and the mastoid
**a, b** Plain axial MRI (SE, 2000/90). Slices at the levels of the internal auditory canal (**a**) and the hypotympanic segments (**b**). Inflammatory changes of the mastoid and the tympanic cavity characterized by increased signal intensities. Strictly inflammatory fluid collections within the tissue show up as mottled shadowing. Involvement of the tympanic cavity, the hypotympanic cavity, and the complete mastoid, as well as the pyramid apex (*arrows*). *i,* internal auditory canal; *B,* superior jugular bulb; *s,* sigmoid sinus

The following MRI characteristics are regarded as typical for epidermoids:

1. Topography
   - located in cerebellopontine angle or posterior cranial fossa
   - intratumoral artery
2. Plain MRI
   - T1 weighting: low signal intensity
   - T2 weighting: increased signal intensity (Fig. 6.22b)
3. Gd-DTPA
   - no significant contrast enhancement

## 6.10 Cholesteatoma and Other Tumors of the Pyramid Apex

MRI yields additional diagnostic information for the evaluation of tumors of the pyramid apex [48, 50, 51]. The most frequent lesion of the apex is primary congenital cholesteatoma, which returns a high signal in all MR sequences (Fig. 6.23 a, b) and displays homogeneously decreased density on CT [42]. For pretherapeutic diagnosis the exact relationship between the tumor and the facial nerve has to be documented using CT and MRI. In occasional cases the pyramid apex is secondarily affected by tumors originating from surrounding structures, such as chordomas of the clivus, trigeminal neuromas, carcinomas of the middle ear, and histiocytoses.

The following features are regarded as for characteristic primary congenital and acquired cholesteatomas:

1. Typical localization
2. Significantly prolonged T2

## 6.11 Tumors of the Posterior Cranial Fossa

Due to the low specificity of MRI signal characteristics of tumors of the posterior cranial fossa, the location of the lesions assumes greater importance [44]. An important criterion for the differentitation of infraaxial tumors is their intraaxial or extraaxial location:

*Intraaxial astrocytoma*
- PNET
- ependymoma
- hemangioblastoma
- plexus chordoma
- lymphoma
- dermoid cyst
- epidermoid
- teratoma

*Extraaxial acoustic neuroma*
- other neuromas
- meningioma
- epidermoid

Astrocytomas, ependymomas, hemangioblastomas and primitive neuroectodermal tumors (medulloblastomas) show solid and cystic components with variably low signal intensity in T1-weighted sequences. Cystic components with higher water or protein content are characterized by high signal intensity in T2-weighted sequences [1, 3, 5–7, 12, 13]. Reliable differentiation between the tumor and the surrounding edema is achieved only after administration of Gd-DTPA.

## 6.12 Overall Efficacy of MRI

Primary tumors such as neuromas, meningiomas, and epidermoids originate from anatomic structures of the cerebellopontine angle and the internal auditory canal [22]. In contrast, secondary tumors extend from neighboring structures into the cerebellopontine angle and the internal auditory canal (glomus jugulare tumors, chondromas, chordomas, cerebellar tumors, metastases, and tumors of the hemopoietic system). In our prospective study facial neuromas ($n = 2$), epidermoids ($n = 2$), and metastases ($n = 3$) were identified correctly by MRI. Two plasmacytomas were wrongly characterized as cholesteatomas and an undifferentiated sarcoma was falsely diagnosed as a meningioma. The advantages of MRI for the evaluation of these tumors are improved specificity and soft tissue contrast together with the capacity to evaluate expansion of processes in all planes [52, 54, 55]. MR techniques yield important information for the tricky differential diagnosis of tumors in this region.

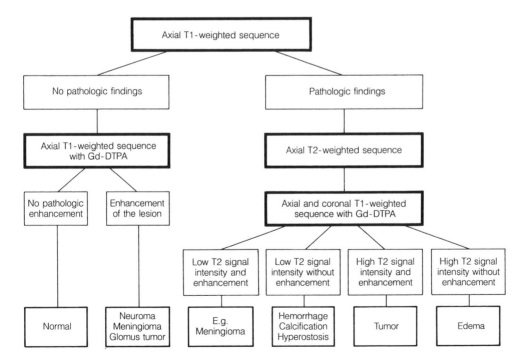

**Fig. 6.24.** Diagnostic strategy: temporal bone, middle skull base, and cerebellopontine angle

## 6.13 Diagnostic Strategy

In spite of the high sensitivity of MRI, CT techniques, especially high-resolution CT, remain important in the diagnosis of conductions of the middle ear [32]. For cartilaginous and osseous structures CT is the modality of choice because of its excellent resolution. For other purposes, though, MRI is now past the stage of clinical testing and can be recommended strongly for specific uses (Table 6.8) [9, 16, 19, 23, 36, 43]. Because of the high diagnostic accuracy of MRI, reliable identification of acoustic neuromas is achieved at an early stage [40, 41]. This enables the surgeon to choose the transtemporal route, which is a much more sparing approach and yields better late results. Above all, diagnostic imaging of the temporal bone, the cerebellopontine angle, and the middle skull base must identify the following primary and secondary tumors (Fig. 6.24):

Primary tumors:  neuroma
        – meningioma
        – epidermoid

Secondary tumors:  Glomus tumor
        – chondroma
        – chordoma
        – cerebellar tumors
        – metastases
        – plasmacytoma
        – osteoma

*References*

1. Bauer M, Baierl P, Vogl T, Wendt T, Lissner J (1986) Efficacy and secondary intracranial tumors before and after radiotherapy. Society of Magnet-Resonance in Medicine, 5th annual meeting, Montreal, Canada. Book of abstracts vol 3, pp 590–591
2. Bauer M, Baierl P, Fink U, Vogl T, Rohloff R (1986) Verlaufskontrolle von primären und sekundären Hirntumoren nach Strahlentherapie mittels Kernspintomographie im Vergleich zur Computertomographie. In: Vogler E, Schneider GH (eds) Digitale bildgebende Verfahren – Integrierte digitale Radiologie. 84th Radiological Symposium, Graz, 3–5 Oct 1985. Schering, Berlin, pp 151–155
3. Bauer M, Vogl T, Krauss B, Nägele N (1987) Plain MR – diagnostic value and potential in comparison to contrast enhanced (Gd-DTPA) MR in tumorous and inflammatory diseases of the brain. In: Lissner J (eds) MR 87 Symposium Garmisch, Schnetztor, Konstanz, pp 133–139
4. Bauer M, Einhäupl K, Heywang S, Vogl T, Seiderer M, Clados D (1987) Magnet resonance imaging of venous sinus thrombosis. AJNR 8:713–715
5. Bauer M, Fenzl G, Vogl T, Fink U, Lissner J (1986) Indications for the use of Gd-DTPA in MR of the CNS. Invest Radiol 5:12
6. Bauer WM, Baierl P, Obermüller H, Bisek H, Valenti M (1985) Comparison of plain and contrast-enhanced MR in intracranial tumors – report on 37 cases confirmed by histology. In: Society of Magnet resonance, 4th annual meeting, London. Book of abstracts, pp 310–311
7. Bauer WM, Baierl P, Vogl T, Obermüller H (1985) Contrast-enhancement in intercranial tumors – a comparison of CT and MR. Radiology 157 (P):126
8. Becker H, Naumann H, Pfalz C (1982) HNO-Heilkunde. Thieme, Stuttgart
9. Beimert U, Grevers G, Vogl T (1988) Zum Stellenwert der digitalen Subtraktionsangiographie bei der Diagnostik von Glomustumoren. Arch Otorhinolaryngol [Suppl II]:100–101
10. Bender A, Bradac GB (1986) Erfahrungen in der radiologischen Diagnostik kleiner Akustikusneurinome. Röntgenblätter 39:36–39
11. Bentson J (1980) Combined gas cisternography and edge enhanced computed tomography of the internal auditory canal. Radiology 136:777–779
12. Blake PR, Carr DH, Goolden AWG (1986) Intracranial Hodgkin's disease. Br J Radiol 59:414
13. Brant-Zawadzki M, Normann D, Newton TH et al. (1984) Magnetic resonance of the brain: the optimal screening technique. Radiology 152:71–77

14. Brasch RC, Weinmann HJ, Wesby GE (1983) Contrast enhanced NMR imaging: animal studies using Gd-DTPA complex. AJR 2:625–630

15. Bydder GM, Steiner RE, Young IR et al. (1982) Clinical NMR imaging of the brain: 140 cases. AJR 139:215–236

16. Carr DH, Brown J, Lenng WL, Pennok JM (1984) Iron and gadolinium chelates as contrast agents in NMR imaging: preliminary studies. Comput Assist Tomogr 8:385–389

17. Daniels DL, Schende JF, Forster T et al. (1985) Surface-coil magnetic resonance imaging of the internal auditory canal. AJR 145:469–472

18. Felix R, Schoerner W, Laniado M, Niendorf HP, Claussen C, Fiegler W, Speck U (1985) Brain tumors: MR imaging with gadolinium-DTPA. Radiology 156:681–688

19. Felix R, Schoerner W, Laniado M, Semmler W (1985) Kontrastmittel in der magnetischen Resonanztomographie. RÖFO 143:9–14

20. Fisch U (1970) Transtemporal surgery of the internal auditory canal. Adv Otorhinolaryngol 17:203–240

21. Fisch U (1977) Die Mikrochirurgie des Felsenbeins. HNO 25:193–197

22. Flannigan BD, Bradley WG, Mazziotta JC (1985) Magnetic resonance imaging of the brainstem: normal structure and basic functional anatomy. Radiology 154:375–383

23. Frahm J, Haase A, Mathai D et al. (1985) FLASH MR imaging: from images to movies. Radiology 157:156 (abstract)

24. Frey KW, Mündnich K (1957) Schichtaufnahmen des Felsenbeins mit polyzyklischer Vermischung bei angeborenen Ohrmißbildungen. RÖFO 87, 164–176

25. Gastpar H (1961) Die Tumoren des Glomus caroticum, Glomus jugulare tympanicum und Glomus vagale. Acta Otolaryngol (Stockh) [Suppl] 167:1–23

26. Glenn WV, Johnston RJ, Morton PE, Dwyer SJ (1975) Image generation and display techniques for CT scan data. Invest Radiol 10:403–416

27. Grevers G, Vogl T (1988) Die arterielle und venöse digitale Subtraktionsangiographie (DSA) – eine aktuelle Studie für die HNO-Heilkunde. Laryngol Rhinol Otol (Stuttg) 67:221–225

28. Grevers G, Vogl T (1988) Zur Bedeutung der digitalen Subtraktionsangiographie bei der Differentialdiagnose zervikaler Schwellungen. Oto-rhinolaryngol 135:12–20

29. Grevers G, Wittmann A, Vogl T, Wiechell R (1989) Untersuchungen zur multiplanaren Darstellung des Felsenbeins – erste Ergebnisse. Laryngol Rhinol Otol (Stuttg) 68:392–395

30. Grevers G, Wilimzig C, Vogl T, Laub G (1991) Eine neue Methode zur 3D-Rekonstruktion im Kopf-Hals-Bereich. Laryngol Rhinol Otol (Stuttg) 1991 (in press)

31. Grevers G, Vogl T, Wilimzig C, Laub G (1991) Zur Aussagefähigkeit der 3D-KST-Rekonstruktion am Beispiel eines Parotisadenoms. Laryngol Rhinol Otol (Stuttg) (in press)

32. Grevers G, Vogl T, Kang K (1989) Radiologische Mittelohrdiagnostik – Möglichkeiten und Perspektiven. Laryngol Rhinol Otol (Stuttg) 68:481–485

33. Hildmann H, Tiedjen KV (1983) Zur Differentialdiagnose des Glomustumors. Laryngol Rhinol Otol (Stuttg) 62:502–504

34. Kazner E, Wende S, Grumme T, Lanksch W, Storchdorph O (1982) Computed tomography in intracranial tumors. Springer, Berlin Heidelberg New York

35. König H, Lenz M, Sauter R (1986) Temporal bone region: high resolution MR imaging using surface coils. Radiology 159:191–194

36. Lenz M, König H, Sauter R, Schrader M (1985) Kernspintomographie des Felsenbeins und des Kleinhirnbrückenwinkels. RÖFO 143:1–8

37. Mafee MF, Valvassai GE et al. (1983) High resolution and dynamic sequential computed tomography. Arch Otolaryngol 109:691–696

38. Mathew GD, Faser GW (1978) Symptoms, findings and methods: a diagnosis in patients with acoustic neuroma. Larnygoscope 88:1893–1903

39. McGinnis BD, Brady TJ, New PF et al. (1983) Nuclear magnetic resonance (NMR). Imaging of tumors in the posterior fossa. Comput Assist Tomogr 7:575–584

40. New PF, Badow TB, Wismer GL et al. (1985) MR imaging of the acoustic nerves and small acoustic neuromas at 0.6 Tesla. AJR 144:1021–1026

41. Nidecker A, Wehrle T, Elke M (1985) Effizienz der Radiodiagnostik von Akustikusneurinomen. RÖFO 142:56–63

42. Plester D, Wende S, Nakayama N (1978) Kleinhirnbrückenwinkeltumoren – Diagnostik und Therapie. Springer, Berlin Heidelberg New York

43. Runge VM, Clanton JA, Price AC, Wehr CJ, Herzer WA, Partain CL, James AE (1985) The use of Gd-DTPA as a perfusion agent and marker of blood-brain barrier disruption. Magn Reson Imaging 3:43–55

44. Schroth G, Thron A, Voigt K (1984) Raumforderungen der hinteren Schädelgrube. RÖFO 141:635–641

45. Stark D, Moss A, Gamsu G, Clark OH, Gooding GAW, Webb WR (1984) Magnetic resonance imaging of the neck, part 1. Radiology 150:447–454

46. Tidwell TJ, Montague ED (1975) Chemodectomas involving the temporal bone. Radiology 116:147

47. Valavanis A, Dabiv K, Hamdi R, Oquz M (1982) The current state of the radiological di-

agnosis of acoustic neuroma. Neuroradiology 23:7–13

48. Valavanis A, Schubinger O, Naidid TP (1987) Clinical imaging of the cerebellopontine angle. Springer, Berlin Heidelberg New York

49. Vogl T, Bauer M, Hahn D, Brüning R, Mees K, Lissner J (1986) Kernspintomographische Untersuchungen bei Verdacht auf Akustikusneurinom: Vorgehen und differentialdiagnostische Überlegungen. RÖFO 145:6

50. Vogl T, Bauer M, Hahn D, Mees K, Brüning R, Lissner J (1987) MR-Imaging of acoustic neuroma: plain and contrast enhanced studies. Magn Reson Imaging 5 [Suppl 1]:112

51. Vogl T, Bauer M, Fenzl G, Mees K, Lissner J (1987) Optimiertes diagnostisches Procedere bei Erkrankungen des Felsenbeins. In: Lemke HU, Rhodes ML, Jaffee CC, Felix R (eds) Computer assisted radiology, CAR. Springer, Berlin Heidelberg New York, pp 17–26

52. Vogl T, Bauer M, Schedel H, Brüning R, Mees K, Lissner J (1988) Kernspintomographische Untersuchungen von Paragangliomen des Glomus caroticum und Glomus jugulare mit Gd-DTPA. RÖFO 148:38–46

53. Vogl T, Mees K, Grevers G (1988) Kernspintomographische Untersuchungen des Oropha-

rynx und Zungengrundes. Nativdiagnostik contra Kontrastmitteluntersuchung. Otorhino-laryngology 135(1):45–48

54. Vogl T, Kellermann O, Randzio J, Kniha H, Requardt H, Tiling R, Lissner J (1988) Ergebnisse der Kernspintomographie des Temporo-mandibulargelenkes mittels optimierter Oberflächenspulen bei 100 Kiefergelenken. RÖFO 149/5:502–507

55. Vogl T, Ballhaus J, Dresel S, Kang K (1989) Gichttophus der Schädelbasis. RÖFO 150 (5):113–114

56. Weber AL, Davis KR, Nadol JB (1982) Chemodectomas of the glomus jugulare, glomus vagale and carotid body. Ann Otol Rhinol Laryngol 91:666–669

57. Yaşargil MG, Fisch U (1969) Mikrochirurgische Exstirpation des Akustikusneurinoms. Arch Otorhinolaryngol 194:243–247

58. Young IR, Hall AS, Pallis CA, Bydder GM, Legg NJ, Steiner RE (1981) Nuclear magnetic resonance imaging of the brain in multiple sclerosis. Lancet 14:1063–1066

59. Young JR, Bydder GM, Hall AS et al. (1983) The role of NMR imaging in the diagnosis and management of acoustic neuroma. AJNR 4:223–224

# 7 Orbit

## 7.1 Clinical Findings

Before the introduction of advanced imaging methods it was barely possible to visualize the orbit and its contents, such as the eyeball, muscles, vessels, optic nerve, and optic chiasm [37]. Conventional plain radiography is helpful in detecting traumatic orbital lesions and in visualizing bony structures, but often fails to identify tumors or inflammatory processes and their extension to neighboring structures [22].

Ultrasonography clearly shows changes of the eyeball in the anterior compartment, but bony structures and the posterior parts of the eye are not demonstrated [25]. Arteriography or venography are used for arteriovenous fistulas or abnormalities, but on the whole these techniques are being replaced by CT and MRI.

The widespread availability of CT and the refinements in image display such as multiplanar imaging and thin-section scanning have been crucial steps forward in the evaluation of orbital disease. Difficulties arise, however, with partial volume artifacts, especially in the region of the optic nerve, and with the radiation dose to the lens [15, 26, 39]. The rapid development over the last few years of safe, high-resolution, cross-sectional imaging methods has considerably influenced the application of MRI to diseases of the orbit. The progressive improvement of image quality is reflected in the literature on orbital imaging [1, 5, 6, 9, 10, 15–17]. The problems imposed by technical limitations such as low spatial resolution and long scanning times have largely been overcome by the introduction of surface coils and the use of higher field strengths [33–35, 38].

## 7.2 Examination Technique

After the procedure has been explained and contraindications to MRI (cardiac pacemaker, metallic foreign body in or near the orbit, makeup) have been excluded, the patient is placed in a relaxed position with eyes open and fixed on one spot during the whole scan time. Table 7.1 lists the sequences used for MRI of the orbit.

Depending on the kind of lesion suspected, the study is started with a surface coil placed over one or both orbits. The depth of imaging is directly related to the diameter of the coil. Different coils in various configurations have been constructed. Surface coils yield a better S/N than head coils but suffer more from motion artifacts. Head coils are used to evaluate deeper structures of both eyes or the chiasm [29–32].

To reduce motion artifacts it is necessary to keep scanning time as short as possible; short TR sequences (500/700, one or two excitations, 256 × 128 matrix) lasting approximately 3 min are preferred. Slice thickness should not exceed 3–5 mm. The field of view has to be small (about 150 mm) to maximize spatial resolution. T2-weighted images with long TR (2000 ms) and long TE (25, 90 ms) are obtained using the head coil.

The basic plane for orbital studies is the axial plane, permitting direct comparison of the two eyes and correlation of MR images with CT. The optic nerve, the cavernous sinus, and the muscles are demonstrated clearly. Images in other planes (coronal and/or sagittal) are obtained to define the extent of a lesion exactly.

GE sequences (300, 500/15, varying flip angle) can be useful in the evaluation of various vascular abnormalities such as capillary heman-

**Table 7.1.** Sequence guide for MRI of the orbit

| No. | Plane | Mode | TR (ms) | TE (ms) | Slice thickness (mm) | Acquisitions |
|-----|-------|------|---------|---------|----------------------|--------------|
| 1. | Sagittal | SE | 200 | 30 | 5 | 1 |
| 2. | Axial | SE | 500 | 15 | 3–5 | 2 |
| 3. | Coronal | SE | 500 | 15 | 3–5 | 2 |
| 4. | Parasagittal | SE | 600 | 15 | 3–5 | 2 |
| 5. | As appropriate (multiecho) | SE | 2000 1600 | 28/90 30–240 | 3–5 | 1 |
| 6. | As appropriate (varying flip angle) | GE | 500 | 15 | 3–5 | 2 |
| After Gd-DTPA | | | | | | |
| 7. | As appropriate | SE | 500 | 15 | 3–5 | 2 |

Field strength 1.5 T, matrix 256 × 128, field of view 120°–180° (surface coil) or >180° (head coil).

gioma or varix. Another advantage of this technique is the demonstration of the T2 effect of calcifications for the diagnosis of retinoblastoma.

Fat suppression techniques are rapidly improving the imaging of the optic nerve and lacrimal gland. Different methods using an inversion recovery sequence are under investigation, including a derivative of the Dixon method called Chopper suppression, chemical shift selected presaturation, and a hybrid method combining a frequency-selective preparatory pulse with an in-phase and an out-of-phase component of the Chopper technique [8, 14].

The administration of contrast medium has become a helpful tool for the differentiation of various tumorous, inflammatory, or degenerative changes of the orbit. The dosage of Gd-DTPA (0.1 mmol/kg body weight) and the selection of pulse sequences (T1 weighting) and parameters are of critical importance [28]. Intravenous injection of the paramagnetic agent shortens T1 and T2. Therefore it is mandatory to obtain T1-weighted images before administration of Gd-DTPA.

## 7.3 Topographic Relations

The structures of the orbit that have to be examined are listed in the checklist in Table 7.2.

**Table 7.2.** Checklist orbit

|  | Normal | Abnormal |
|--|--------|----------|
| Aqueous humor | | |
| Vitreous | | |
| Ciliary body | | |
| Lens | | |
| Choroid/retina | | |
| Medial rectus muscle | | |
| Lateral rectus muscle | | |
| Superior rectus muscle | | |
| Inferior rectus muscle | | |
| Superior oblique muscle | | |
| Inferior oblique muscle | | |
| Levator palpebrae muscle | | |
| Lacrimal gland | | |
| Optic nerve/chiasm | | |
| Superior orbital fissure/ orbital apex | | |
| Superior ophthalmic vein | | |
| Ophthalmic artery | | |
| Cavernous sinus | | |
| Intraextraconal fat tissue | | |

## 7.3.1 Eyeball

The eyeball is best visualized on axial and sagittal images using a special developed surface coil. Differentiation of lens, ciliary body, vitreous, choroid/retina, and sclera is possible (Fig. 7.1a). The lens, containing two thirds water and one third protein is of intermediate signal intensity on T1-weighted images, surrounded by the darker anterior chamber and vitreous. A loss of signal of the lens is seen on T2-weighted scans, where increased signal intensity of the anterior chamber and the vitreous corresponds to the high water content (98.5%). Processes of the sclera (low signal on all images) are best delineated in T2-weighted sequences. Choroid and retina are demarcated by their higher signal intensity on T1- and T2-weighted images.

## 7.3.2 Nerves

The ophthalmic nerve (branches: lacrimal, frontal, and nasociliary nerves) arises from the trigeminal ganglion and passes through the superior orbital fissure into the orbit. In coronal projection the frontal nerve is delineated as a hyperintense structure on T1-weighted images. The oculomotor nerve, which also traverses the superior orbital fissure, is mainly responsible for the movements of the extraocular muscles, except the superior oblique and lateral rectus muscles. The trochlear nerve, innervating the superior oblique muscle, arises in the dorsal part of the CNS and also passes through the superior orbital fissure. The abducens nerve supplies only the lateral rectus muscle. It runs through the superior orbital fissure accompanied by the superior ophthalmic vein.

The optic nerve, as part of the white matter, is surrounded by three meningeal layers containing the sclera at the posterior aspect of the eyeball. In a sinuous intraconal course medially and dorsally toward the orbital apex the nerve traverses the optic canal alongside the ophthalmic artery and passes into the middle cranial fossa to reach the optic chiasm. The intracanalicular and prechiasmatic portions

of the nerve are particularly well demonstrated on MRI compared with CT (Fig. 7.1a–c). On T1- and T2-weighted sequences the optic nerve shows signal intensity similar to that of normal white matter. Well-defined areas of hypointensity bordering the nerve are caused by chemical shift artifact.

The chiasm, which demonstrates signal intensity similar to that of the optic nerve is best delineated in sagittal or coronal T1-weighted images. A lesion at the chiasm level classically produces bitemporal hemianopsia or heteronymous field defects. After crossing of the fibers the information is guided over the lateral geniculate body to the optic radiation (retrochiasmal part). Injuries to the visual pathway usually produce homonymous hemianopsia.

## 7.3.3 Blood Vessels

The superior ophthalmic vein (Fig. 7.1a), the largest and most often visualized intraorbital vein, passes serpiginously from the trochlea of the superior oblique muscle to the apex of the orbit and through the superior orbital fissure to drain with the supraorbital and angular veins into the cavernous sinus.

The ophthalmic artery (Fig. 7.1a), arising from the internal carotid artery, traverses the optic canal cranially to the optic nerve.

Normal vascular structures, especially the ophthalmic artery, may show signal void on SE sequences, depending on pulse sequence parameters, velocity of flow, and type of flow (laminar, turbulent).

## 7.3.4 Muscles and Fatty Tissue

The motion of the eye is coordinated by six skeletal extraocular muscles. The four rectus muscles (superior, inferior, lateral, medial) arise from a tendinous ring (annulus of Zinn) and form a cone. The superior oblique muscle, the largest of the six, is supplied by the trochlear nerve, the lateral rectus muscle by the abducens nerve, and all others by the oculomotor nerve. The inferior oblique muscle is

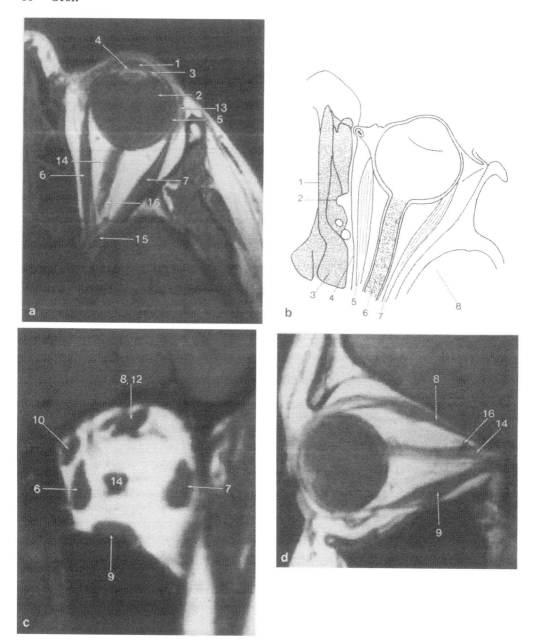

**Fig. 7.1 a–d.** Normal topography of the orbit
**a** Plain axial MRI (SE, 500/15). *1*, Anterior chamber; *2*, vitrous; *3*, ciliary body; *4*, lens; *5*, sclera; *6*, medial rectus muscle; *7*, lateral rectus muscle; *8*, superior rectus muscle; *9*, inferior rectus muscle; *10*, superior oblique muscle; *12*, levator palpebrae muscle; *13*, lacrimal gland; *14*, optic nerve; *15*, ophthalmic vein; *16*, ophthalmic artery

**b** Diagram of the topographic relations of the orbit in the axial plane. *1*, Ethmoid bone; *2*, ethmoid sinus; *3*, sphenoid sinus; *4*, periorbital space; *5*, medial rectus muscle; *6*, optic nerve; *7*, lateral rectus muscle; *8*, middle cranial fossa
**c** Plain coronal MRI (SE, 500/15). For explanation of numbers see **a**
**d** Plain parasagittal MRI (SE, 500/15). For explanation of numbers see **a**

the only one to arise not from the apex of the orbit but from the orbital plate of the maxilla near the nasolacrimal duct.

All muscles of the orbit are well delineated on T1-weighted sequences by their low signal intensity compared with the surrounding fat tissue (Fig. 7.1 a – c). In coronal or parasagittal images differentiation of the superior rectus muscle and the levator palpebrae muscle is possible.

Orbital fatty tissue, intra- and extraconal, exhibits high signal intensity on T1-weighted images and intermediate signal intensity on T2-weighted images. The soft tissues surrounding the anterior aspect of the orbit (upper and lower eyelid) are demarcated well from the bony structures.

### 7.3.5  Lacrimal Gland

The lacrimal gland appears as an inhomogeneous area of intermediate signal intensity depending on the separation of single secretory lobuli by fatty tissue. This gland is well demonstrated on axial scans lying in the lacrimal fossa, extraconal and superolateral to the anterior orbit (Fig. 7.1 a).

### 7.3.6  Bony Borders

The bony orbit is formed by the lacrimal, palatine, zygomatic, maxillary, ethmoid, sphenoid, and frontal bones. The orbital septum (a fibrous sheath lined by periosteum) divides the orbit into a preseptal and a postseptal compartment, influencing the spread of infection. The cortical bony structures show a low signal intensity on T1-weighted images. By virtue of the short T1 of fatty tissue and fat-bearing bone marrow good soft tissue contrast is achieved on MRI.

## 7.4  Ocular Lesions

### 7.4.1  Congenital Lesions

*Coats' disease* is a primary vascular anomaly of the retina in which teleangiectatic vessels exude lipoproteinaceous serum into the subretinal space, causing retinal detachment. This phenomenon is also seen in other diseases such as trauma, macular degeneration, PHPV (persistent hyperplastic primary vitreous), and tumors, depending on the amount of exudation and organization of subretinal materials. Coats' disease mainly affects at an early age. In MRI the signal intensity is increased on T1- and T2-weighted images due to the dense subretinal lipoproteinaceous exudate [30].

*Retinoblastoma* is the most common autosomal dominant tumor in children [36, 39]. The malignant aggressive tumor consists of undifferentiated embryonal retinal cells and is usually detected up to the 4th or 5th year of life. Retinoblastoma is bilateral in up to 25% of cases, dense ocular calcification – better demonstrated on CT – and retinal hemorrhage are common. Exact staging of the disease (infiltration of surrounding structures) is essential for decisions on therapeutic strategy (irradiation, enucleation). Retinoblastomas appear bright on T1-weighted and dark on T2-weighted images. In the case of hemorrhage signal intensities may vary enormously.

---

Retinoblastoma:
- most common ocular tumor in children
- bilateral in 25% of cases
- signal intensity high with T1 weighting, low with T2 weighting, moderate with T1 weighting and Gd-DTPA
- calcification better detected on CT

---

### 7.4.2  Traumatic Lesions

Traumatic lesions of the orbit caused by foreign bodies may only be examined if the objects concerned are nonferromagnetic. Exact localization of these objects (wood, glass) on MR images is possible on the basis of their lower signal intensity.

Hyperacute hemorrhage (first few hours) shows intermediate signal on T1-weighted images and intermediate or bright signal on T2-weighted images. In the acute phase (hours to 4 days) signal loss on T2-weighted images depends on the formation of deoxyhemoglobin. Differentiation from melanin, which decreases T1 and T2 values by the paramagnetic effect, is essential, although hemorrhage may dominate in melanoma [31]. In the subacute stage (days to weeks) the bright signal corresponds to the methemoglobin. In chronic hemorrhage (weeks to months) a dark hemosiderin rim is seen on T2-weighted images.

### 7.4.3 Inflammation

Intraocular and intraconal inflammation usually occurs as the result of spread of infection from adjacent structures, e.g., after foreign body penetration or other trauma of the paranasal sinuses. Anterior septal cellulitis or scleritis and encapsulated abscess are the most common findings. Clinically, periorbital pain, proptosis, edema, and diplopia are often found in acute processes. Thickening and increased attenuation of the wall of the eyeball characterize the acute phase, while contraction and thickening of the eyeball are indicative of the chronic stage, when the sclera gives a low-intensity signal on T1- and T2-weighted images in posterior scleritis or phthisis bulbi. The latter is often caused by mechanical irritation of the eyeball.

### 7.4.4 Tumors

*Retinoblastoma*: see Sect. 7.4.1
*Uveal melanoma* (Fig. 7.2) is the most common ocular neoplasm in adults and occurs between 50 and 70 years of age. It is often associated with retinal detachment. The two conditions are difficult to distinguish on CT, but the relaxation times and signal intensities on T1- and T2-weighted MRI and the use of Gd-DTPA help to differentiate them

**Table 7.3.** Signal characteristics of various orbital lesions

| Lesion | Signal | | |
| --- | --- | --- | --- |
| | T1 | T2 | T1 with Gd-GTPA |
| Dermoid | Moderate-high | Moderate-high | Moderate |
| Encephalocele | Low | High | Low |
| Epidermoid | Low | High | Moderate |
| Glioma | Low | High | Low |
| Graves' disease | Low | Low | Low-moderate |
| Hemangioma | Low | High | Moderate-high |
| Lipoma | High | Low | High |
| Lymphoma | Low | High | Moderate-high |
| Melanoma, uveal | Moderate-high | Low | High |
| Meningioma | Isointense | Moderate | High |
| Metastases | Low | Moderate | High |
| Mucocele | High | High | Moderate-high |
| Optic neuritis | Isointense | High | Moderate-high |
| Phthisis bulbi | Low | Low | Low |
| Post irradiation lesion | Low | Moderate-high | Low |
| Pseudotumor | Low | Low | Moderate |
| Retinoblastoma | High | Low | Moderate |
| Tolosa-Hunt syndrome | Low | Low | Moderate |
| Vascular lesions | Low | Low | Low |

when ophthalmoscopic examination fails. Melanomas have an isointense high signal on T1-weighted images and a low signal on T2-weighted images (Table 7.3) [13, 21, 27, 31]. Retinal lesions are hyperintense both with short TR/TE and with long TR/TE. The signal intensity of malignant melanoma mainly depends on the melanin, which has paramagnetic properties: the higher the concentration of melanin, the greater the shortening of T1 and T2. Exact division into histologic types of melanoma, e.g., malignant epitheloid cell form or benign spindle cell form, is not yet possible. Most important for differential diagnosis are metastases from tumors of the kidney, breast, gastrointestinal tract, or lung. Metastatic lesions usually have an isointense low signal on T1-weighted images and a moderate to high signal on T2-weighted images (Table 7.3). Accompanying diagnostic signs include bony destruction, irregular shape, infiltration to extraocular tissue, and calcification.

*Benign tumors* such as choroidal osteoma, choroidal nevi, medulloepithelioma, retinal gliosis and choroidal hemangiomas (astrocytic retinal hamartoma associated with phakomatoses) are very rare. The first three can be similar in intensity to melanoma. The latter, in the small number of cases examined, are characterized by marked enhancement after administration of Gd-DTPA, comparable to retrobulbar cavernous hemangioma.

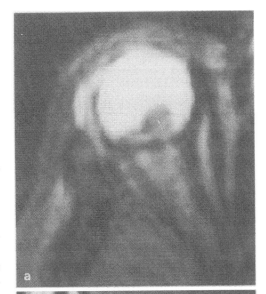
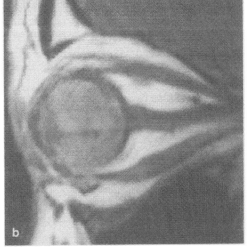
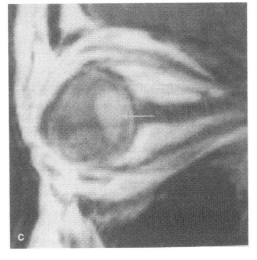

▷

Fig. 7.2 a–c. Malignant melanoma in a 48-year-old man
a Plain axial MRI (SE, 2000/90). A low-signal-intensity mass (*arrow*) is seen on the T2-weighted image. The surrounding vitreous body appears as a high-signal-intensity structure
b Plain parasagittal MRI (SE, 500/15)
c Parasagittal MRI (SE, 500/15) with Gd-DTPA. Comparative analysis of the plain and Gd-DTPA-enhanced images demonstrates the biconvex lesion with enormous enhancement after administration of Gd-DTPA (*arrow*)

Uveal melanoma:
- most common ocular tumor in adults
- signal intensity high with T1 weighted, low with T2 weighted, high with T1 weighted and Gd-DTPA; depending on the paramagnetic properties of melanin

ous stages. Acute occlusion of the central retinal vein without bleeding is best controlled by ophthalmologic means. After radiotherapy the optic nerve may be enlarged or atrophic with homogeneous high signal on T2-weighted images.

## 7.5 Optic Nerve/Sheath Lesions

Various clinical patterns and symptoms, such as impaired vision, visual field defects, proptosis, headaches, and strabismus arouse suspicion of optic nerve lesions. The course of the optic nerve is depicted better on MRI than on CT, and images in the appropriate plane are useful to discriminate changes of the nerve such as atrophy or enlargement. The former usually occurs in chronic inflammatory or late tumors changes, while enlargement is seen in a great number of tumorous and nontumorous diseases.

### 7.5.1 Nontumorous Enlargement

In pseudotumor or the advanced stages of Graves' disease thickening of the optic nerve may be present [2, 11, 12]. In Graves' disease the nerve is well demarcated from the surrounding enlarged intraorbital muscles. Increased intracranial pressure causes widening of the subarachnoid space around the optic nerve. The patient's history and clinical examination help to identify the cause. Arachnoid hyperplasia can also be associated with endocrine ophthalmopathy (Graves' disease) on optic nerve glioma, and can be differentiated from the tumor by virtue of the similar signal intensity to the CSF. Optic neuritis is found in many systemic (lymphoma, sarcoidosis, diabetes, hyperthyroidism), viral, or bacterial infections, but may also be idiopathic or toxic. If multiple sclerosis is suspected, T2-weighted MRI can be used to investigate the periventricular area, which is usually involved.
Blood surrounding the optic nerve is depicted by the signal intensities differing in the vari-

### 7.5.2 Tumorous Enlargement

MR is the method of choice for differentiating the two most common tumors of the optic nerve and sheath, glioma and meningioma. In younger patients, optic glioma is usually a benign, slow-growing tumor with low recurrence rates and high survival rates, in contrast to older patients [20]. Bilateral involvement is strongly indicative of neurofibromatosis. Tumors, arising from glial cells (rarely from oligodendrocytes) may involve any part of the visual pathway. Florid growth and calcification are rare. In posterior enlargement of the optic nerve the optic canal is widened. The MRI signal intensities are low on T1-weighted images, high on T2-weighted images, and there is no significant enhancement on administration of Gd-DTPA (Table 7.3).
Meningioma (Fig. 7.3) is found in older women and, like optic glioma, is associated with neurofibromatosis. The tumor arises from arachnoid cells in the dural sheath or reaches the orbit via various foramina. The optic canal is normal in size, and calcification of the lesion is common. Bony structures may be involved. The meningioma shows isointense moderate signal intensity on T1- and T2-weighted images. After administration of contrast medium there is marked enhancement of the tumorous lesions (Table 7.3), enabling detection of even small lesions at the orbital apex, the sphenoid, or clinoid process with high sensitivity. Sclerosis, calcification, and bony destruction are better evaluated with CT.
Other conditions that should be considered in the differential diagnosis of optic nerve tumors include optic meningoceles, drusen, schwannomas, hemangioblastomas, and choristomas. Metastases or extensions of ocular

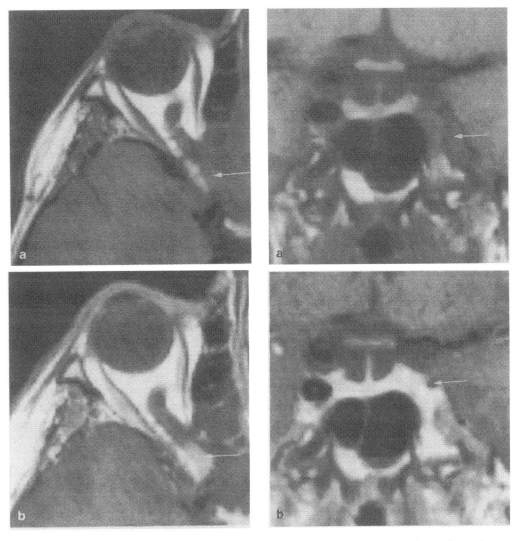

**Fig. 7.3 a, b.** Meningioma of the optic nerve
**a** Plain axial MRI (SE, 500/15). The retrobulbar part of the optic nerve appears with low signal intensity. Soft tissue mass (*arrow*) near the foramen measuring 10 × 7 mm
**b** Axial MRI (SE, 500/15) with Gd-DTPA. Marked enhancement of the optic nerve (*arrow*) near the foramen. These findings are characteristic for a meningioma in contrast to optic nerve glioma. No significant widening of the optic canal

**Fig. 7.4 a, b.** Tolosa-Hunt syndrome in a 56-year-old woman
**a** SE, TR/TE = 500/15. Plain coronal MRI (SE, 500/15)
**b** Coronal MRI (SE, 500/15) with Gd-DTPA. On the plain image **a** low-intensity mass (*arrow*) is seen in the area of the cavernous sinus and Meckel's cave. The contrast-enhanced image better demonstrates the soft tissues and the narrowed internal carotid artery (*arrow*) on the left side

tumors to the optic nerve can also simulate primary tumors.

---

Optic nerve glioma vs meningioma:
Glioma:
– widening of optic canal
– no significant enhancement after Gd-DTPA
– bilateral involvement – neurofibromatosis?
Meningioma:
– normal size of optic canal
– marked enhancement after Gd-DTPA

---

## 7.6 Intra- and Extraconal Lesions

### 7.6.1 Pseudotumor

Pseudotumor (idiopathic orbital inflammatory syndrome, IOIS) presents as a nonspecific, unilateral process usually infiltrating the retrobulbar space with displacement of the eyeball, the optic nerve, or the muscles [4]. The etiology of pseudotumor is not yet known, but probably immunologic antigen-antibody reactions are responsible for this disease, which is managed well with steroids. Clinical features such as pain or periorbital edema, difficult to distinguish from neoplasm, are dominant. Radiologically, various lesions show features such as amorphous masses, muscle involvement, scleral thickening, or infiltration of surrounding structures. Diagnosis must rely on the course, with alternating exacerbations and remissions. The changes may be intra- or extraconal, although bony destruction or invasion of the sinus is very rare. The signal intensity of pseudotumors is low on T1- and T2-weighted images (Table 7.3)

### 7.6.2 Tolosa-Hunt Syndrome

Tolosa-Hunt syndrome is defined as a type of orbital pseudotumor involving the orbital apex and spreading to the optic chiasm. The internal carotid artery is usually compressed, causing painful ophthalmoplegia. Signal intensities are similar to those of other orbital pseudotumors (Fig. 7.4). Infiltration of retrobulbar fat prolongs T1 and shortens T2, thus decreasing signal intensity. In contrast, true focal masses exhibit increased intensity of T2-weighted images, which enables differentiation from pseudotumors (Table 7.3). Other inflammatory changes such as myositis, dacryoadenitis, periscleritis, or perineuritis can be caused by bacterial, viral, or mycotic infections or by granulomatous disease. Preseptal or subperiosteal inflammation, diffuse orbital spread, or scleral thickening may be found. Clinically, acute periorbital inflammation is distinguished by the abrupt onset, in contrast to pseudotumor, and by the history of sinus problems or trauma. In some cases antibiotic treatment is helpful, but in others surgical intervention may be necessary.

### 7.6.3 Graves' Disease

Graves' disease, still a poorly understood endocrine ophthalmopathy (Fig. 7.5), usually bilaterally affects and enlarges the extraocular muscles. Predominantly the inferior and medial rectus muscles are involved, followed by the superior and lateral rectus muscles. The muscle bellies show uniform involvement, but the tendons are spared, yielding the well-known tapering appearence that distinguishes this disease from other infiltrative muscle processes. Histopathologically and on MRI (low signal intensity on T1- and T2-weighted images), Graves' disease resembles orbital pseudotumor (Table 7.3). An increase in signal intensity on T2-weighted images is thought to indicate the activity of Graves' disease. A common sign is the increased volume of retrobulbar fat tissue.

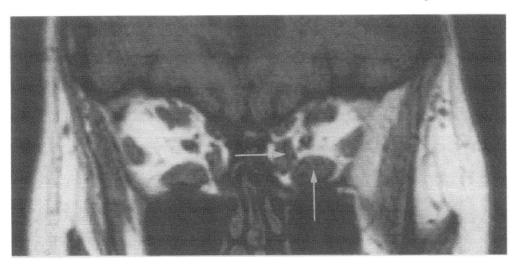

**Fig. 7.5.** Graves' disease. Plain coronal MRI (SE, 500/15). Diffuse enlargement of all rectus muscles, especially the inferior and medial rectus muscles, on the left side (*arrows*). Volume increase of the retroorbital fat tissue

---

Graves' disease:
- bilaterally involvement of inferior and medial rectus muscles
- retrobulbar fat tissue volume increased
- signal characteristics: low on T1 and T2, no significant enhancement after application of contrast medium

### 7.6.4 Lymphoma

Lymphomas must be considered in the differential diagnosis of pseudotumor and Graves' disease. Involvement of the orbit may be primary or secondary to systemic disease. Differentiation of benign reactive lymphoid hyperplasia and malignant lymphoma is important. The latter commonly affects adults aged 50–70 years. These tumors are characterized by aggressive diffuse growth and, often, bony destruction. On MRI, lymphomas show low signal on T1-weighted scans and high signal on T2-weighted scans. There is significant enhancement after Gd-DTPA administration (Fig. 7.6, Table 7.3).

### 7.6.5 Malignant Lesions

The MRI signal characteristics of malignant lesions permit differentiation from pseudotumor and Graves' disease. Metastatic lesions, sometimes from an unknown primary, may be found. Erosion or destruction of the bony walls of the orbit is common in cases of primary carcinoma or secondary sarcoma [18, 22]. Occasionally calcification is seen. Rhabdomyosarcoma and neuroblastoma predominantly occur in childhood and show signal intensities comparable to those of lymphoma. Malignancies such as osteosarcoma and chondrosarcoma arising in surrounding structures (paranasal sinuses, nasal cavity, nasopharynx) may invade the orbital structures, and have an inhomogeneous appearance on MRI.

### 7.6.6 Benign Lesions

Among the benign orbital tumors, cavernous hemangiomas (Fig. 7.7) are most common in adults, while capillary hemangiomas, with a high perfusion rate, often occur in childhood.

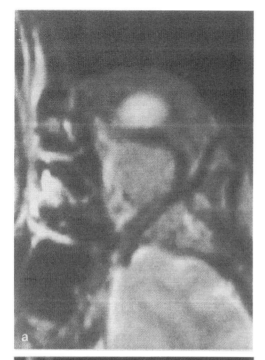

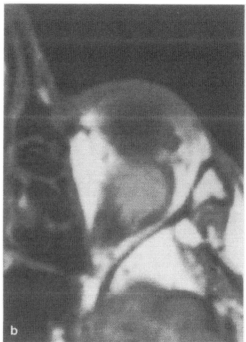

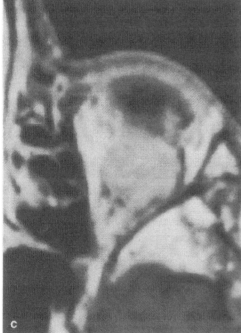

**Fig. 7.6a–c.** Lymphoma
**a** Plain axial MRI (SE, 2000/90). Ill-defined mass inferior to the eyeball with intermediate to high signal intensity. No infiltration of surrounding structures
**b** Plain axial MRI (SE, 500/15). In the T1-weighted sequence the tumor appears hypointense in comparison with orbital fat
**c** Axial MRI (SE, 500/15) with Gd-DTPA. Moderate increase in signal intensity of the lymphoma

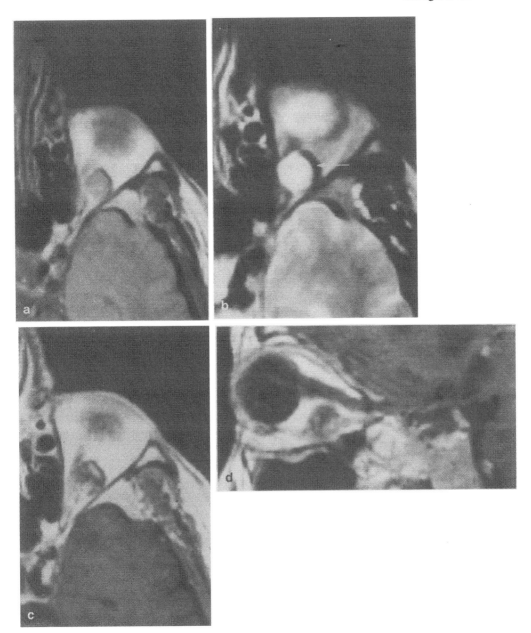

**Fig. 7.7a–d.** Cavernous hemangioma
**a** Plain axial MRI (SE, 500/15)
**b** Plain axial MRI (SE, 2000/90)
**c** Axial MRI (SE, 500/15) with Gd-DTPA
**d** Sagittal MRI (SE, 500/15) with Gd-DTPA. Well-demarcated lesion, beneath the optic nerve with low signal intensity on the T1-weighted image (**a**) and high signal intensity on the T2-weighted image (**b**). After injection of Gd-DTPA, inhomogeneous moderate to high enhancement of the lesion (**c**, **d**). The ventrolateral low-intensity rim might correspond to a tumor capsule (**c**)

Depending on the vascular supply, these lesions appear dark to intermediate on T1-weighted images and bright on T2-weighted images, with strong enhancement after Gd-DTPA administration (Table 7.3). Some authors describe a tumor capsule delineating the process from the surrounding structures. Other osseous lesions involving the orbit include osteomyelitis, fibrous dysplasia, and osteoma. Fibrous dysplasia gives an intermediate signal on T1- and T2-weighted images and shows no enhancement after administration of Gd-DTPA. The bony structure is replaced by fibrous tissue usually in the lateral superior wall of the orbit. Nonuniform marked sclerosis and thickening is a common finding. Os-

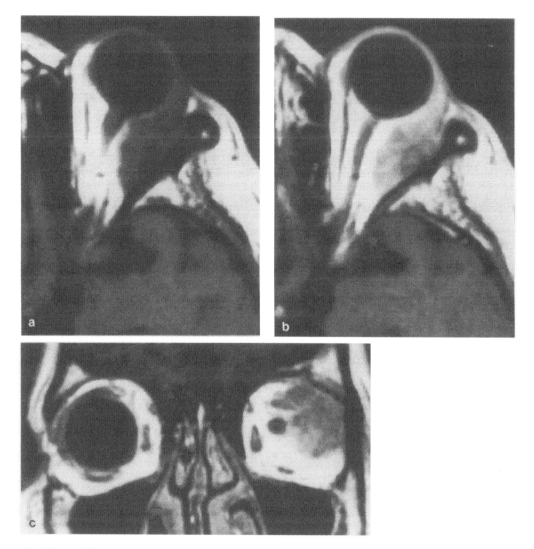

**Fig. 7.8 a–c.** Pleomorphic adenoid carcinoma of the lacrimal gland in a 70-year-old man
**a** Plain axial MRI (SE, 500/15)
**b** Axial MRI (SE, 500/15) with Gd-DTPA

**c** Coronal MRI (SE, 500/15) with Gd-DTPA. Hypointense enlargement of the lacrimal gland with dislocation of the eyeball is seen on the plain image (**a**). On the contrast enhanced images (**b, c**), involvement of the muscles. The inhomogeneous mass is better delineated after Gd-DTPA

teomas arising in the bony paranasal sinuses are characterized by uniform calcification, best visualized on CT.

Osteopetrosis, eosinophilic granuloma, and osteoblastoma are very rare in the orbit.

### 7.6.7 Vascular Lesions

Lymphangiomas, as extraconal processes, have no capsule and tend to hemorrhage; this differentiates them from hemangiomas. Other angiomas include venous malformation and varices. Signal void is seen in high flow systems, while thrombosis or slow flow is characterized by a rise in signal intensity. The radiologic appearance is changed by jugular compression or the Valsalva maneuver, which increase the size of the lesion. Angiomas are often accompanied by phleboliths. Additionally, dilatation of the superior ophthalmic vein strongly suggests carotid cavernous fistula.

### 7.6.8 Lacrimal Gland Lesions

Lesions of the lacrimal gland are located extraconally in the superior temporal quadrant of the orbit [3, 24, 37]. Changes are detected easily by palpation, and the location is sometimes specific for certain diseases. Benign lesions include lymphoid hyperplasia, Sjögren's syndrome, pseudotumor, pleomorphic adenoma, and cystic processes like dermoid cyst and epidermoid tumor. Sharp margins and lack of infiltration are taken to indicate benignity. Dermoid cysts account for more than 50% of lacrimal gland tumors and are of epithelial origin. On MRI they show fat-like signal intensity on T1- and T2-weighted images with a homogeneous internal pattern and fat-fluid levels. Differential diagnosis should include epidermoid tumors, characterized by low signal intensity on T1-weighted images and bright appearance on T2-weighted images. Mucoceles stand out clearly by virtue of their high signal intensity on T1- and T2-weighted images (Table 7.3). These lesions may be congenital and primary (lacrimal sac) or secondary to acquired paranasal sinus lesions (lacrimal gland). The latter show progression in size caused by fluid accumulation,

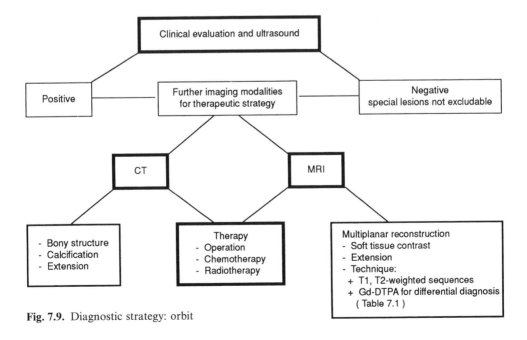

**Fig. 7.9.** Diagnostic strategy: orbit

leading to bony expansion with thinning and loss of peripheral margins.

Malignant lacrimal gland lesions usually infiltrate adjacent tissues and exhibit bony destruction, an inhomogeneous pattern, and unsharp margins. Low signal intensity on T1-weighted images, high signal intensity on T2-weighted images and marked enhancement after administration of Gd-DTPA are common (Table 7.3). Calcifications are not well detected on MRI. Characteristic signal intensities for different malignant tumors have not yet been described.

## 7.7 Summary

MRI is a very sensitive method for detecting lesions of the orbit and the surrounding structures. Ultrasound and CT are very helpful tools in primary diagnosis of various diseases; CT, in particular, is better than MRI in identifying bony erosions or destruction and in confirming calcification [7, 19]. Certain lesions show characteristic signal intensities on T1- and T2-weighted images (Table 7.3). The contrast medium Gd-DTPA is indicated in many cases, yielding more accurate diagnosis and higher specificity. The diagnostic strategy shown in Fig. 7.9 is recommended for MRI of the orbit.

*References*

1. Atlas SW, Grossman RI, Axel L et al. (1987) Proton spectroscopic phase dependent MR imaging of orbital lesions. Radiology 64: 510–514
2. Atlas SW, Grossman RI, Savino PI et al. (1987) Surface-coil MR of orbital pseudotumor. AJNR 8:141–146
3. Balchunas WR, Quencer RM, Byrne SF (1983) Lacrimal gland and fossa masses: evaluation by computed tomography and A-mode echography. Radiology 149:751–758
4. Bernardino ME, Zunn RD, Citrin CM, Davis DO (1977) Scleral thickening: a sign of orbital pseudotumor. AJR 129:703–706
5. Bilaniuk LT, Schenk JF, Zimmermann RA et al. (1985) Ocular and orbital lesions: surface coil MR imaging. Radiology 156:669–674
6. Bilaniuk LT, Atlas SW, Zimmermann RA (1987) Magnetic resonance imaging of the orbit. Radiol Clin North Am 25:509–528
7. Bradley WG Jr, Schmidt PG (1986) Effect of methemoglobin formation on the MR appearance of subarachnoid hemorrhage. Radiology 156:99–103
8. Brateman L (1986) Chemical shift imaging: a review. AJR 146:971–980
9. Daniels DL, Herfkens R, Gager WE et al. (1984) Magnetic resonance imaging of the optic nerves and chiasm. Radiology 152:79–83
10. Daniels DL, Kneeland JB, Shimakawa A et al. (1986) MR imaging of the optic nerve and sheath: correcting the chemical shift misregistration effect. AJNR 7:249–253
11. Enzmann DR, Donaldson SS, Kriss JP (1979) Appearance of Graves' disease on orbital computed tomography. J Comput Assist Tomogr 3:815–819
12. Forbes GS, Sheedy PF, Waller RR (1980) Orbital tumors evaluated by computed tomography. Radiology 136:101–111
13. Gomori JM, Grossman RI, Shields JA et al. (1986) Choroidal melanomas: correlation of NMR spectroscopy and MR imaging. Radiology 158:443–445
14. Gomori JM, Grossman RI, Shields JA et al. (1986) Ocular MR imaging and spectroscopy: an ex vivo study. Radiology 160:201–205
15. Grossmann I (1987) CT and MRI of the orbit. Basic review and recent advances in head and neck radiology. Department of Radiology/Harvard Medical School/Massachusetts General Hospital Eye and Ear Infirmary, Boston
16. Han JS, Benson JE, Bonstelle CT et al. (1984) Magnetic resonance imaging of the orbit: a preliminary experience. Radiology 150:755–759
17. Hawkes RC, Holland GN, Moore WS et al. (1983) NMR imaging in the evaluation of orbital tumors. AJNR 4:254–256

18. Hesselink JR, Davis KR, Weber AL et al. (1980) Radiological evaluation of orbital metastases with emphasis on computed tomography. Radiology 137:363–366
19. Holland BA, Kucharczyk W, Brandt-Zawadzki M et al. (1985) MR imaging of calcified intracranial lesions. Radiology 157:353–356
20. Holman RE, Grimson BS, Drayer BP, Brennan MW (1985) Magnetic resonance imaging of optic gliomas. Am J Ophthalmol 100:596–601
21. Jimbow K, Miyake Y, Homma K et al. (1984) Characterization of melanogenesis and morphogenesis of melanin and melanosomes in malignant melanoma. Cancer Res 44:1128–1134
22. Jones ES, Jakobiec FA (1979) Diseases of the orbit. Harper and Row, Hagerstown
23. Kelly WM, Paglen PG, Pearson JA et al. (1986) Ferromagnetism of intraocular foreign body causes unilateral blindness after MR study. AJNR 7:243–245
24. Lee DA, Campbell RJ, Waller RR, Ilstrup OM (1985) A clinicopathologic study of primary adenoid cystic carcinoma of the lacrimal gland. Ophthalmology 92:128–134
25. Li KC, Poon PY, Hinton P et al. (1984) MR imaging of orbital tumors with CT and ultrasound correlations. J Comput Assist Tomogr 8:1039–1047
26. Mafee MF, Goldberg MF, Valvassori GE, Capek V (1982) Computed tomography in the evaluation of patients with persistent hyperplastic primary vitreous (PHPV). Radiology 145:713–717
27. Mafee MF, Peyman GA, Grisolano JE et al. (1986) Malignant uveal melanomas and simulating lesions: MR evaluation. Radiology 160:773–780
28. Markl AA, Riedel KG, Oeckler R et al. (1986) MR imaging of orbital disease using surface coils and contrast agents. Radiology 161:286

29. Mödder U, Zanella FE (1990) Diseases of the eyeball, orbit and accessory structures. In: Huk WJ, Gademann GF, Friedmann G (eds) Magnetic resonance imaging of central nervous system diseases. Springer, Berlin Heidelberg New York
30. Okabe H, Kizosawa M, Yamada S, Yamada K (1986) Nuclear magnetic resonance imaging of subretinal fluid. Am J Ophthalmol 102:640–646
31. Peyman GA, Mafee MF (1987) Uveal melanoma and similar lesions: the role of magnetic resonance imaging. Radiol Clin North Am 25:471–486
32. Peyster PG, Augsburger JJ, Shields AJ et al. (1988) Intraocular tumors: evaluation with MR imaging. Radiology 168:773–779
33. Sobel DF, Mills C, Char D et al. (1984) NMR of the normal and pathologic eye and orbit. AJNR 5:345–350
34. Sullivan JA, Harms SE (1986) Surface coil MR imaging of orbital neoplasms. AJNR 7:29–34
35. Sullivan JA, Harms SE (1987) Characterization of orbital lesions by surface coil. MR imaging. Radiographics 7:9–28
36. Wells RG, Sty JR, Gonnering RS (1989) Imaging of the pediatric eye and orbit. Radiographics 9:1023–1043
37. Wright JE, Stewart WB, Krohel GB (1979) Clinical presentation and management of lacrimal gland tumors. Br J Ophthalmol 63:600–606
38. Wright RM, Swietek PA, Simmons ML (1985) Eye artifacts from mascara in MRI. AJNR 6:652
39. Zimmermann RA, Bilaniuk LT (1979) Computed tomography of the evaluation of patients with bilateral retinoblastomas. J Comput Tomogr 3:251–257

# 8 Nasopharynx and Paranasal Sinuses

## 8.1 Clinical Findings

Most diseases of the nose and paranasal sinuses are of inflammatory origin and do not require sophisticated diagnostic or therapeutic management. In some cases, however, there are complications of paranasal sinus infections involving the orbit (complicated ethmoid or frontal sinusitis) or the meninges (pyocele of the frontal sinus). These complications require immediate surgical intervention. A large number of benign and malignant tumors of the nose and paranasal sinuses have been reported. Malignant tumors of these sites account for 0.2%–0.8% of all malignancies in human beings: that means, for instance, that one new case of maxillary sinus carcinoma is diagnosed per 200 000 persons per annum. The majority of the malignomas (75%) are squamous cell carcinomas and adenocarcinomas. Malignant tumors of mesenchymal origin make up 15%. In children, histiocytosis and rhabdomyosarcoma are observed quite frequently. The most common symptoms in patiens suffering from tumors of the nose and paranasal sinuses are unilateral nasal obstruction (48%), facial or palatal swelling (41%), facial pain (41%), nasal discharge (37%), and epistaxis (35%).

The nasopharynx contains a wide variety of cell types. Therefore many kinds of lesions may occur, ranging from embryologic abnormalities to benign and malignant neoplasms. Squamous cell carcinomas and lymphoepithelial tumors make up 75% of the nasopharyngeal malignancies in adults. In children, lymphomas and plasmocytomas are the predominant malignant tumors. In nasopharyngeal malignancies, the clinical presentation does not always immediately indicate the diagnosis. Hearing loss, due to impairment of Eustachian tube function, and enlargement of cervical lymph nodes are the most common initial symptoms. Nasal obstruction and bleeding may also appear in nasopharyngeal carcinoma, but occur in only about 30% of patients.

*Diagnostic Procedures.* Patients suffering from diseases of the nose, paranasal sinuses, or nasopharynx can be examined by either indirect nasopharyngoscopy or direct flexible or rigid fiberoptic examination. The development of endoscopic devices has eased the early detection of small tumors of the nasopharynx. In the case of impaired Eustachian tube function or serous otitis media of unknown origin, careful endoscopic evaluation of the nasopharynx is obligatory.

Inflammatory diseases of the paranasal sinuses require investigation by ultrasound or roentgenology.

*Demands on the Radiologist.* Complications of inflammatory diseases of the ethmoid and frontal sinuses, i.e., involvement of the orbit and the meninges of the anterior cranial fossa might require surgical therapy immediately. Therefore it is important to know the extent and localization of the inflammation. In the case of a pyocele of the frontal sinus, the topographic relations of the cele and the surrounding structures, as well as the degree of concomitant inflammation of bone and soft tissue, can be helpful in preoperative planning. In malignant tumors of the nose, paranasal sinuses, and nasopharynx, it is essential for treatment planning to know the extent of the lesion and the infiltration of the surrounding tissues. Due to their location, tumors of the paranasal sinuses and nasopharyngeal space are often hard to detect by rhinoscopy or even endoscopy. Furthermore, a variety of tumors of the nasopharyngeal space grow in the submucosal tissue layer and will not be detected by rhinoscopic or endoscopic examination. To improve the prognosis of these tumors, however, it is essential to establish the diagnosis as early as possible.

In benign tumors with a rich blood supply, such as angiofibroma of the nasopharynx, identification of the supplying vessels is absolutely necessary in order to plan an appropriate surgical approach.

## 8.2 Examination Technique

All MR examinations are performed at a field strength of 1.0 T or 1.5 T on a 1.5 T superconducting magnet (Siemens Magnetom). Images are acquired using a 30-cm head coil. Sections 5 or 8 mm thick are recommended in two or three planes depending on the extent of the tumor.

After a sagittal survey image performed for the purpose of craniocaudal orientation, images are obtained in the axial plane with a long (3000/25, 90) and a short (500/25) SE sequence, and in the coronal plane with a short (500/25) SE) sequence with same parameters. Following contrast medium injection, images are obtained in the axial plane with a short SE sequence and, in most cases, also in the coronal plane. In some cases, during and after injection of Gd-DTPA a very short sequence (30/13) with a flip angle of 30° is performed every minute over a period of at least 8 min in order to measure the change in signal intensity. Gd-DTPA at a concentration of 0.1 mmol/l is used in a dose of 0.2 ml/kg body weight.

## 8.3 Topographic Relations

### 8.3.1 Nasopharynx

The nasopharynx represents the upper part of the pharynx and is continuous with the nasal cavity ventrally. The roof is formed by the sphenoid bone; caudally, the anatomic mar-gin of the nasopharynx is situated at the level of the soft palate. These anatomic relations are well demonstrated on sagittal and coronal images (Fig. 8.1 c). The pharyngeal recess (fossa of Rosenmüller) extends laterally in direction to the parapharyngeal space (PPS), directly adjacent to the opening of the eustachian tube. This region is often the origin of malignant neoplasms. The posterior part of the eustachian tube forms the cartilaginous torus tubarius. Laterally lies the levator veli palatini muscle, which, with the pharyngobasilar fascia, forms the margin to the PPS. The pharyngobasilar fascia is a tough fascial tissue connecting the pharynx with the skull base and containing holes for the transmission of the eustachian tube. Infiltration of this fascia is a sure sign of infiltrative growth of a neoplasm in the nasopharynx [2, 3].

In T1-weighted images, superficial structures such as the pharyngeal recess and the torus tubarius are well delineated (Fig. 8.1 a, b), as are the pterygoid muscles (Table 8.1). Due to the fact that mucosa shows a higher enhancement after Gd-DTPA administration than do the surrounding tissues, the levator and tensor veli palatini muscles, as well as the pharyngobasilar fascia, the tube openings, and the pharyngeal recess are better differentiated in Gd-DTPA-enhanced T1-weighted sequences (Fig. 8.1 b, Table 8.1). MRI detects infiltration or encasement of the internal carotid artery and the jugular vein, as well as tumor supply vessels. However, if the vessels supplying the tumor cannot be identified with certainty, angiography should be performed.

The multiplanar capability of MRI means that the extension of a lesion, as well as its relations to the surrounding tissues, particularly the trigeminal, glossopharyngeal, and vagus nerves can be demonstrated in all three orientations. The bony structures of the skull base are demonstrated to better advantage with Gd-DTPA because of the enhancement of bone marrow. After administration of the contrast medium the cavernous sinus and the skull base veins with their slow flow, appear as structures of high signal intensity, whereas rapidly flowing arterial blood appears dark due to the flow-void phenomenon.

**Table 8.1.** The usefulness of different MRI pulse sequences in evaluating tumor infiltration

| Location | T1 weighted plain | Spin density | T2 weighted plain | T1 weighted, Gd-DTPA |
|---|---|---|---|---|
| *Superficial structures* | | | | |
| Pharyngeal recess | 2 | 3 | 2 | 3 |
| Torus tubarius | 2 | 3 | 2 | 3 |
| *Muscles* | | | | |
| Levator veli palatini muscle | 2 | 2 | 1 | 3 |
| Tensor veli palatini muscle | 2 | 2 | 1 | 3 |
| Medial/lateral pterygoid muscle | 2 | 3 | 2 | 3 |
| Longus colli muscle | 2 | 3 | 2 | 3 |
| *Deep structures* | | | | |
| Parapharyngeal space | 2 | 3 | 2 | 3 |
| Infratemporal fossa | 2 | 2 | 2 | 3 |
| Sphenoid bone, skull base | 2 | 2 | 2 | 2 |
| Carotid artery | 2 | 2 | 2 | 3 |
| Cavernous sinus | 2 | 2 | 2 | 3 |
| Eustachian tube | 1 | 2 | 1 | 2 |
| Pharyngobasilar fascia | 1 | 1 | 1 | 2 |
| Walls of maxillary sinus | 1 | 2 | 1 | 2 |

Grading of visualization: 1, satisfactory; 2, good; 3, excellent. T1-weighted, 500/25; spin density, 3000/25; T2 weighted, 3000/90. Gd-DTPA was administered in a dose of 0.2 ml or 0.1 mmol/1 per kilogram body weight.

**Table 8.2.** Checklist nasopharynx and face

| | | Normal | Abnormal |
|---|---|---|---|
| Muscles | Tensor veli palatini muscle | | |
| | Levator veli palatini muscle | | |
| | Medial/lateral pterygoid muscle | | |
| Fascias | Pharyngobasilar fascia | | |
| Torus tubarius | | | |
| Pharyngeal recess | | | |
| Bone | Styloid process | | |
| | Bony walls of sinuses | | |
| Vessels | Internal carotid artery | | |
| | Jugular vein | | |
| | Cavernous sinus | | |
| Lymphatic tissue | | | |
| Trigeminal nerve | | | |
| Space | Infratemporal fossa | | |
| | Parapharyngeal space | | |
| | Pterygopalatine fossa | | |

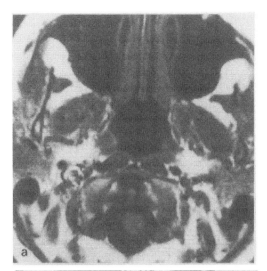

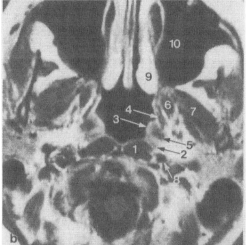

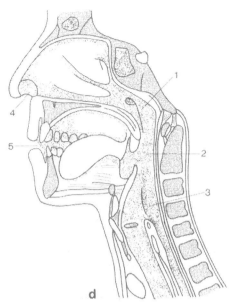

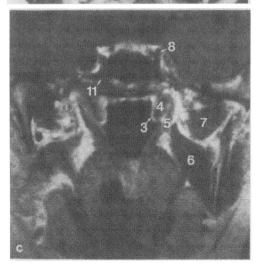

**Fig. 8.1a–d.** Normal topography of nasopharyngeal structures. Normal anatomic structures can be identified on MRI in the axial and coronal planes, particularly after administration of Gd-DTPA: *1*, Longus colli muscle; *2*, pharyngeal recess; *3*, torus tubarius; *4*, levator veli palatini muscle; *5*, tensor veli pterygoid muscle; *6*, medial pterygoid muscle; *7*, lateral pterygoid muscle; *8*, internal carotid artery; *9*, nasal mucosa; *10*, maxillary sinus; *11*, intracranial part of internal carotid artery

**a** Plain axial MRI (SE, 500/17)

**b** Axial MRI (SE, 500/17) with Gd-DTPA

**c** Coronal MRI (SE, 500/17) with Gd-DTPA

**d** Diagram of the topographical relations in the median sagittal plane. *1*, Nasopharynx; *2*, oropharynx; *3*, hypopharynx; *4*, entrance to nasal cavity; *5*, entrance to oral cavity

The walls and the roof of the nasopharynx are coated with lymphatic tissue. In the case of hypertrophy the extension of this tissue may lead to obstruction of the opening of the eustachian tube and to hearing loss. On MRI the lymphatic tissue appears bright compared to muscle.

### 8.3.2 Parapharyngeal Space

The PPS, which is separated from the nasopharynx by the pharyngobasilar fascia, is a common site of extension of nasopharyngeal neoplasms. It is a fat-filled triangular space bordered anterolaterally by the pterygoid muscles and posterolaterally by the parotid gland. Medially, the PPS is bordered by the levator and tensor veli palatini muscles. Caudally, it extends to the oropharynx, where it is in continuity with the digastric space. The PPS is divided into two compartments by the styloid process. The posterior PPS (carotid space) contains the internal carotid artery, the internal jugular vein, the glossopharyngeal, vagus, accessory, and hypoglossal nerves, and lymphatic tissue. Metastatic or inflamed lymph nodes are commonly found. Laterally, the infratemporal fossa is seen, bordered by the maxillary sinus and the zygomatic arch and divided into the masticator space and the parotid space.

### 8.3.3 Nose and Paranasal Sinuses

The paranasal sinuses are air-filled cavities surrounded by bone. The bony margins of the nose and the paranasal sinuses are formed cranially by the ethmoid bone; caudally, the nose is bordered by the hard palate, which is of medium signal intensity on MRI due to the bone marrow content. Both axial and coronal images are suitable for evaluating of the paranasal sinuses: both show adjacent structures such as the medial and lateral pterygoid muscles. The thin bony walls of the paranasal sinuses give no signal, so on MRI the surrounding fat and muscle tissue forms the borders of the sinuses. The thinnest bone lies along the posteromedial boundary of the antrum and has been called the membranous wall of the antrum. The infraorbital nerve, artery, and vein can be found in a groove in the posterior portion of the roof of the antrum. This groove becomes a canal anteriorly and later exits to the cheek as a foramen.

## 8.4 Lesions of the Nasopharynx

### 8.4.1 Squamous Cell Carcinoma

Some 80% of squamous cell carcinomas of the nasopharynx arise at the lateral walls; the pharyngeal recess is a particularly common site of origin. In almost all patients suffering

**Table 8.3.** Comparison of MR and CT for lesions of the nasopharynx and paranasal sinuses

|  | MR (plain) | MR (Gd-DTPA) | Value of MR relative to CT |
|---|---|---|---|
| *Nasopharynx* |  |  |  |
| Squamous cell carcinoma | 2 | 3 | + |
| Lymphoepithelial, adenoid-cystic carcinoma | 2 | 3 | + |
| Angiofibroma | 3 | – [a] | + |
| *Paranasal sinuses* |  |  |  |
| Squamous cell carcinoma | 2 | 2 | 0 |
| Meningioma | 1 | 3 | 0 |
| Esthesioneuroblastoma | 2 | 3 | + |
| Oropharyngeal tumors | 2 | 3 | + |
| Other (lymphoma, neurinoma, cyst) | 2 | 3 | + |

Grading of visualization: 1, satisfactory; 2, good; 3, excellent.
[a] Gd-DTPA could not be given (patient under 18 years of age).

from squamous cell carcinomas, infiltration
of the levator and tensor veli palatini muscles
and a destruction of the pharyngobasilar fascia are found. These tumors typically grow
into the PPS, the nasal cavity, and the sinuses
and infiltrate the longus colli muscles dorsally
[1, 11]. Because of eustachian tube obstruction 90% of the patients with squamous cell
carcinomas of the nasopharynx exhibit fluid
in the mastoid cells. Squamous cell carcinomas can also invade the sphenoid and
cavernous sinuses and extend from there into
the nasal cavity. Indistinct margins and necrotic areas are characteristic for these tumors
(Fig. 8.2). Low-intensity nonenhancing regions within the tumor mass can be considered to represent necrosis. Discrete crossing of
the midline by the tumor can be diagnosed
with confidence only on contrast-enhanced
images, but may be suspected on plain images.
In rare cases, squamous cell carcinomas of the
nasopharynx also invade the parotid space.
Often the poststyloid compartment of the PPS
is infiltrated, showing encasement and compression of the internal carotid artery. The
glossopharyngeal, vagus, accessory, and hypoglossal nerves are sometimes involved, and
extensive lymph node metastasis may be seen.
Subtle extension of these tumors to the ptery-

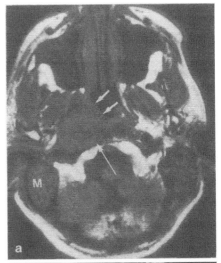
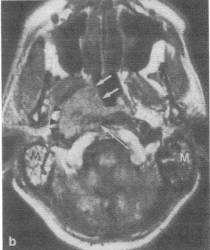
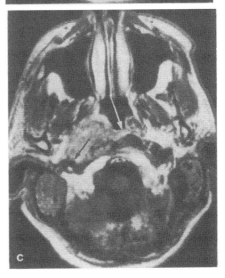

Fig. 8.2 a–c. Primary squamous cell carcinoma of
the nasopharynx
a Plain axial MRI (SE, 500/23). Before Gd-DTPA
administration, the tumor is demonstrated with the
same signal intensity as muscle. It can not be seen
whether the midline has been crossed
b Plain axial MRI (SE, 1600/23). A space-occupying lesion of medium signal intensity is seen on the
right side in the nasopharynx. Infiltration of the
parapharyngeal space (short arrows) and of the
longus colli muscle (long arrow). Mastoiditis on the
right (M)
c Axial MRI (SE, 500/23) with Gd-DTPA. Inhomogeneous contrast medium enhancement of the tumor, less than that of mucosa. Incomplete encasement of the internal carotid artery on the right
(black arrow), infiltration of the right longus colli
muscle and torus tubarius. The levator and tensor
veli palatini muscles are destroyed, and the tumor
extends to the parapharyngeal space. Transgression
of the midline (white arrow), infiltration of the left
pharyngeal recess

goid muscles can best be judged on images
with Gd-DTPA enhancement, because the signal intensity of squamous cell carcinomas in
the plain image is about the same as that of
muscle. Squamous cell carcinomas show a
moderate increase in signal intensity after Gd-
DTPA administration. The T1 and T2 relaxation times are moderate [10]. The enhancement factor after administration of Gd-DTPA
is 1.6 (Table 8.4). Gd-DTPA improves the diagnostic information in all cases of squamous
cell carcinoma of the nasopharynx (Fig. 8.2,
Table 8.3). Indeed, exact delineation of the
lesion is often rendered possible only by administration of the contrast medium [8, 9].

### 8.4.2 Lymphoepithelial
### and Adenoid-Cystic Carcinomas

The rare lymphoepithelial and adenoid-cystic
carcinomas grow more aggressively and infiltrate the skull base earlier than do squamous
cell carcinomas. This behavior is typically
found already in small lesions originating
from the lateral or posterior wall of the
nasopharynx (Fig. 8.3, 8.4). On contrast-enhanced images these tumors show quite distinct margins with small necrotic areas. Adenoid-cystic and lymphoepithelial carcinomas
have a high enhancement factor of about 2,
due to the rich vascularization, and exhibit
moderate T1 and moderate to high T2 values
(Table 8.4).

### 8.4.3 Juvenile Angiofibroma

In young, male patients nasopharyngeal angiofibromas are occasionally found that display no signs of malignancy. However, some
of these tumors show infiltrative growth.
Originating from the roof of the nasopharynx, they grow along the mucosa into the
nasal cavity (Fig. 8.5). Even in very large tumors necrosis is usually not seen, due to the
high degree of vascularization. The margins
are frequently distinct. Particularly T2-
weighted images provide good diagnostic information (Table 8.4).

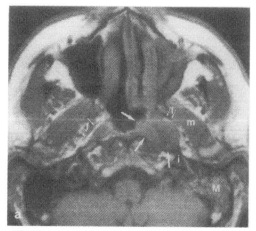

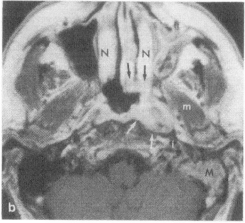

**Fig. 8.3 a–e.** Adenoid-cystic carcinoma of the nasopharynx
**a** Plain axial (SE, 500/25). Lesion in the area of the
left pharyngeal recess, signal intensity similar to
muscle. Exact delineation not possible. *m*, Pterygoid muscle; *M*, mastoiditis; *i*, internal carotid artery; *f* pharyngobasilar fascia
**b** Axial MRI (SE, 500/25) with Gd-DTPA. Inhomogeneous enhancement of the tumor, good lateral
delineation, pharyngobasilar fascia not destroyed.
No infiltrations of the longus colli muscles. Due to
the higher enhancement of the nasal mucosa (*N*),
delineation from tumor is possible (*black arrows*).
Central areas of low signal intensity represent necrosis (*white arrows*). **c–e** see p. 107

An intracranial extension can be reliably excluded on axial images, whereas infiltration of
the orbit is diagnosed on coronal images [7].
Juvenile angiofibromas enhance by a factor of
2.3 after administration of Gd-DTPA due to
their rich vascularization.

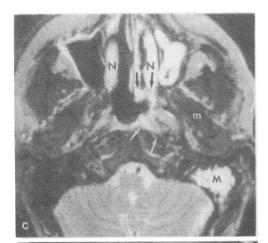

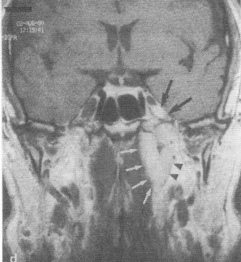

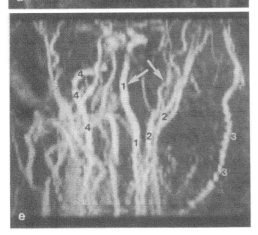

**Fig. 8.3. c** Plain axial MRI (SE, 3000/90). The tumor appears with high signal intensity. However, the delineation of surrounding tissues is not as good as in the Gd-DTPA enhanced image (**b**). Mastoiditis on the left, due to the obstruction of the tube opening by tumor tissue in the pharyngeal recess. Inflammatory changes in the left maxillary sinus
**d** Coronal MRI (SE, 500/25) with Gd-DTPA. Lesion of high signal intensity (*white arrows*) with central necrosis and infiltration of the cavernous sinus (*black arrows*). No infiltration of the sphenoid sinus. Exact delineation of the parapharyngeal fatty tissue (*arrowheads*)
**e** MR angiography, arterial phase. The internal carotid artery is displaced medially (*1*) and the external carotid artery laterally (*2*). The extent of the lesions is marked by *arrows*. Additionally some veins are visible. *3*, jugular vein; *4*, internal carotid artery
◁

**Fig. 8.4** see p. 108

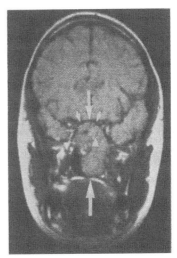

**Fig. 8.5.** Juvenile angiofibroma. Plain coronal MRI (SE, 500/23). Tumor in the sphenoid sinus and the nasal cavity on the left. Distinct margins without bony destruction. In the central part structures of low signal intensity are seen, representing vessels (*arrowhead*). The *arrows* show the margins of the lesion

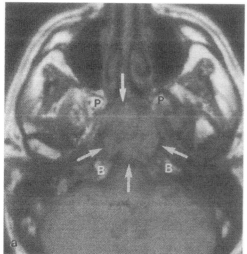

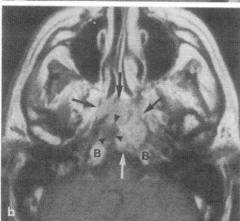

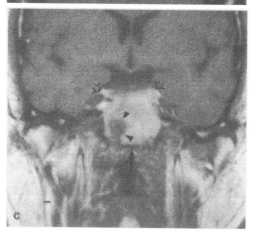

**Fig. 8.4 a–c.** Lymphoepithelial carcinoma of the nasopharynx
**a** Plain axial MRI (SE, 500/25). Lesion on the roof of the nasopharynx with medium signal intensity and diffuse extension (*arrows*). Good delineation of the nodular lesion from the fatty tissue of the skull base (*B*) and of the parapharyngeal space (*P*)
**b** Axial MRI (SE, 500/25) with Gd-DTPA. Inhomogeneous contrast enhancement. Indistinct margins, the pharyngobasilar fascia is destroyed on both sides. Infiltration of the sphenoid bone. Tumor necrosis is seen on the right (*arrow heads*)
**c** Coronal MRI (Se, 500/25) with Gd-DTPA. Destruction of the bony skull base and of the cavernous sinus on both sides (*open arrows*)
◁

**Fig. 8.5** see p. 107

**Fig. 8.6 a–f.** Lymphoid hyperplasia    ▷
**a** Plain axial MRI (SE, 500/25). Homogeneous lesion with a signal intensity similar to that of mucosa. *m*, Longus colli muscle; *f*, pharyngobasilar fascia
**b** Axial MRI (SE, 500,25) with Gd-DTPA. Medium contrast enhancement of the lesion, which is homogeneous and symmetrical in the lumen of the nasopharynx and the pharyngeal recess. No infiltrations. Septation of the lymphoid tissue (*s*) is a typical feature of lymphoid hyperplasia on MRI
**c** Plain axial MRI (SE, 3000/90). The T2-weighted image shows a homogeneous lesion (*arrows*) with high signal intensity; however, the typical septations are not seen. Inflamed mucosa of the nasal cavities (*N*)
**d** Coronal MRI (SE, 500/25) with Gd-DTPA. In the coronal plane the lesion is sharply bordered and symmetrical in the roof of the nasopharynx. The septations are seen well
**e, f** Axial MRI (turbo-FLASH, 30/13 flip angle 6°), plain and with Gd-DTPA. Turbo-FLASH enables exact dynamic recording of contrast medium enhancement due to the extremely short acquisition time, 5 s. Due to the short TR, vessels appear with high signal intensity. *N* nasal mucosa; *i*, internal carotid artery

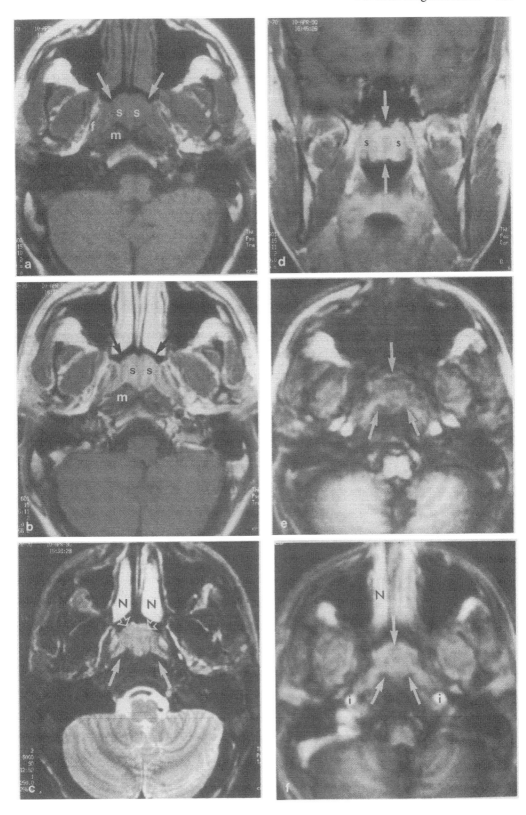

### 8.4.4 Lymphoid Hyperplasia and Lymphomas

The nasopharynx is, after the tonsillar region, the second most frequent site of lymphoid hyperplasia in the head and neck. In children this disease is common and causes respiratory disturbances. Among adults lymphoid hyperplasia is often found in those suffering from chronic infections, such as HIV-positive patients.

Lymphoid hyperplasia displays a high signal intensity on T1- and T2-weighted MRI (Fig. 8.6), with symmetric extension within the lumen of the nasopharynx. The characteristic septations are best seen on Gd-DTPA-enhanced T1-weighted images (Fig. 8.6b).

The most important differential diagnosis is lymphoma (Fig. 8.7). Nasopharyngeal lymphomas are mostly of the non-Hodgkin type. Their growth is asymmetric, usually without infiltration of surrounding tissues [4]. The signal intensity of nasopharyngeal lymphoma on T1- and T2-weighted images is very similar to that of lymphoid hyperplasia. The enhancement after administration of contrast medium is moderate and homogeneous without the septations that are typical for lymphoid hyperplasia (Fig. 8.7b) [9, 10].

## 8.5 Lesions of the Parapharyngeal Space

In healthy subjects the normal PPS appears symmetric [5]. Lesions infiltrating or displacing the PPS usually arise in surrounding structures such as the nasopharynx, parotid gland, or skull base. In most cases MRI enables conclusions as to the origin of a lesion. Most of the lesions involving the PPS are carcinomas of the nasopharynx, which destroy the pharyngobasilar fascia and infiltrate the pterygoid muscles. Aggressive malignant tumors of the parotid gland infiltrate the PPS laterally. In more than 80% of these tumors the pharyngobasilar fascia can still be delineated and primary infiltration from a nasopharyngeal lesion can therefore be excluded.

The only primary lesions that arise in the PPS are tumors of the minor salivary gland. On T1-weighted images these neoplasms display

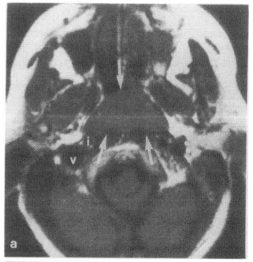

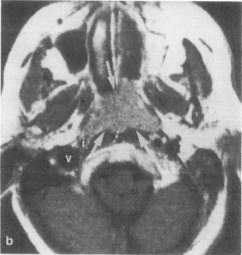

**Fig. 8.7 a, b.** Non-Hodgkin lymphoma of the nasopharynx
**a** Plain axial MRI (SE, 500/17). Large lesion, filling the nasopharynx completely. Tumor appears to be isointense to muscles. No evident signs of infiltration of surrounding tissues. Parapharyngeal space without infiltrations. *i,* Internal carotid artery; *V,* jugular vein
**b** Axial MRI (SE, 500/17) with Gd-DTPA. Inhomogeneous uptake of contrast medium by the lymphoma. In contrast to lymphoid hyperplasia no septations are visible

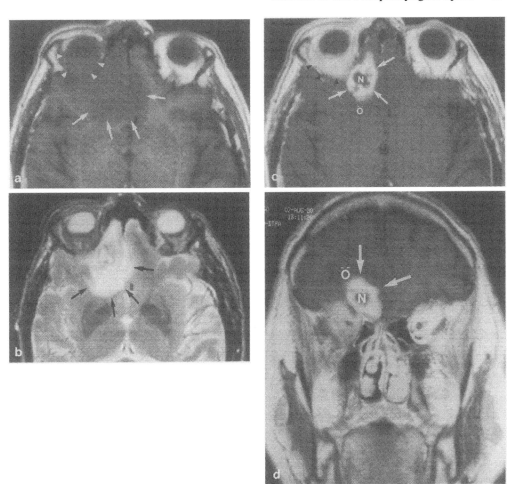

medium signal intensity and moderate Gd-DTPA enhancement. In T2-weighted sequences they are brighter than surrounding tissues and have an inhomogeneous internal pattern representing necrosis or calcification [5].

For diagnosing all malignant lesions of the nasopharynx plain and Gd-DTPA-enhanced T1-weighted images should be obtained in the axial plane. Additionally, coronal T1-weighted images should be obtained to demonstrate skull base extension. Optimal diagnostic information can be achieved by combining these sequences with axial T2-weighted images to depict surrounding edema accompanying inflammatory changes.

**Fig. 8.8a–d.** Squamous cell carcinoma of the paranasal sinuses with infiltration of the orbit and the skull base
**a** Plain axial MRI (SE, 500/17). Lesion of low signal intensity in the right intracranial parts of the orbit (*arrowheads*). Inhomogeneous signal intensity of the right frontal lobe (*arrows*)
**b** Plain axial MRI (SE, 2000/90). A 4 × 4 cm region of high signal intensity (*arrows*), representing edema. The tumor itself appears with medium signal intensity in the orbit
**c, d** Axial and coronal MRI (SE, 500/17) with Gd-DTPA. The tumor in the orbit shows marked enhancement after Gd-DTPA administration. The halo-like contrast medium enhancement represents the cerebral infiltration (*white arrows*), histologically proven to be an abscess with central necrosis (*N*). The edema (*ö*) does not show any enhancement

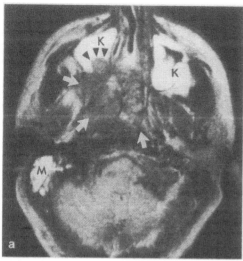

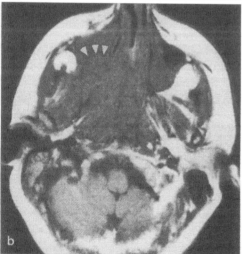

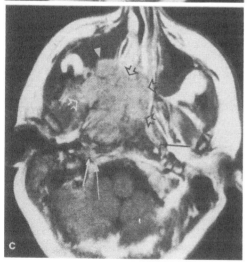

## 8.6 Lesions of the Nose and Paranasal Sinuses

### 8.6.1 Inflammatory Changes

Inflammatory changes of the nose and paranasal sinuses are common incidental findings in MR examinations of the head. The following manifestations must be differentiated:

– Hyperplasia of the mucosa
– Polyps
– Retention cysts
– Mucoceles
– Retained fluid

Most of these changes appear bright in T2-weighted sequences. Mucosal hyperplasia is seen as a diffuse bulge coating the sinuses, whereas polyps appear as space-occupying lesions. Plain T1-weighted sequences do not allow differentiation of mucosa and fluid, while after administration of Gd-DTPA the mucosa shows slight enhancement but the fluid does not. Retention cysts of the sinuses show a very high signal intensity in T2-weighted sequences but are hypointense on T1-weighted images. After administration of Gd-DTPA the wall of the cyst shows enhancement but the contained fluid does not. An abscess (Fig. 8.8) shows the

◁
**Fig. 8.9 a–c.** Squamous cell carcinoma of the nasal cavity and infiltration of the nasopharynx
**a** Plain axial MRI (SE, 2000/90). Large tumor of the paranasal sinuses originating on the posterior wall of the right maxillary sinus (*arrowheads*). Infiltrations of the nasopharynx, the parapharyngeal space, and the longus colli muscle. Fluid retention in both maxillary sinuses (*K*), mastoiditis on the right (*M*). Unsatisfactory delineation of surrounding structures
**b** Plain axial MRI (SE, 500/17). Also in the plain T1-weighted sequence, unsatisfactory contrast between tumor and inflamed mucosa (*arrowheads*)
**c** Axial MRI (SE, 500/17) with Gd-DTPA. Marked enhancement of the tumor after administration of Gd-DTPA. Good delineation possible (*open arrows*). Infiltration of the pyramid (*white arrows*) and of the parapharyngeal space (*black arrow*)

typical ring-like appearance with marked enhancement at the margins. T2-weighted images allow exact demonstration of accompanying edema.

### 8.6.2 Squamous Cell Carcinoma

Most tumors of the nose and parapharyngeal sinuses are squamous cell carcinomas of the maxillary sinuses. The incidence of these lesions is higher in the wake of chronic inflammatory changes. For that reason, early symptoms of a neoplasm are often overlooked, so that the diagnosis is not made until a late stage, when the tumor is already eroding the bony walls. These tumors show MRI characteristics resembling those of primary nasopharyngeal carcinomas (Fig. 8.9): a moderate increase in signal intensity after the administration of Gd-DTPA and moderate T1 and T2 values (Table 8.4). On plain T1-weighted images and on spin-density images it is difficult or impossible to distinguish tumor masses in the maxillary sinus from inflammatory changes and fluid. Differentiation is possible on enhanced MR but is also readily achieved on T2-weighted images, on which fluid appears bright and tumor is usually of lower intensity. Infiltration of the longus colli muscle by the posterior part of the tumor is best assessed after administration of contrast medium. Discrimination between inflammation and the anterior part of the tumor is also possible with contrast enhancement. Infiltration of the bony walls of the maxillary sinuses is seen to better advantage on CT, but the extent of the tumor can be judged more accurately on MRI.

A further advantage of contrast-enhanced MRI is the discrimination between solid tumors and fluid-containing cystic processes (Figs. 8.9, 8.10).

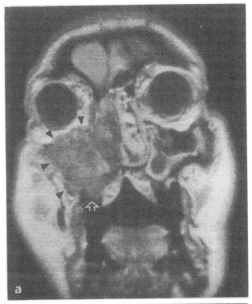

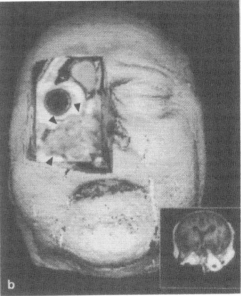

**Fig. 8.10a, b.** Squamous cell carcinoma of the right maxillary sinus
**a** Coronal MRI (SE, 500/25) with Gd-DTPA. Extensive space-occupying lesion in the region of the right maxillary sinus, showing complete destruction of the bony margins and infiltration of the left nasal cavity and the caudal and medial parts of the orbit (*arrowheads*)
**b** 3D turbo-FLASH with Gd-DTPA. Reconstruction of the head by means of a 3D sequence. The window cut in the tumor region demonstrates the relationship of the lesion to the face

**Table 8.4.** Characteristics of the most common nasopharyngeal lesions

| | Growth | Relaxation times | Relative enhancement with Gd-DTPA | Features |
|---|---|---|---|---|
| Primary squamous cell carcinoma | Aggressive growth, early skull base infiltration | Medium T1, medium T2 | Moderate (1.6) | Indistinct margins, necrosis |
| Lymphoepithelial and adenoid-cystic carcinoma | Aggressive growth, early skull base infiltration | Medium T1 medium T2 | Moderate (2.0) | Quite distinct margins, necrosis |
| Angiofibroma | Origin from roof of nasopharynx, mucosal infiltration | Prolonged T1, medium T2 | Marked (2.3) | Distinct margins, highly vascularized, no necrosis |
| Paranasal sinus carcinoma | Infiltration and destruction of paranasal sinuses, skull base infiltration | Low T1, prolonged T2 | Moderate (1.8) | Indistinct margins, inhomogeneous |
| Esthesioneuro-blastoma | Origin from olfactory nerve, growth to sphenoid sinus and nasopharynx | Prolonged T1, prolonged T2 | Marked (2.3) | Distinct margins, inhomogeneous |

### 8.6.3 Rare Lesions

A rare but important neoplasm is esthesioneuroblastoma, originating from the neuroectoderm of the olfactory nerve. These lesions grow across the cribriform lamina, infiltrate the sphenoid sinus as well as the maxillary sinus, and extend intracranially to the anterior cranial fossa. On MRI, esthesioneuroblastomas have an inhomogeneous internal pattern, prolonged T1 and T2, and high Gd-DTPA enhancement (factor 2.3). The MRI appearance of esthesioneuroblastomas closely resembles that of meningiomas of this region. The site of origin of meningiomas is common the brain or the skull base, but they spread into the paranasal sinuses and the nasopharynx by eroding the bony skull base. Characteristically, they are isointense to gray matter. Meningiomas often exhibit the MRI features of necrosis or calcifications but no signs of infiltrative growth. Due to the disturbance of the blood-brain barrier, the administration of Gd-DTPA leads to an increase in signal intensities by a factor of 2.3, providing excellent diagnostic information on coronal and axial images.

In the preoperative diagnosis of meningiomas, CT and MRI with Gd-DTPA are of equal value; however, the topographic relations are better demonstrated on MRI. A variety of other lesions – hamartoma (Fig. 8.11), lipoma, papilloma, melanoma – are occasionally found in the nose and paranasal sinuses. Analysis of topography, signal intensity, contrast enhancement, and morphology can help establish the diagnosis. Meningoencephalocele (Fig. 8.12) may also be encountered [11].

---

Lesions of the nose and paranasal sinuses can best be identified using plain and Gd-DTPA-enhanced T1-weighted images in combination with T2-weighted images in the axial and coronal planes. Gd-DTPA in T1-weighted sequences allows exact delineation of tumor margins. T2-weighted sequences differentiate inflammatory changes and fluid from solid tumors. In inflammatory changes where no tumor is suspected Gd-DTPA need not be administered.

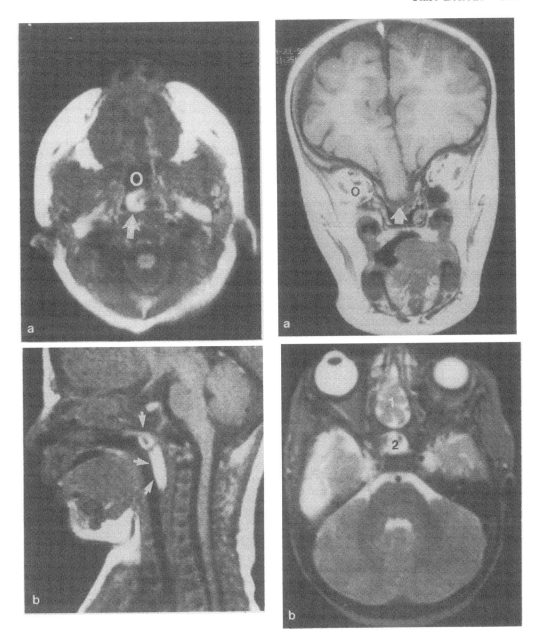

**Fig. 8.11 a, b.** Hamartoma of the nasopharynx in an infant
**a** Plain axial MRI (SE, 500/17). Documentation of a round lesion with high signal intensity in the naso- and oropharynx. Distinct margins, homogeneous internal pattern (*arrow*) *O,* oropharynx
**b** Plain median sagittal MRI (SE, 500/17). Exact delineation of surrounding tissues. The tumor is seen to extend from the roof of the nasopharynx to the oropharynx. Signal intensity similar to that of fat

**Fig. 8.12 a, b.** Meningoencephalocele in the nasopharynx
**a** Plain coronal MRI (SE, 500/25). The frontal lobe with the associated dura extends to the sphenoid sinus and the nasopharynx (*arrows*). No displacement of nasopharynx. Orbits (*O*) not infiltrated
**b** Plain axial MRI (SE, 3000/90). In the axial T2-weighted image frontal lobe is seen surrounded by cerebrospinal fluid in the sphenoid sinus (*1*) and the ethmoid sinus (*2*)

## 8.7 Value of MRI
## and Diagnostic Procedure

Multisequence MRI is superior to CT in most cases for the differential diagnosis of tumors and inflammatory changes in the nasopharynx and paranasal sinuses [6]. The MR examination must incorporate T2-weighted sequences to demonstrate inflamed tissue and fluid-containing spaces. Further improvement was achieved with the introduction of the paramagnetic contrast medium Gd-DTPA. Normal mucosa shows a moderate to marked increase in signal intensity after Gd-DTPA administration, yielding better delineation of small structures such as the veli palatini muscles and the pharyngobasilar fascia. Whereas tumor and inflammation usually display similar signal intensity on plain T1-weighted images, after Gd-DTPA administration tumors usually enhance to a lesser degree than inflammatory changes. Cystic lesions with high signal intensities on T2-weighted images exhibit no central increase in intensity after Gd-DTPA, but the cyst walls show a slight increase. Another advantage of Gd-DTPA is its ability to demonstrate the degree of vascularization of a lesion. Different tumors show increases in signal intensity varying from a factor of 1.6 to a factor of 2.3 after administration of Gd-DTPA. The highest values being measured for angiofibromas. Necrosis is demonstrated as usually centrally located areas of lower signal intensity. Despite the good soft tissue contrast on MRI, the diagnosis of superficial mucosal infiltrations is difficult due to the enhancement of both normal mucosa and tumor tissue after administration of Gd-DTPA. In these cases the subtraction technique proves helpful, because the tumors enhance to a lesser degree than normal mucosa.

An important reason for the superiority of MRI over CT in the differential diagnosis of lesions of the nasopharynx and paranasal sinuses is the contrast medium Gd-DTPA, which allows not only exact delineation of tumors but also differentiation between tumor types on the basis of enhancement patterns. Evaluation of T1 and T2 is also sometimes helpful; however, its usefulness is limited by the very high standard deviation.

In conclusion, the diagnostic procedure shown in Fig. 8.13 is recommended. The pri-

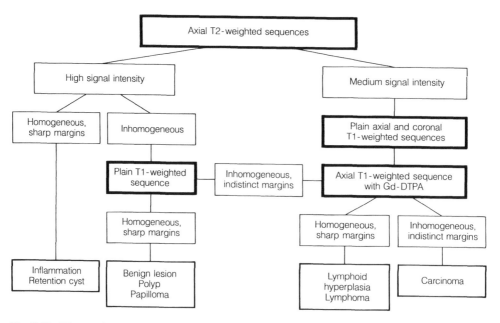

**Fig. 8.13.** Diagnostic strategy: nasopharynx and paranasal sinuses

mary diagnostic tool should be MRI, plain and with Gd-DTPA. CT with contrast medium may be performed additionally to demonstrate small osseous structures.

In the future, three-dimensional imaging will further improve preoperative staging, while MRI combined with MR spectroscopy will allow better follow-up of the response to treatment.

## References

1. Mancuso AA, Hanafee WN (1985) Computed tomography and magnetic resonance imaging of the head and neck, 2nd edn. Williams and Wilkins, Baltimore
2. Mancuso AA, Bohmann L, Hanafee WN, Maxwell D (1980) Computed tomography of the nasopharynx: normal and variants of normal. Radiology 137:113–121
3. Mödder U, Steinbrich W, Heindel W, Lindemann J, Brusis T (1985) Indikationen zur Kernspintomographie bei Tumoren des Gesichtsschädels und Halsbereiches. Digitale Bilddiagn 5:55–60
4. Silver JA, Mawad ME, Hilal SK et al. (1983) Computed tomography of the nasopharynx and related spaces. I. Anatomy. Radiology 147:725–731 II. Pathology. Radiology 147:733–738
5. Som PM, Braun JF, Shapiro MD, Reed DL, Curtin HD, Zimmermann RA (1987) Tumors of the parapharyngeal space and upper neck. Radiology 164:823
6. Teresi LM, Lufkin RB, Hanafee WN et al. (1987) MR imaging of the nasopharynx and floor of the middle cranial fossa. I. normal anatomy. Radiology 164:811–816. II. malignant tumors. Radiology 164:817–821
7. Vogl T (1989) KST: Gesichtsschädel/Oropharynx. KST: Felsenbein. KST: Hals. In: Lissner J (ed) Klinische Kernspintomographie. Enke, Stuttgart, pp 266–283
8. Vogl T, Mees K, Grevers G (1987) Die diagnostische Wertigkeit der Kernspintomographie bei Raumforderungen des Pharynx. Laryngol Rhinol Otol (Stuttg) 66:543–546
9. Vogl T, Dresel S, Schedel H, Markl A, Grevers G, Stelzer S, Lissner J (1989) KST des Nasopharynx mit Gd-DTPA: Wertigkeit und differentialdiagnostische Kriterien. RÖFO 150(5):516–522
10. Vogl T, Dresel S, Kang K, Hahn D, Grevers G, Lissner J (1990) Nasopharyngeal and adjacent tumors, MRI with Gd-DTPA. AJNR 11:187–194
11. Zonneveld FW, van der Meulen JC, van Akkerveeken PF, Koornneef L, Vaandrager JM, van der Horst CM (1988) Dreidimensionale Bildgebung durch Verarbeitung von CT-Daten und klinische Anwendungen in der Orthopädie und Chirurgie des Gesichtsschädels. Röntgenstrahlen 59:28–39

# 9 Salivary Glands

## 9.1 Clinical Findings

Diseases of the major salivary glands can basically be divided in two groups, nonneoplastic diseases and tumors.

*Nonneoplastic Diseases.* Various types of lesions have to be considered. Acute suppurative sialadenitis, for instance, may involve either the parotid or the submandibular glands. The majority of cases, however, occur in the parotid gland; this is thought to be because of the reduced bacteriostatic activity of parotid gland saliva. In chronic recurrent sialadenitis, which is also more common in the parotid gland, the primary pathogenic event is believed to be a decreased secretion rate.

Sjögren's syndrome can affect the salivary glands. This disease is characterized by destruction of the exocrine glands with xerostomia and xerophthalmia. Sjögren's syndrome is the second most common autoimmune disease after rheumatoid arthritis.

Another important nonneoplastic disorder is mumps, which is thought to be the most common cause of parotid swelling. The disease is due to a viral infection and occurs mainly in children aged 4–6 years.

Sialolithiasis is a common disease in the submandibular gland; 80% of salivary calculi are found in this gland. The disease can lead to recurrent sialadenitis if the calculi are not removed.

Sialadenosis is a nonspecific term used to describe noninflammatory, nonneoplastic enlargement of a salivary gland. In most cases the parotid gland is involved. The pathogenic mechanism is still unknown, but the disease may be observed in association with endocrinologic and metabolic disorders.

Rare nonneoplastic diseases affecting the salivary glands include actinomycosis, tuberculosis, sarcoidosis, and uveoparotid fever. Salivary gland enlargement as a side effect of a number of drugs must also be considered in the differential diagnosis.

*Tumors.* Some 80% of salivary gland tumors occur in the parotid gland, compared to 10% in the submandibular gland, 10% in the minor salivary glands, and 1% in the sublingual gland. On the other hand, only 30% of parotid gland tumors are malignant, compared to 50% in the submandibular gland, 50% in the minor salivary glands, and 80% in the sublingual gland. Salivary gland tumors make up 15% of all tumors of the head and neck and represent the most complex and diverse group of tumors encountered by the oncologist in this region.

The benign pleomorphic adenoma is the most common of all salivary gland neoplasms, and occurs mainly in the parotid gland. Warthin's tumor (papillary cystadenoma lymphomatosum) is another common lesion that is almost exclusively confined to the parotid gland, though cases involving the submandibular gland have been reported. Other benign tumors of the salivary glands are oncocytomas and monomorphic adenomas. The latter have to be distinguished from pleomorphic adenomas.

The recommended treatment for benign tumors is excision of the lesion (Warthin's tumor) or partial/total removal of the gland (pleomorphic adenoma).

Malignant salivary gland tumors are characterized by rapid growth, pain and – at an advanced stage – facial paresis and skin infiltration. One may also find involvement of cervical lymph nodes. Mucoepidermoid carcinoma is the most common malignancy of the parotid gland, while adenoid-cystic carcinoma is most commonly found in the submandibular gland and the minor salivary glands. Other, less common malignant tumors of the salivary glands are acinus cell carcinoma, adenocarcinoma, carcinoma in pleomorphic adenoma, squamous cell carcinoma, undifferentiated carcinoma, and salivary duct carcinoma.

The therapeutic approach in all salivary gland malignomas depends on the histologic pattern.

*Diagnostic Procedures.* The diagnostic management includes physical examination (inspection and bimanual palpation) and ultrasound. If Sjögren's syndrome is suspected, a variety of diagnostic procedures (ENT and ophthalmological examination as well as internal medicine investigations) have to be carried out. The diagnostic value of needle biopsies of the parotid gland is controversial. Conventional roentgenology of the floor of the mouth, as well as sialography, may be indicated if sialolithiasis of the submandibular gland is suspected. However, sialography must not be performed in acute inflammation of the gland.

*Demands on the radiologist.* In many patients, enlargement of a salivary gland occurs without any other symptoms. It is desirable in these cases to establish the size and tissue homogeneity of the glands. In the cases of inhomogeneous enlargement, one must check for infiltration of the surrounding tissue. Progressive growth of a malignant parotid gland tumor, for instance, can lead to infiltration of the skull base and the vessels of the parapharyngeal space, thus worsening the patient's prognosis significantly; in such cases the demonstration of extensive, infiltrative growth might influence the therapeutic management.

## 9.2 Examination Technique

All examinations presented here were carried out on a 1.5-T MR unit (Siemens Magnetom) operating at 1.0 or 1.5 T. A head coil with a diameter of 25 cm is used on all patients. First, a sagittal survey image is obtained to establish craniocaudal orientation (300/13, one acquisition). Thereafter, axial images were obtained using long (3000/25, 90) and short (500/25) SE sequences, with two acquisitions at a matrix size of $256 \times 256$ pixels. With a field of view of 30 cm and a zoom factor of 1.3, the pixel size was 0.9 mm $\times 0.9$ mm. Coronal images were acquired with a short SE sequence using the same parameters. After injecting Gd-DTPA, axial and in most cases coronal images were obtained. Slice thickness was 5 mm in all cases. A quantity of 0.2 ml/kg body weight of a solution of Gd-DTPA at a concentration of 0.1 mmol/l was injected using the bolus technique. In some cases subtraction images were made.

## 9.3 Topographic Relations

### 9.3.1 Parotid Gland

In the salivary glands a lot of anatomic details have to be distinguished in a relatively small area. Fat and muscle can easily be differentiated by virtue of their different relaxation times. The parenchyma of the parotid gland has a higher signal intensity than muscle on T1-weighted images and a lower intensity than fat. The most important anatomic structures are directly adjacent to the parotid gland and the masseter muscle and include the facial vein and artery and the retromandibular vein (Table 9.1). The facial nerve and the parotid duct are seen as areas of lower signal intensity within the gland (Fig. 9.1). The facial nerve leaves the skull base at the stylomastoid foramen and passes through the buccal fat pad before entering the parotid gland. This fat pad is normally seen on MRI and is important in the evaluation of perineural tumor spread. The main trunk of the facial nerve runs lateral to the retromandibular vein and external carotid artery, or between these two structures, and divides into its two major branches at the posterior margin of the mandibular ramus.

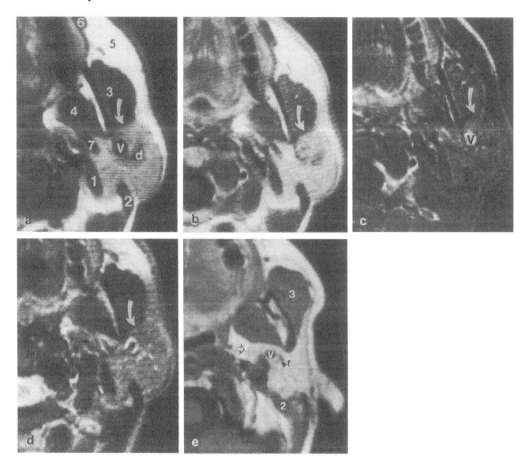

**Fig. 9.1 a–g.** Normal topography of the parotid gland and surrounding tissues using different MRI sequences and Gd-DTPA. *V,* Retromandibular vein; *f,* facial nerve; *d,* parotid duct; *1,* digastric muscle; *2,* sternocleidomastoid muscle; *3,* masseter muscle; *4,* pterygoid muscle; *5,* buccal fat pad; *6,* buccinator muscle; *7,* facial vein; *curved arrow,* border of the parotid gland; *open arrow,* parapharyngeal space

**a** Plain axial MRI (SE, 500/17)
**b** Axial MRI (SE, 500/17) with Gd-DTPA
**c** Subtraction image (**b** − **a**)
**d** Plain axial MRI (SE, 3000/90)
**e** Axial MRI (SE, 500/17) with Gd-DTPA. Demonstration of the intraglandular facial nerve
**f, g** see p. 121

The location of small parotid tumors is described as superficial, deep, above or below the main trunk of the facial nerve. (There is no anatomic division of the parotid gland into a superficial and a deep lobe, but lesions lateral to the nerve are said to be in the superficial lobe and those medial to the nerve in the deep lobe.) The parotid gland is bordered ventrally by the ptyergoid muscles, the styloid process, the carotid arteries, the jugular vein, and the parapharyngeal space, dorsally by the sterno-

cleidomastoid muscle and the posterior belly of the diagastric muscle. Another important boundary for describing the primary location of a lesion is the pharyngobasilar fascia, dividing the parotid gland and the parapharyngeal space from the nasopharynx.

Lesions located in the prestyloid space anterior to the styloid process must be diagnosed as primary lesions of the parotid gland. Lesions in the poststyloid space are described as primary parapharyngeal lesions. Tumors trans-

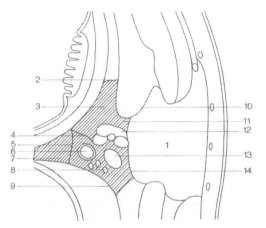

**Fig. 9.1. f** Topographic relations of the parapharyngeal space in the axial plane. *1*, parotid gland; *2*, parapharyngeal fascia; *3*, lateropharyngeal space; *4*, stylopharyngeal fascia; *5*, sagittal septal line between retro- and parapharyngeal space; *6*, internal carotid artery; *7*, retropharyngeal space; *8*, vagal nerve, accessory nerve, hypoglossal nerve; *9*, prevertebral lamina; *10*, masseteric fascia; *11*, connection between parotid gland and lateropharyngeal space; *12*, styloid process and muscle; *13*, internal jugular vein; *14*, border between parotid gland and parapharyngeal space

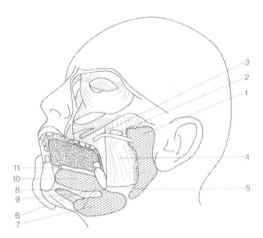

**Fig. 9.1. g** Topographic relations of the parotid gland. *1*, Parotid gland; *2*, accessory parotid gland; *3*, parotid duct; *4*, masseter muscle; *5*, masseteric fascia; *6*, submandibular gland; *7*, submandibular duct; *8*, mylohyoid muscle; *9*, anterior belly of digastric muscle; *10*, sublingual gland; *11*, major sublingual duct

**Table 9.1.** Checklist: salivary gland

*Parotid gland*

|  | Normal | Abnormal |
|---|---|---|
| Buccal fat pad |  |  |
| Pterygoid muscle |  |  |
| Masseter muscle |  |  |
| Buccinator muscle |  |  |
| Sternocleidomastoid muscle |  |  |
| Digastric muscle |  |  |
| Facial artery and vein |  |  |
| Retromandibular vein |  |  |
| Facial nerve |  |  |
| Parotid duct |  |  |
| External carotid artery |  |  |
| Internal jugular vein |  |  |

*Submandibular gland*

|  | Normal | Abnormal |
|---|---|---|
| Mylohyoid muscle |  |  |
| Genioglossus muscle |  |  |
| Geniohyoid muscle |  |  |
| Lingual artery |  |  |
| Facial vein |  |  |

*Sublingual gland*

|  | Normal | Abnormal |
|---|---|---|
| Geniohyoid muscle |  |  |
| Genioglossus muscle |  |  |
| Mandible |  |  |
| Lingual septum |  |  |
| Lingual artery |  |  |

gressing the fascia dividing the prestyloid and poststyloid spaces, are very probably malignant – except in patients in whom this fascia has already been surgically divided, in which case benign lesions can also cross from one compartment to the other.

The parotid duct passes anteriorly from the midportion of the gland around the anterior aspect of the masseter muscle, penetrates the buccal fat pad and the buccinator muscle, and finally drains into the mouth opposite the second upper molar.

After administration of Gd-DTPA the normal parenchyma of the parotid gland shows enhancement of about 130%. The facial nerve and its main trunk do not enhance to the same degree as parotid tissue and therefore can be identified as structures of lower signal intensity (Fig. 9.1). The examination has to be carried out in at least two planes. In the axial plane, the superficial structures and their relationship to surrounding areas are demonstrated. Coronal images document the extension of a lesion to the skull base as well as its relation to the major vessels.

### 9.3.2 Submandibular and Sublingual Glands

The paired submandibular glands are located beneath the floor of the mouth in the submandibular trigone bordered by the digastric muscle and the mandible. The main portion of the submandibular gland is indented by the lingual artery along its lateral border and the common facial vein along its posterolateral border. The submandibular duct originates from the anteromedial border of the gland and runs over the posterior surface of the mylohyoid muscle. It lies adjacent to the floor of the mouth until it reaches the region of the frenulum of the tongue, where it finally exits into the mouth through a small papilla. On MRI the submandibular duct is seen only if dilated.

The sublingual glands can be identified between the mandible and the tongue, adjacent to the mylohyoid muscle and lateral to the geniohyoid/genioglossus muscle complex. The lingual and hypoglossal nerves pass close enough to the submandibular and sublingual glands to be potential pathways of perineural extension. The MRI signal characteristics and the contrast medium dynamics of both glands are similar to those of the parotid gland.

MRI was originally thought to be equivalent or inferior to CT in diagnosing lesions of the salivary glands [3, 12–14, 17]. Nowadays, however, it is known to be superior, for various reasons [1, 5, 8]. It is important to choose the correct sequence parameters, to examine both sides [1, 8, 15], and to obtain images in at least two planes.

## 9.4 Inflammatory Changes

### 9.4.1 Parotitis

Inflammatory processes of the parotid gland result in prolonged T2 relaxation times but only slightly increased T1 relaxation times. Acute parotitis appears as an enlarged gland with high signal intensity on T2-weighted images. Occasionally, the subcutaneous fat tissue and the masseter muscle also appear to be infiltrated by inflammation (Table 9.2, Fig. 9.2). Furthermore, the retromandibular vein usually appears compressed.

Administration of Gd-DTPA leads to diffuse enhancement with no further diagnostic information (Table 9.2). The caudal and cranial extent of the gland is readily appreciated on plain coronal images. In T2-weighted sequences the accompanying inflammatory infiltration of surrounding tissues is seen well. Thus, Gd-DTPA does not necessarily have to be administered; the best information can be obtained using plain T1- and T2-weighted sequences (Table 9.3).

### 9.4.2 Sjögren's Syndrome

The parotid gland shows characteristic internal patterns and abnormalities in gland size in all patients with Sjögren's syndrome (SS). An inhomogeneous nodular structure limited to the organ itself can always be seen (Fig. 9.3). This honeycomb-like morphology is more or less distinct depending on the stage (Table 9.4). This is also valid for the size of the gland and the accompanying inflammatory infiltration of surrounding tissues, particularly of the masseter muscle. In advanced stages the retromandibular vein, which passes through the parotid gland, is medialized, and involved cervical lymph nodes are frequently discovered. T2 is prolonged in over 70% of cases due to the inflammatory changes, whereas T1 appears to be unchanged in more than 90% of cases. The administration of Gd-DTPA does not add any significant morphological information; the best evaluation is obtained via plain T2-weighted images.

**Table 9.2.** MRI characteristics of the most common lesions of the parotid gland

|  | Margins, infiltration (best shown by) | Internal structure | T1 (ms) | T2 (ms) | Contrast medium enhancement |
|---|---|---|---|---|---|
| Parotitis | Inflammatory infiltration of surrounding tissues (T2 weighted) | Homogeneous | 1283 (I) ±352 | 103 (I) ±38 | 190% ±26% |
| Sjögren's syndrome | Distinct margins (T2 weighted) | Inhomogeneous honeycomb like | 1305 (I) ±249 | 82 (I) ±35 | 118% ±21% |
| Adenoma | Distinct margins (T2, Gd-DTPA), displacement of vessels | Homogeneous, necrosis | 3900 (I) ±1749 | 101 (I) ±41 | 184% ±55% |
| Cysts | Distinct margins (T2 weighted, Gd-GTPA without infiltrations | Homogeneous | 907 (D) ±213 | 113 (I) ±27 | 8% ±5% |
| Warthin's tumor | Distinct margins (Gd-DTPA) | Homogeneous | 517 (D) ±326 | 61 (N) ±17 | 39% ±14% |
| Squamous cell carcinoma | Infiltrative growth (Gd-DTPA) | Inhomogeneous, necrosis | 1467 (I) ±431 | 84 (N) ±26 | 90% ±29% |
| Adenocarcinoma | Indistinct margins, infiltrative growth (Gd-DTPA) | Diffuse | 2592 (I) ±1375 | 50 (N) ±11 | 83% ±16% |
| Adenoid-cystic carcinoma | Very indistinct margins, infiltrative growth (Gd-DTPA) | Homogeneous, necrosis | 2070 (I) ±897 | 80 (N) ±23 | 97% ±31% |
| Lymphoma | Distinct margins (Gd-DTPA) | Homogeneous | 2950 (I) ±1585 | 76 (N) ±37 | 86% ±19% |
| Tumor recurrence | Indistinct, diffuse margins (Gd-DTPA) necrosis | Inhomogeneous | 1310 (I) ±328 | 58 (N) ±19 | 172% ±43% |
| Postoperative fibrosis | Diffuse margins (Gd-DTPA) | Inhomogeneous | 1190 (N) ±403 | 61 (N) ±26 | 11% ±6% |

D, decreased; N, normal; I, increased.

**Table 9.3.** Comparison of different pulse sequences in lesions of the parotid gland

|  | T1 weighted, plain | Spin density | T2 weighted, plain | T1 weighted Gd-DTPA |
|---|---|---|---|---|
| Parotitis | 2 | 2 | 3 | 2 |
| Sjögren's syndrome | 1 | 2 | 3 | 3 |
| Adenoma | 2 | 2 | 3 | 3 |
| Cysts | 1 | 2 | 3 | 3 |
| Warthin's tumor | 2 | 2 | 2 | 3 |
| Adenocarcinoma | 1 | 2 | 2 | 3 |
| Adenoid-cystic carcinoma | 2 | 2 | 2 | 3 |
| Squamous cell carcinoma | 2 | 2 | 2 | 3 |
| Lymphoma | 1 | 2 | 2 | 3 |
| Tumor recurrence | 1 | 2 | 1 | 3 |
| Postoperative fibrosis | 1 | 2 | 1 | 3 |

Grading of visualization: 1, satisfactory; 2, good; 3, optimal.

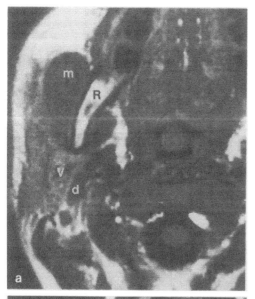

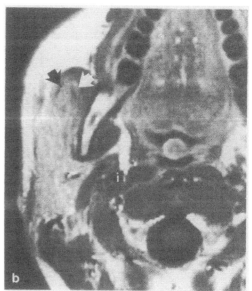

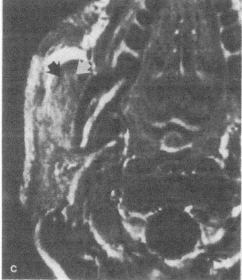

**Fig. 9.2 a–c.** Acute parotitis
**a** Plain axial MRI (SE, 500/25). Enlarged parotid gland on the right with displacement of the masseter muscle (*m*). *V*, retromandibular vein; *d*, digastric muscle; *R*, ramus mandibulae; *i*, internal carotid artery
**b** Axial MRI (SE, 500/25) with Gd-DTPA. Marked enhancement of the right parotid gland after administration of contrast medium. Inflammatory infiltration of the masseter muscle (*arrows*) shows up as an area of marked contrast medium uptake
**c** Plain axial MRI (SE, 1600/90). Inhomogeneous internal pattern of the parotid gland with high signal intensity in the posterior parts of the masseter muscle, as seen in the Gd-DTPA-enhanced image

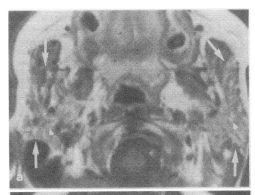

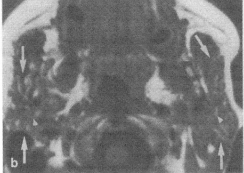

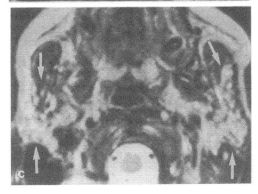

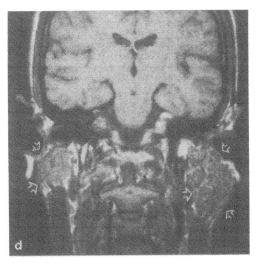

**Fig. 9.3 a–d.** Sjögren's syndrome, stage III
**a** Axial MRI (SE, 500/25) with Gd-DTPA. After
contrast medium administration quite marked enhancement is documented in both parotid glands.
The typical honeycomblike internal pattern is seen
in this image
**b** Plain axial MRI (SE, 500/25). Enlarged parotid
glands on both sides showing an inhomogeneous
internal pattern. (*arrows*). Normal tissue is inter-
spersed with areas of higher signal intensity (*arrowheads*)
**c** Plain axial MRI (SE, 3000/90). The typical criteria
for Sjögren's syndrome are also seen in the T2-
weighted sequence. The glands appear with high
signal intensity and nodular, honeycomblike internal pattern. Inflammatory changes of the masseter
muscle posteriorly
**d** Plain coronal MRI (SE, 500/25). The exact topographic relations of both glands are seen, and the
typical morphology is demonstrated

**Table 9.4.** Stages of Sjögren's syndrome

|  | Appearance of parenchyma | Size of gland |
|---|---|---|
| Stage 0 | Normal | Normal |
| Stage I | Reticular | Normal |
| Stage II | Small nodular | Normal or slightly enlarged |
| Stage III | Medium nodular | Slightly to moderately enlarged |
| Stage IV | Large nodular | Greatly enlarged |

Patients suffering from SS have a higher risk for developing lymphomas. The lymphomas we found in two of our patients showed the typical appearance of lymph node conglomerations with quite homogeneous internal signal intensity.

Acute inflammatory changes of the salivary glands show a diffuse increase of signal intensity on T2-weighted images with matching changes in surrounding tissues. Sjögren's syndrome and chronic parotitis exhibit a typical honeycomb-like, inhomogeneous internal pattern.
Gd-DTPA is of no significant diagnostic benefit in inflammatory diseases of the salivary glands.

## 9.5 Benign Lesions

Some 90% of all salivary gland tumors are found in the parotid gland, and most of these are histologically benign. Tumors of the submandibular and sublingual glands are malignant in a higher proportion of cases.

### 9.5.1 Pleomorphic Adenoma

Pleomorphic adenomas, the most frequent benign tumors of the salivary glands, usually grow slowly and without symptoms and are found more often in middle-aged patients. In the parotid gland these lesions occur in both the superficial lobe and the deep lobe. On

T1-weighted images adenomas appear as areas of low signal intensity within the parenchyma of the gland (Fig. 9.4). The margins are distinct and without infiltration (Table 9.3). On T2-weighted images the adenomatous tissue shows high signal intensity, representing fluid-containing spaces and displays a slightly inhomogeneous internal pattern. Adenomas exhibit the highest T1 times of all salivary gland tumors, benign or malignant, and their T2 times is also prolonged. After contrast medium administration, adenomas appear heterogeneous with areas of low signal intensity representing necrosis. Some patients exhibit small intraglandular tumors causing displacement of the retromandibular vein and the facial nerve, while others have tumors with marked expansive growth pattern that displace the soft tissues medially. In the latter the facial nerve usually can not be identified.

### 9.5.2 Lymphoepithelial Cysts

Cysts of the salivary glands are commonly found in patients suffering from chronic infections such as HIV and in patients with obstruction of the excretory duct. There is usually a history of recurrent painful swelling of that side of the face. One side is consistently affected and the gland is extensively enlarged. Lymphoepithelial cysts always have distinct borders.
On plain T1-weighted images, the delineation of cysts from normal glandular tissue is difficult due to the same signal intensity of both structures (Table 9.3). After administration of Gd-DTPA, however, the normal glandular tissue enhances but the cyst does not, making the lesion stand out more clearly. On T2-weighted images the cysts appear with increased signal intensity (Table 9.2).
Some authors [3, 8] have stated that no reliable differentiation of lymphoepithelial cysts and adenomas seems possible, but in our opinion these lesions can always be distinguished. In both cases Gd-DTPA improves the visualization of the lesion and its effect on adjacent structures. Though cysts and adenomas often look similar in plain T1-weighted

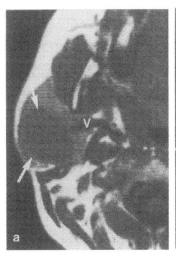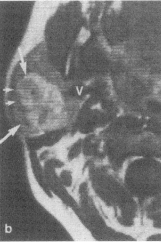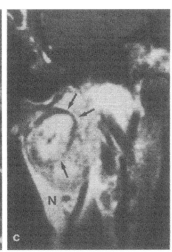

**Fig. 9.4 a–c.** Pleomorphic adenoma of the right parotid gland
**a** Plain axial MRI (SE, 500/25). Homogeneous intraglandular lesion of low signal intensity in the right parotid gland. Distinct borders (*arrows*). *V*, retromandibular vein
**b** Axial MRI (SE, 500/25) with Gd-DTPA. After administration of Gd-DTPA inhomogeneous enhancement is seen. The lateral margin seems to be indistinct (*small arrows*). However, the tumor appears to be without signs of infiltration. Compression and displacement of the retromandibular vein (*V*)
**c** Coronal MRI (SE, 500/25) with Gd-DTPA. The coronal image shows that the caudal and cranial parts of the lesion are also localized within the parotid gland (*arrows*). Inhomogeneous internal pattern with margins of low signal intensity, representing a capsule. *N*, normal parenchyma

sequences (Fig. 9.5), they can be differentiated on combined plain T2-weighted and Gd-DTPA-enhanced T1-weighted images.

The best results can be obtained using T1-weighted sequences with Gd-DTPA in combination with plain T2-weighted sequences (Table 9.3).

### 9.5.3 Warthin's Tumor

Warthin's tumors usually grow slowly and painlessly and may be multiple and bilateral. The lesions always show distinct margins and, after administration of Gd-DTPA, high signal intensity in central areas with less enhancement at the periphery (Table 9.2). Plain images reveal decreased T1 times and normal T2 times. No infiltrative growth is to be seen; the tumor is usually limited to the parotid space. The retromandibular vein and the facial nerve are often displaced medially, sometimes laterally, but are not compressed or infiltrated. T1-weighted images after administration of

Gd-DTPA are significantly more informative than plain T2-weighted images (Table 9.3). Gd-DTPA images confirm the presumed benign nature of these lesions by showing the distinct margins and the lack of infiltration. Other rare benign tumors such as neuromas, lipomas, and fibromas are usually also sharply demarcated from surrounding tissues.

Almost all benign lesions of the salivary glands can be diagnosed preoperatively on the basis of their characteristic appearances on plain T1- and T2-weighted images and their contrast medium enhancement.

If a cystic lesion appears homogeneous and exhibits high signal intensity on T1- and T2-weighted images, Gd-DTPA need not be given.

In inhomogeneous lesions with low signal intensity, however, Gd-DTPA has to be administered to exclude malignancy.

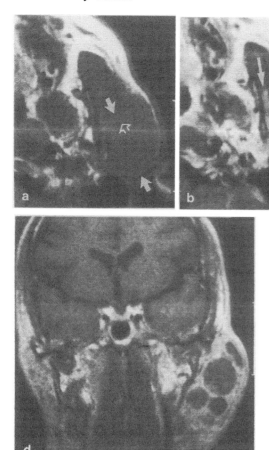

**Fig. 9.5 a–d.** Lympho-epithelial cyst in an HIV-positive patient

**a** Plain axial MRI (SE, 500/25). Space-occupying lesion of the left parotid gland (*white arrows*) showing a signal intensity similar to that of gland tissue and muscles (*open arrow*)

**b** Axial MRI (SE, 500/25) with Gd-DTPA. The normal gland tissue shows medium enhancement, whereas the cyst does not enhance. Additionally, a small cyst is seen (*black arrow*). The parenchyma and the masseter muscle of the gland appears to be inflamed (*white arrows*). The retromandibular vein is completely compressed

**c** Plain axial MRI (SE, 1600/90). Lesion of high signal intensity, representing a fluid-containing cyst

**d** Coronal MRI (SE, 500/25) with Gd-DTPA. Multiple areas of low signal intensity after Gd-DTPA administration in an enlarged left parotid gland. All cysts show distinct margins within the gland tissue

**Fig. 9.6 a–e.** Adenocarcinoma of the left parotid gland

**a** Plain axial MRI (SE, 500/25). Lesion of the left parotid gland with indistinct margins (*small arrows*). *White arrow*, jugular vein; *i*, internal carotid artery; *v*, retromandibular vein

**b** Axial MRI (SE, 500/25) with Gd-DTPA. After Gd-DTPA the lesion shows an inhomogeneous internal pattern and displacement of the retromandibular vein (*black arrow*). Displacement of the masseter muscle and extension of the tumor to the parapharyngeal space (*white arrow*)

**c** Coronal MRI (SE, 500/25) with Gd-DTPA. The ▷ coronal sequence demonstrates the relationship of the tumor to the major vessels (*open arrows*). The retromandibular vein is displaced laterally (*black arrow*)

**d** Plain axial MRI (FLASH, 30/13, flip angle 30°)

**e** Axial MRI (FLASH, 30/13, flip angle 30°) with Gd-DTPA. Fast FLASH sequences permit measurement of contrast medium enhancement over time. Good delineation of the lesion and of the extension to the parapharyngeal space (*small arrow*)

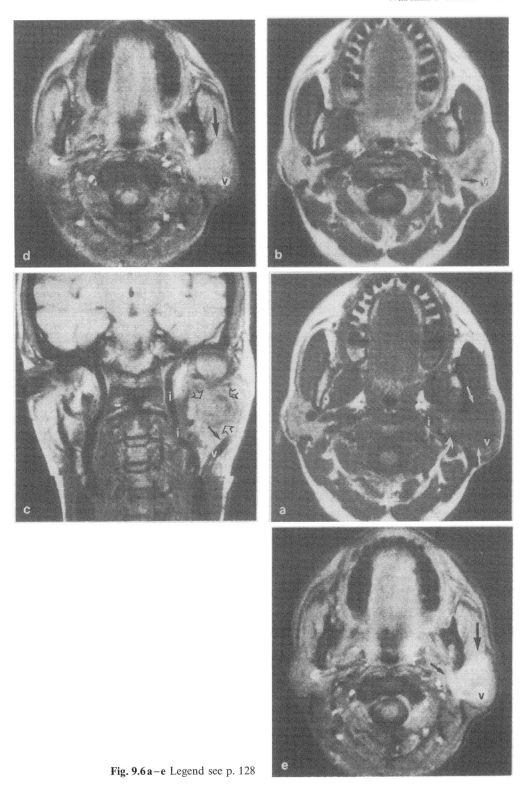

**Fig. 9.6 a–e** Legend see p. 128

## 9.6 Malignant Lesions

### 9.6.1 Adenocarcinoma

Adenocarcinomas are among the most common malignant tumors of the parotid gland. Pathologically they are divided into high-, intermediate-, and low-grade lesions [2, 6]. Low-grade adenocarcinomas resemble adenomas on MRI. The margins of intermediate- and high-grade adenocarcinomas can not be clearly appreciated in plain T1-weighted sequences, but after Gd-DTPA administration a diffuse, infiltrative growth pattern can be recognized (Table 9.2). Due to these infiltrations, the facial nerve can often be identified only by using contrast-enhanced T1-weighted sequences. The nerve usually can not be seen on T2-weighted plain images. The retromandibular vein is always either compressed or infiltrated (Fig. 9.6). Adenocarcinomas can extend to the mandible with parapharyngeal growth and infiltration of the pterygoid muscles and the major vessels, best seen in Gd-DTPA-enhanced T1-weighted sequences. Adenocarcinomas display increased T1 relaxation times and normal T2 relaxation times.

### 9.6.2 Adenoid-Cystic Carcinoma

These lesions are found not only in the parotid but also in the smaller submandibular and sublingual glands. Characteristically, they grow along the sheath of the facial nerve and show a high rate of recurrences (Fig. 9.7). Adenoid-cystic carcinomas display more aggressive growth than adenocarcinomas. They spread diffusely to the parapharyngeal space as well as to the lateral facial skeleton and infiltrate the neck muscles, the masseter muscle, and the mandible (Table 9.2). In some cases the disease is in such an advanced stage that no more normal glandular tissue can be

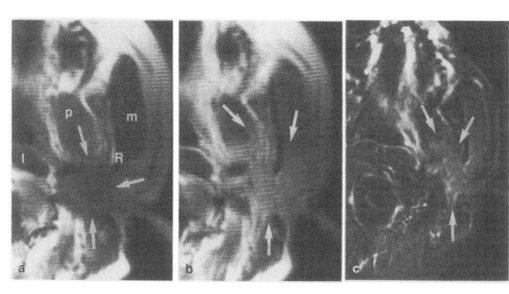

**Fig. 9.7a–c.** Adenoid-cystic carcinoma, recurrent lesion after parotidectomy
**a** Plain axial MRI (SE, 500,25). Lesion of low signal intensity. No evidence of normal gland tissue. Scarring due to the operation. *p*, Pterygoid muscles; *m*, masseter muscle; *l*, longus colli muscle; *R*, mandibular ramus
**b** Axial MRI (SE, 500/25) with Gd-DTPA. Diffuse infiltrations of the tumor appear after administration of contrast medium. Infiltrative growth to the longus colli muscles and encasement of the major vessels. Infiltration also of the masseter and pterygoid muscles (*arrows*)
**c** Subtraction image (**b** – **a**). The subtraction image shows significant enhancement of the lesion. Excellent delineation of the infiltration to surrounding muscle tissue (*arrows*)

identified. In plain T1- and T2-weighted sequences the muscles often appear not to be infiltrated, but after Gd-DTPA administration the infiltration of surrounding muscles is clearly visualized and the best overall results are achieved (Table 9.3). Usually the retromandibular vein is compressed and the facial nerve undetectable. The T1 times and T2 times of adenoid-cystic carcinomas resemble those of adenocarcinomas and are therefore not helpful in differentiating the two types of tumors.

### 9.6.3 Squamous Cell Carcinoma

The rare squamous cell carcinoma has an indistinct growth pattern (Fig. 9.8) and a quite heterogeneous internal appearance (Table 9.2). After Gd-DTPA administration these tumors show areas of low signal intensity representing necrosis, which is not apparent on plain T2-weighted images. Small infiltrations of surrounding muscles and the precise margins of the tumor are best recognized on Gd-DTPA-enhanced T1-weighted images. Squamous cell carcinomas display increased T1 and normal T2 times.

### 9.6.4 Lymphoma

Lymphomas are also among the rarer space-occupying lesions of the salivary glands. Non-Hodgkin's lymphomas are found more frequently in patients with a history of Sjögren's syndrome. Lymphomas can be divided in two different groups with different appearances on MRI. In the first group small conglomerations of lymph nodes are visible at the medial margin of the parotid gland. The surrounding glandular tissue displays no signs of tumorous infiltration on plain or Gd-DTPA-enhanced images (Fig. 9.9) (Table 9.2). The lymph nodes appear hypointense on T1-weighted and hyperintense on T2-weighted plain images. In the second group enlarged lymph nodes completely displace the normal tissue of the parotid gland.

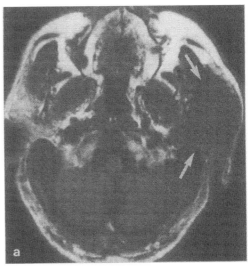
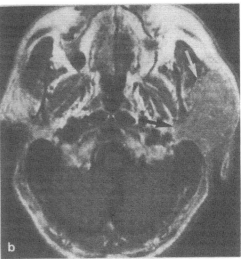

Fig. 9.8a, b. Squamous cell carcinoma of the left parotid gland
a Plain axial MRI (SE, 500/25). Homogeneous lesion of the left parotid gland with low signal intensity, isointense to muscles
b Axial MRI (SE, 500/25) with Gd-DTPA. Medium enhancement after Gd-DTPA administration. Inhomogeneous internal pattern, infiltration of the masseter muscle (*white arrow*). Destruction of the temporomandibular joint and extension to the parapharyngeal and retromaxillary space (*black arrow*). The retromandibular vein and facial nerve are not delineated

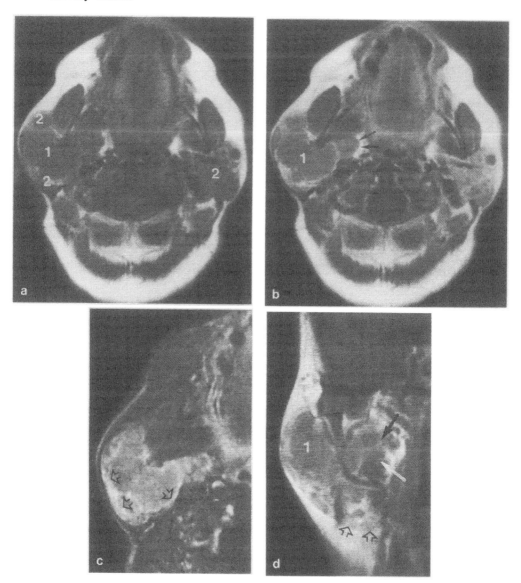

**Fig. 9.9 a–d.** Non-Hodgkin's lymphoma in a patient suffering from Sjögren's syndrome

**a** Plain axial MRI (SE, 500/25). Homogeneous lesion of the right parotid gland, showing medium signal intensity and bright margins (*1*). Speckled internal pattern of the remaining normal gland tissue of both parotid glands (*2*)

**b** Axial MRI (SE, 500/25) with Gd-DTPA. Low enhancement after Gd-DTPA administration. Documentation of lymph node conglomerates extending to the parapharyngeal space (*arrows*). Displace-

ment of the pterygoid muscles, compression of the retromandibular vein

**c** Subtraction image. The margins show marked contrast medium enhancement (*arrows*). Speckled enhancement of the normal parenchyma, representing the typical changes of Sjögren's syndrome

**d** Coronal MRI (SE, 500/25) with Gd-DTPA. Documentation of the extension medially and laterally to the pharynx (*solid arrows*). Inhomogeneous lymph nodes (*open arrows*)

These tumors typically show small extensions to the parapharyngeal space, best seen in Gd-DTPA-enhanced T1-weighted sequences (Table 9.3). The contrast medium enhancement is comparable to that of squamous cell carcinoma. The central portions of the lymphomas show homogeneous enhancement; the enhancement at the margins is significantly greater. These tumors show the highest T1 relaxation time of any salivary gland tumors with the exception of adenomas: T2 is unchanged. Differentiation of Hodgkin's and non-Hodgkin's lymphomas is not usually possible on MRI.

### 9.6.5 Recurrent Lesions

MRI has an important part to play in the follow-up of patients treated for tumors of the salivary glands, particularly the parotid gland and the submandibular gland.

In the early postoperative stage it is not possible to differentiate between residual tumor, bleeding, and fibrosis on the basis of T1, T2, and Gd-DTPA enhancement [10]. After a period of at least 3 months though, discrimination between tissues seems to be possible. The T1 and T2 of fibrosis resemble those of normal muscle. Fibrosis enhances only slightly after administration of Gd-DTPA.

Tumor recurrences show a typical appearance (Fig. 9.10). In plain T1- and T2-weighted sequences recurring tumor can not be easily differentiated, but after administration of Gd-DTPA it presents an enormous uptake of the contrast medium on T1-weighted images, allowing exact evaluation of the diffuse tumor infiltration to the pterygoid muscles and the parapharyngeal space. The findings can be confirmed using MR angiography and specially designed surface coils.

It is not possible to differentiate malignant from benign lesions on the basis of relaxation times alone. Indistinct tumor margins, clinical impairment of facial nerve function, failure to identify this nerve, and infiltration of the retromandibular vein are signs of malignancy. Gd-DTPA has to be administered in patients suspected to have a malignant tumor. However, distinction between different histological entities is rarely possible.

In follow-up, a recurrent lesion can be differentiated from postoperative fibrious tissue on the basis of T1, T2, and Gd-DTPA enhancement.

## 9.7 Value of MRI and Diagnostic Procedure

In most cases it is possible to distinguish between benign and malignant lesions by using a combination of plain T2-weighted sequences and plain and Gd-DTPA-enhanced T1-weighted images. Indistinct margins are taken as a sure sign of malignancy [8, 12], but heterogeneous internal patterns and zones of necrosis can also be seen in benign lesions [18]. The internal structure and vascularization of a tumor are better demonstrated after Gd-DTPA administration. Due to the high standard deviations, the T1 and T2 values do not allow reliable differentiation of malignant lesions [4, 8, 12, 16].

Plain MRI is often unsatisfactory for diagnosing small lesions because of the difficulty in distinguishing the lesion from high-signal normal gland tissue [12]. After administration of Gd-DTPA, however, the signal intensities differ significantly, permitting documentation of the patterns of infiltration.

In postoperative follow-up, marked Gd-DTPA enhancement must be taken to signify a recurrence. In fibrous areas only slight enhancement is found. MRI is useful for the diagnostic examination of lymph nodes because of the ability to image the cervical lymph chains in different planes [11].

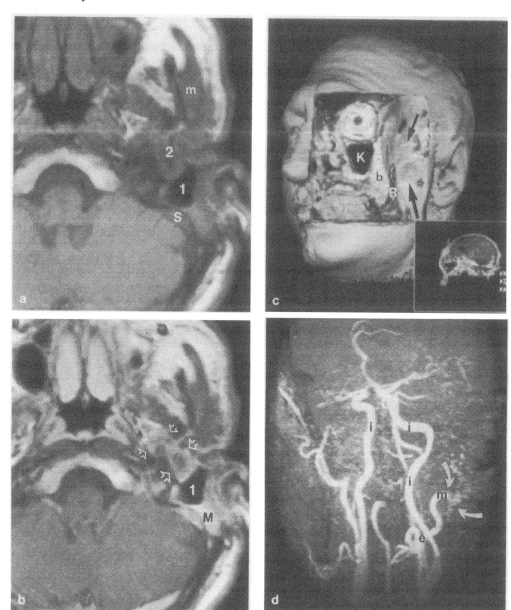

**Fig. 9.10 a–d.** Recurrence of aggressive fibromatosis in the left parotid space
**a** Plain axial MRI (SE, 500/17). In plain images the area of resection appears with low signal intensity in the deep parotid space (*1*). Anteriorly a lesion is seen in the retromaxillary space (*2*). *m*, masseter muscle; *S*, sigmoid sinus
**b** Axial MRI (SE, 500/17) with Gd-DTPA. After Gd-DTPA administration two halo-like lesions are delineated in the retromaxillary space, showing marked enhancement (*arrows*). This significant enhancement is evidence of recurrence. Postoperative fibrosis is excluded. *M*, mastoiditis
**c** 3D turbo-FLASH, ray tracing. In the reconstruction the relationship of the lesion in the infratemporal fossa is demonstrated. *K*, maxillary sinus; *b*, buccal fatty tissue; *R* ramus of mandible
**d** MR angiography, arterial with venous saturation. Normal appearance of the internal carotid artery on both sides (*i*). The maxillary artery (*m*) is operatively occluded on the left side (*arrows*). *e*, External carotid artery

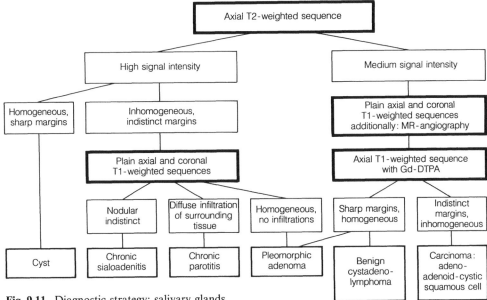

**Fig. 9.11.** Diagnostic strategy: salivary glands

For diagnostic purposes, plain MRI of the parotid gland is superior to CT due to the lack of beam-hardening artifacts and the better soft tissue contrast [9]. In contrast to other authors [7, 8], we have found the administration of Gd-DTPA helpful in establishing which of various possible neoplasms is present. Additionally, the contrast medium improves the delineation of lesions that are isointense to normal glandular tissue on plain MRI [19].

The procedure shown in Fig. 9.11 is recommended for the diagnosis of lesions of the parotid gland.

## References

1. Bohndorf K, Lönnecken I, Zanella F, Laufermann L (1987) Der Wert von Sonographie und Sialographie in der Diagnostik von Speicheldrüsenerkrankungen. ROFO 147(3):288–293
2. Bryan RN, Miller RM, Ferreyro RJ et al. (1982) Computed tomography of the major salivary glands. AJR 139:547–554
3. Casselmann JW, Mancuso AA (1987) Major salivary gland masses: comparison of MR imaging and CT. Radiology 165:183–189
4. Castelijns JA, Doornbos J, Verbeeten B, Vielvoje GJ, Bloem JL (1985) Magnetic resonance imaging of the normal larynx. Comput Assist Tomogr 9(5):919–925
5. Curtin HP, Wolfe P, Syndermann N (1983) Facial nerve between the stylomastoid foramen and parotid: CT-imaging. Radiology 149:165–169
6. Dillon WP (1986) Applications of magnetic resonance imaging to the head and neck. Semin US CT MR 7:202
7. Gademann G, Semmler G, Bachert-Baumann P, Zabel H-J, van Kaick G, Lorenz W-J (1987) 31P-spectroscopy follow up studies of human tumor after chemotherapy. Society of Magnetic Resonance in Medicine, 6th Annual Meeting and Exhibition. Book of abstracts, p 506
8. Gademann H, Haels J, Semmler W, von Kaick G (1988) KST bei Erkrankungen der Parotis. Laryngol Rhinol Otol (Stuttg) 67:211–216
9. Hansson LG, Johansen CC, Biörklund A (1988) CT sialography and conventional sialog-

raphy in the evaluation of parotid gland neoplasm. J Laryngol Otol 102:163–168

10. Hart H, Beimert U, Vogl T (1989) Vestibularer Schwindel als Initialsymptom eines Parotisrezidivtumors. HNO-Information 1:S 94

11. Holliday RA, Cohen WP, Schinella RA, Rothstein SG, Pursky MS, Jacobs JM, Som PM (1988) Benign lymphoepithelial parotid cysts and hyperplasic cervical adenopathy in AIDS risk patients. A new CT appearance. Radiology 168:439–441

12. Mancuso AA, Hanafee WN (1985) Computed tomography and magnetic resonance imaging of the head and neck, 2nd edn. Williams and Wilkins, Baltimore

13. Mann W, Wachter W (1988) Ultraschalldiagnostik der Speicheldrüsen. Laryngol Rhinol Otol (Stuttg) 67:S 192–201

14. Schäfer SB, Maravilla KR, Close LG, Burms DK, Merkel MA, Richards AS (1985) Evaluation of NMR versus CT for parotid masses: a preliminary report. Laryngoscope 95:945–950

15. Smith FW, Deans HE, McLay KA, Rayner CW (1988) Magnetic resonance imaging of the parotid glands using inversion-recovery sequences at 0.08 Tesla. Br J Radiol 61:480–491

16. Som PM, Braun JF, Shapiro MD, Reed DL, Curtin HD, Zimmermann RA (1987) Tumors of the parapharyngeal space and upper neck. Radiology 164:823

17. Som PM, Shugar JMA, Sacher M, Stallmann AL, Biller HF (1988) Benign and malignant parotid pleomorphic adenomas: CT and MR studies. Comput Assist Tomogr 12:65–69

18. Teresi LM, Lufkin RB, Warthan DG, Abemayor E, Hanafee WN (1987) Parotid masses: MR imaging. Radiology 163:405–409

19. Vogl T, Dresel S, Kang K, Grevers G, Riederer A, Späth M, Lissner J (1989) Kernspintomographie der Glandula parotis: Nativdiagnostik und Gd-DTPA. Digitale Bilddiagn 5:59–68

20. Vogl T, Dresel S, Späth M, Grevers G, Wilimzig C, Schedel H, Lissner J (1990) MR imaging of the parotid gland: plain and Gd-DTPA enhanced studies. Radiology 177:667–674

# 10 Oral Cavity and Oropharynx

## 10.1 Clinical Findings

The entrance to the *oral cavity* is formed by the lips. The upper lip features the philtrum in the midline. The corners of the lips are called the commissures.

In the oral cavity, the slit-like oral vestibule is bordered by the lips, the cheeks, the teeth, and the alveolus. Within the oral vestibule, the upper and lower labial frenula run from the lips to the alveolus. The cheeks are bordered anteriorly by the labial commissures, posteriorly by the ascending ramus of the mandible, and inferiorly and superiorly by the lower and upper vestibular sulci. The palate is divided into the posterior soft palate, with the uvula in the middle of the free posterior border, and the anterior bony hard palate. The fibrous aponeurosis of the soft palate is formed by the tensor palatini, levator palatini, palatoglossus, and palatopharyngeus muscles. The lingual frenulum divides the floor of the mouth into two sides, each containing the duct of the submandibular gland and the sublingual fold, which overlies the sublingual gland. The dorsal surface of the tongue is covered with the various papillae, while the ventral surface is coated by a smooth mucous membrane.

The bones relating to the oral cavity are the maxilla, the mandible, the palatine bone, and the zygomatic bone. The maxilla consists of a body and four processes, the frontal, palatine, zygomatic, and alveolar. The first three of these processes come into contact with the bones of the same names, while the alveolar process forms the foundation for the maxillary teeth. The maxilla contains the maxillary sinus. The two maxillae meet at the intermaxillary suture. The mandible consists of a horizontal body and two vertical rami. At the upper rim of the rami are anteriorly the coronoid process and posteriorly the condylar process. The latter articulates with the glenoid fossa of the temporal bone to form the temporomandibular joint. On the medial side of the rami the inferior dental foramen opens into the inferior dental canal, which ends at the mental foramen after running through the body of the mandible. The alveolar margin lies at the upper border of the mandible and contains the sockets for the roots of the mandibular teeth. In the midline the lower portion of the mandible forms the mental protuberance or chin. The palatine bones with their horizontal plates form the posterior part of the bony palate and articulate with the palatal process of the maxilla. The zygomatic bone consists of maxillary, frontal, and temporal processes.

The temporal, masseter, lateral pterygoid, and medial pterygoid muscles are the muscles of mastication. The temporal muscle arises from the lateral aspect of the skull up to the inferior temporal line and inserts on the coronoid process of the mandible. The masseter muscle arises from the zygomatic arch and inserts into the mandibular ramus. The inferior head of the lateral pterygoid muscle arises from the lateral pterygoid plate and the superior head from the greater wing of the sphenoid. The anterior head of the medial pterygoid muscle arises from the palatine bone and the posterior head from the lateral pterygoid plate; they both insert into the pterygoid tuberosity of the mandible. The muscles of the tongue can be divided into intrinsic and extrinsic muscles. The muscle fibers of the intrinsic muscles can be separated into transverse, longitudinal, and vertical groups. The extrinsic muscles of the tongue consist of the genioglossus, hyoglossus, styloglossus, and palatoglossus muscles.

The *oropharynx* extends between the soft palate and the epiglottis, including the tonsillar sinuses with the palatine tonsils. It is bordered anteriorly by the posterior third of the tongue and posteriorly by the midline wall of the pharyngeal constrictor muscles. The anterior border is marked by the V-shaped terminal sulcus of the tongue, which represents the position of the circumvallate papillae anteriorly. Another landmark is the foramen cecum at the apex of the terminal sulcus. This is the point from which the thyroid gland starts migrating down during development. At the posterior part of the tongue lie the lingual valleculae, two small fossae between the median glossoepiglottic fold and the paired lateral glossoepiglottic folds. The median glossoepiglottic fold runs between the base of the tongue and the top of the epiglottis, while the lateral glossoepiglottic folds extend between the lateral surface of the tongue and the lateral and inferior margins of the epiglottis. On the posterior third of the tongue are found raised, circular papilliform masses, the lingual tonsils, with a single opening at each side. The sinus of the palatine tonsil is formed by the middle constrictor muscle in the lateral pharyngeal wall and completed anteriorly by the palatoglossal fold and posteriorly by the palatopharyngeal fold, which are formed by the underlying palatoglossus and palatopharyngeus muscles. Superiorly the palatine tonsil is adjacent to the soft palate and inferiorly it extends to the inferior limit of the middle constrictor muscle. Between the eustachian tube and the base of the tongue the pharyngeal mucosa is filled with lymphatic tissue, including lymphatic nodules. This lymphatic tissue, including the palatine, lingual, pharyngeal, and tubal tonsils, is named Waldeyer's lymphatic ring, and represents the first line of immunologic defense.

In the pathology of the oropharynx and oral cavity one basically has to distinguish between inflammatory and tumorous lesions. The most common anatomic structure to be affeced in this region is the palatine tonsil. A wide variety of viral and bacterial pathogens can cause acute tonsillitis, and the severity of the disease depends on the virulence of the infecting organism and on the resistance of the patient. In some cases, suppurative infections of the tonsils can be complicated, thus resulting in a peritonsillar abscess. This infection penetrates the tonsillar capsule and extents into the connective tissue space between the capsule and the posterior wall of the tonsillar sinus. It can cause severe, life-threatening complications if it penetrates the constrictor muscle to reach the adjacent parapharyngeal space, which contains the carotid sheath.

Cancer of the oral cavity and oropharynx is rather uncommon. Nevertheless, the incidence of tumors of the upper aerodigestive tract is increasing steadily. Alcohol and tobacco abuse are blamed for this increase and are thought to explain the change of the male to female ratio from 10:1 to 4:1. The most common benign tumor of the oropharynx and oral cavity is simple papilloma. This lesion may be single or multiple and usually does not cause any symptoms. Even though these tumors rarely cause irritation and are mainly discovered incidentally, excision should be at least considered, because cases of malignant transformation have been reported. Other benign lesions are mucous retention cysts and minor salivary gland tumors. In addition, tumors of mesenchymal origin such as lipomas, fibromas, neuromas, and hemangiomas may occur in this region.

The most common malignant tumor of the oral cavity and oropharynx is squamous cell carcinoma. The majority of these carcinomas arise in the tonsillar sinus. Deep extension may result in fixation to or erosion of the mandible as well as infiltration of the pterygoid musculature. Infiltration of the parapharyngeal space can also cause loss of function of the caudal cranial nerves. Other relatively common sites of cancer growth within the oropharynx and oral cavity are the tongue, the base of the tongue, the vallecula, the palatine arch, the pharyngeal wall, the anterior floor of the mouth, and the gingiva.

Other malignancies that have been described include adenoid-cystic carcinomas, mucoepidermoid carcinomas, adenocarcinomas, and malignant pleomorphic adenomas, as well as

Hodgkin's and non-Hodgkin's lymphomas and, occasionally, sarcomas.

*Diagnostic Procedures.* Patients with diseases of the oral cavity and oropharynx will be examined by either direct inspection or endoscopy. If a lesion is suspicious of a malignant process, a biopsy specimen will be taken; in addition, the upper airway and the upper digestive tract (direct laryngoscopy, tracheoscopy, bronchoscopy, and esophagoscopy) must be inspected to exclude multiple carcinomas. The risk of multiple primary cancer is generally increased in patients with malignant tumors of the upper aerodigestive tract. Additionally, as in the management of all malignant tumors of the head and neck, the patient must be palpated for cervical lymph nodes. Sometimes ultrasound examination can be helpful in the detection of impalpable cervical lymph nodes.

*Demands on the Radiologist.* In the oral cavity and oropharynx the use of imaging should be restricted mainly to tumors. Radiologic evaluation may also be necessary in occasional cases of complicated parapharyngeal abscess when concomitant inflammation of the parapharyngeal space is suspected, in order to exclude inflammatory spread to the parapharyngeal space and the carotid sheath.

The tumor margins as well as the grade of infiltration affect the treatment of malignancies of the oropharynx and oral cavity. In tumors of the anterior floor of the mouth or the tonsils, infiltration of the mandible is an important point; in the tongue, it is important to know whether the tumor has crossed the midline. In oropharyngeal cancer (tonsillar carcinoma) the extension of the tumor towards the tongue, the mandible, and the parapharyngeal space influences the therapeutic approach.

In tumors of the base of the tongue and the vallecula, too, the grade of infiltration determines whether surgical intervention is still appropriate. If surgery seems to be reasonable, the extent of the procedure will depend on the size of the lesion and on the depth of infiltration.

## 10.2 Examination Technique

Images are acquired using SE pulse sequences on a 1.0 T and 1.5 T superconducting magnet. One of two different receiver coils is used, depending on the site of the tumor. A specially designed pharnyx and neck surface receiver coil, individually adapted to the patient's anatomy, is used for lesions of the base of the tongue and the vallecula. For the body of the tongue and the tonsil area with the parapharyngeal space, the head coil covers the region of interest optimally. Also depending on the location of the process, either sagittal or coronal images are obtained. Sagittal images are preferred for lesions of the tongue base and the vallecula, whereas for examinations with the head coil, coronal images are better for demonstrating tumors. Axial scans are mandatory for every examination of the oropharyngeal area. After a short sagittal sequence for craniocaudal orientation, axial images with long (3000/25, 90) and short (500/17) repetition times must be obtained. Next, the paramagnetic contrast medium Gd-DTPA should be administered, followed by another T1-weighted sequence with the same parameters. The dosage of the contrast medium is 0.1 mmol/l, corresponding to 0.2 ml/kg body weight. The examination concludes with a last T1-weighted sequence in the second plane. In all planes the slices are 5 mm thick with no gaps. In extremely large lesions, slice thickness can be increased to 8 mm.

Subtraction of pre- from post-Gd-DTPA images proves very helpful in some cases.

## 10.3 Topographic Relations

Detailed knowledge of the intricate anatomy of the oral cavity and oropharynx is necessary (Table 10.1).

Topographically, this area is divided into the oral cavity with the body of the tongue, the tonsillar region with the parapharyngeal space, and the floor of the mouth with the valleculae epiglotticae.

The oral cavity and the body of the tongue are delineated cranially by the hard and the soft palate and caudally by an imaginary horizontal line extending back from the tongue (Fig. 10.1). The tonsils and the parapharyngeal space occupy the lateral borders of the oral cavity. Tumors often spread beyond the area of the tonsils because the soft tissue between the oral cavity and the skull base offers no resistance. The oropharyngeal space posterior to the tongue constitutes the third topographic area, delineated anteriorly by the floor of the mouth with the mylohyoid and geniohyoid muscles and caudally by the glossoepiglottic folds including the valleculae.

**Table 10.1.** Checklist: oral cavity oropharynx

| Oral cavity | Normal | Abnormal | Oropharynx | Normal | Abnormal |
|---|---|---|---|---|---|
| Mucosa | | | Mucosa | | |
| Lymphatic tissue | | | Lymphatic tissue | | |
| | | | Palatine tonsil | | |
| *Extrinsic tongue muscles* | | | Epiglottis | | |
| | | | Pharyngobasilar fascia | | |
| Genioglossus muscle | | | Digastric muscle | | |
| Hyoglossus muscle | | | Prevertebral muscles | | |
| Styloglossus muscle | | | retropharyngeal lymph | | |
| Mylohyoid muscle | | | nodes | | |
| Geniohyoid muscle | | | Preepialottic space | | |
| | | | Parapharyngeal space | | |
| *Intrinsic tongue muscles* | | | Palate | | |
| | | | Internal carotid artery | | |
| Palate, uvula | | | External carotid artery | | |
| Lingual septum | | | Jugular vein | | |
| Sublingual gland | | | | | |
| Submandibular gland | | | | | |
| Mandible, maxilla | | | | | |
| Lingual artery, vein | | | | | |
| Submandibular lymph nodes | | | | | |
| Submental lymph nodes | | | | | |

▷

**Fig. 10.1 a–f.** Normal topography of the oral cavity and oropharynx

**a** Plain axial MRI (SE, 1600/70). Exact delineation of the floor of the mouth, the tongue base muscles, the tonsils, and the parapharyngeal space. *1*, Genioglossus muscle; *2*, stylohyoglossus muscle; *3*, mylohyoid muscle; *4*, sternocleidomastoid muscle; *5*, parotid gland

**b** Plain median sagittal MRI (SE, 500/17). The anatomic relations of the intrinsic tongue base muscles (*1*), epiglottis (*arrow*), oropharynx (*2*), nasopharynx (*3*), and uvula (*4*)

**c** Plain coronal MRI (SE, 500/17) See diagram in **f**: *a*, superior surface of tongue; *b*, piriform recess; *c*, vocal fold; *d*, infraglottic cavity; *e*, masseter muscle; *f*, facial artery, vein; *g*, thyroid cartilage; *h*, cricoid cartilage

**d** Topographic relations of the oropharynx in the coronal plane. *1*, Soft palate; *2*, tongue base; *3*, epiglottis; *4*, vallecula; *5*, lateral fold; *6*, thyroid artery; *7*, tonsillar gland; *8*, lateral fold; *9*, lymphoid tissue; *10*, thyroid vein; *11*, small vessels

**e** Plain coronal MRI (SE, 500/17). Demonstration of the anterior part of the digastric muscle (*1*), the geniohyoid muscle (*2*), the oral cavity (*3*), the turbinates (*4*), and the lingual septum (*arrow*)

**f** Diagram of the topography of the oral cavity and oropharynx in the coronal plane (see **c**)

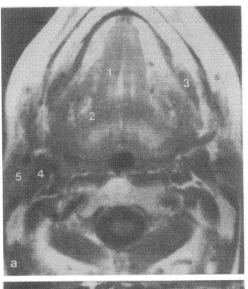

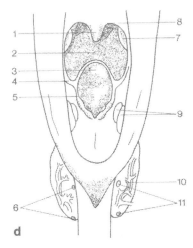

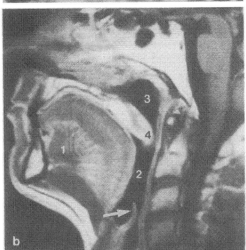

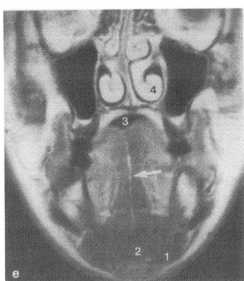

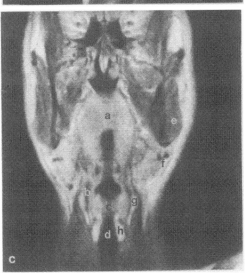

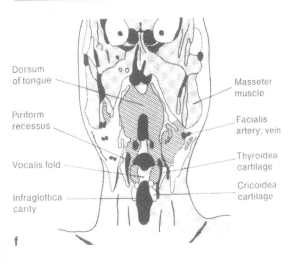

Dorsum of tongue

Piriform recessus

Vocalis fold

Infraglottica carity

Masseter muscle

Facialis artery; vein

Thyroidea cartilage

Cricoidea cartilage

**Table 10.2.** The value of different MRI sequences for representing anatomic details

|  | T1 weighted, plain | T2 weighted | T1 weighted Gd-DTPA |
|---|---|---|---|
| Mandible | 2 | 2 | 2 |
| Genioglossus muscle | 2 | 1 | 2 |
| Hyoglossus, styloglossus muscles | 2 | 1 | 2 |
| Mylohyoid muscle | 1 | 2 | 3 |
| Geniohyoid muscle | 1 | 2 | 3 |
| Pterygoid muscle, medial/lateral | 2 | 2 | 3 |
| Masseter muscle | 2 | 2 | 3 |
| Lingual artery branches | 2 | 2 | 3 |
| Palatine tonsil | 2 | 2 | 3 |
| Soft palate | 2 | 2 | 3 |
| Hard palate | 2 | 1 | 2 |

Grading of visualization: 1, satisfactory; 2, good; 3, optimal.

The posterior border of the whole oropharynx is represented by the constrictor muscle of the pharynx with its superior, medial and inferior parts. All muscles are visualized with intermediate signal intensity on MRI; however, the surrounding fatty and connective tissue can serve to distinguish single muscles or parts of muscles. The complete pharyngeal cavity is coated by mucosa, which shows a characteristic high enhancement in T1-weighted sequences after administration of contrast medium. The tonsils consist of lymphatic tissue and therefore can easily be discerned on plain T2-weighted images. Due to the flow phenomenon, blood vessels are of low signal intensity, so that branches of the lingual artery can be identified in the body of the tongue.

Osseous structures containing medullary tissue, such as the mandible and the hard palate, are visualized as areas of high signal intensity surrounded by the low signal of the cortex.

The tongue consists of nine pairs of intrinsic muscles with intermediate signal intensity. After administration of Gd-DTPA the intrinsic muscles show significant enhancement, whereas the extrinsic muscles, such as the mylohyoid, geniohyoid, and digastric muscles, take up contrast medium only modestly (Table 10.2).

## 10.4 Squamous Cell Carcinoma

### 10.4.1 Tumor Classification (modified from [1])

TX  Primary tumor can not be assessed

T0  No evidence of primary tumor

Tis  Carcinoma in situ

T1  Tumor 2 cm or less in greatest dimension

T2  Tumor more than 2 cm but not more than 4 cm in greatest dimension

T3  Tumor more than 4 cm in greatest dimension

T4  Tumor more than 4 cm in greatest dimension with extension to bone, muscle, skin, antrum, or neck (not root of tongue)

NX  Regional lymph nodes cannot be assessed

N0  No regional lymph node metastasis

N1  Metastasis in a single ipsilateral lymph node, 3 cm or less in greatest dimension

N2a Metastasis in a single ipsilateral lymph node, more than 3 cm but not more than 6 cm in greatest dimension

N2b Metastasis in multiple ipsilateral lymph nodes, none more than 6 cm in greatest dimension

N2c Metastasis in bilateral or contralateral lymph nodes, none more than 6 cm in greatest dimension

N3  Metastasis in a lymph node more than 6 cm in greatest dimension

### 10.4.2 Tonsils and Parapharyngeal Space

Carcinomas of the tonsils and parapharyngeal space usually grow initially along nerve and vessel sheaths and muscle bundles. The most frequent site is the anterior part of the tonsils, followed by the posterior part of the tonsils with the posterior wall of the pharynx. These tumors infiltrate cranially the soft palate, caudally the lateral wall of the pharynx and the tongue base, and laterally the parapharyngeal space and the mandible.

Infiltration of the parapharyngeal space and of the body of the tongue are evident in more than 70% of small mucosal tumors (T2). In more extensive lesions, infiltration of the longus colli muscles and displacement of the pharynx are visible. T1 tumors and superficial lesions are very difficult to detect on MRI. Tumors of stages T2–T4 can be diagnosed correctly with adequate examination quality. Axial and coronal images are necessary for exact documentation of the craniocaudal and lateral extent of the lesion.

In T1-weighted sequences squamous cell carcinomas appear iso- or hypointense to the extrinsic muscles. Due to the destruction of the internal patterns of the intrinsic muscles infiltrations are already evident on plain images. On T2-weighted images the signal intensity of the lesion is higher than that of muscle.

After administration of Gd-DTPA there is significant enhancement of the signal intensity of the carcinoma (150%) compared to the intrinsic tongue muscles. In most cases the delineation of tumors is improved by using Gd-

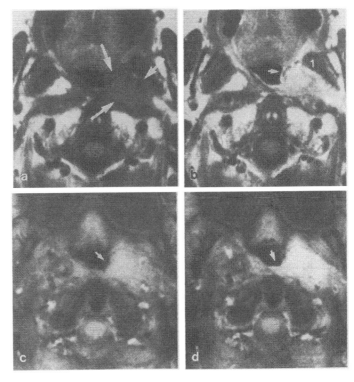

**Fig. 10.2 a–d.** Tonsil carcinoma, stage T3, N1

**a** Plain axial MRI (SE, 500/30). An area of lower signal intensity is seen in the left tonsil region (*arrows*)
**b** Axial MRI (SE, 500/30) with Gd-DTPA. Medium enhancement of the lesion and the infiltrations after Gd-DTPA administration. Exact delineation of the medial pterygoid muscle (*1*)
**c** Plain axial MRI (FLASH, 30/12, flip angle 40°)
**d** Axial MRI (FLASH, 30/12, flip angle 40°) with Gd-DTPA. Using the fast imaging technique the infiltration is demonstrated, particularly in the nerve-vessel sheath (*arrow*)

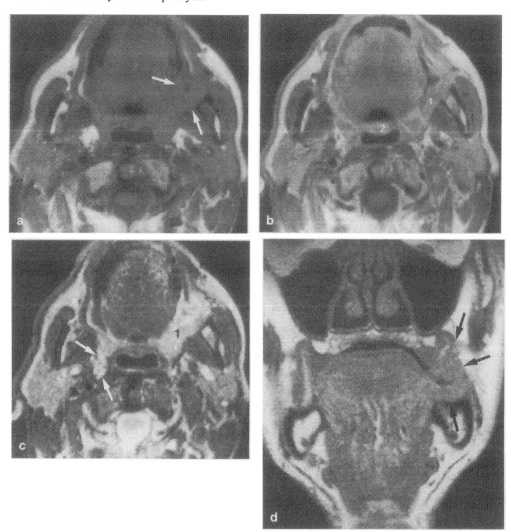

**Fig. 10.3a–d.** Squamous cell carcinoma of the buccal mucosa with infiltration of the mandible, stage T4

**a** Plain axial MRI (SE, 500/25). Homogeneous lesion (*arrows*) in the left cheek, no exact delineation possible

**b** Axial MRI (SE, 500/25) with Gd-DTPA. Low contrast medium enhancement (*1*) without significant diagnostic information. Infiltration of the mandible on the left, the dorsal tongue, and the soft palate (*2*)

**c** Plain axial MRI (SE, 3000/90). The lesion appears with high signal intensity in the T2-weighted image (*1*), with exact delineation of surrounding muscle tissue. The mandible is not seen to be infiltrated in this sequence, and the pharyngeal mucosa appears intact. The facial soft tissues on the left are infiltrated (*arrows*)

**d** Coronal MRI (SE, 500/25) with Gd-DTPA. In the coronal image, the relationship of the tumor (*arrows*) to muscles and tongue is demonstrated

**Table 10.3.** The value of different MRI sequences in the diagnosis of squamous cell carcinoma

|  | T1 weighted, plain | T1 weighted Gd-DTPA | T2 weighted, plain |
|---|---|---|---|
| Tonsils and oropharynx |  |  |  |
| >1.5 cm | 2 | 3 | 3 |
| <1.5 cm | 1 | 3 | 2 |
| Oral cavity/body of tongue |  |  |  |
| >1.5 cm | 2 | 3 | 2 |
| <1.5 cm | 1 | 3 | 2 |
| Base of tongue |  |  |  |
| >1.5 cm | 2 | 3 | 3 |
| <1.5 cm | 1 | 3 | 2 |

Grading of visualization: 1, satisfactory; 2, good; 3, optimal.

DTPA (Fig. 10.2, Table 10.3). Diagnostically important is the differentiation of lymphatic tissue of the tonsils and the tongue base from a tumor infiltration. Symmetrical homogeneity and the typical location are essential identifying features of hyperplastic lymphatic tissue.

### 10.4.3 Oral Cavity and Body of Tongue

Squamous cell carcinomas of the tongue usually start causing clinical symptoms in stage T2. Their growth is of a very destructive and infiltrative kind, so they tend to show a necrotic inner structure. Exact visualization of infiltration is impossible using only plain T1- and T2-weighted sequences, but after administration of Gd-DTPA the enhancement even of small infiltrations enables clear delineation from normal muscle. In particular, the contrast agent yields an immense improvement in the diagnostic value of MRI for tumors of a lower stage (T2). However, tumors at the mucosal level staged T1 can not be diagnosed with sufficient confidence by means of MRI. Tumors of stage T3 and T4 show only a slight displacement of normal anatomic structures due to the infiltrative character of the tumors

(Figs. 10.3, 10.4). Nevertheless, osseous structures of the mandible and the hyoid bone are eroded at an advanced stage.

The best diagnostic results have been obtained using axial and coronal T1-weighted sequences. Gd-DTPA is indispenable for exact tumor staging in this area. Additional subtraction images before and after administration of contrast medium are very helpful in case of doubt. In T1- and T2-weighted sequences the tumor had a higher signal intensity than the muscles of the tongue. However, only in the case of questionable malignancy of cystic and inflammatory lesions do T2-weighted sequences add relevant information; generally such sequences are not necessary. Lesions of the tongue are examined using the head coil. Although other authors have achieved good results with a surface receiver coil, a head coil is of great advantage in assessing infiltration of the posterior pharyngeal wall or extension into the cranial nasopharynx.

### 10.4.3.1 Characteristic Tumor Growth

*Stage T1.* It is still more or less impossible to diagnose tumors of stage T1 in the body of the tongue. There are no characteristic symptoms, and not even the imaging techniques with the highest resolution and best soft tissue contrast are able to demonstrate tumorous infiltration of that size with sufficient reliability. Only if the tumor is macroscopically visible at the back or the side of the tongue is a clinical diagnosis possible.

*Stage T2.* Tumors staged T2 require the complete range of diagnostic MR techniques. Usually, Gd-DTPA-enhanced T1-weighted sequences allow clear definition of tumorous masses infiltrating the muscles of the tongue. The subtraction technique demonstrates subtle infiltrations. The tumors are between 2 and 4 cm in diameter, infiltrating intrinsic and extrinsic muscles of the tongue. Clinical symptoms include swallowing difficulties and sometimes asymmetric displacement or narrowing of the pharyngeal cavity.

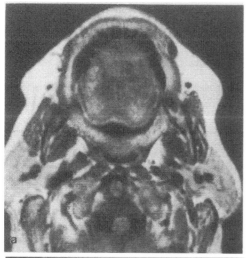

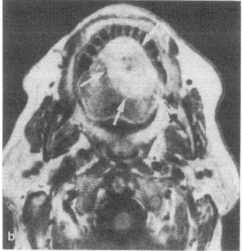

**Fig. 10.4a, b.** Carcinoma of the tongue (stage T3) crossing the midline
**a** Plain axial MRI (SE, 500/30). Inhomogeneous appearance of the tongue muscles. No evidence of tumor growth
**b** Axial MRI (SE, 500/30) with Gd-DTPA. Marked enhancement in the area of tumorous infiltration *(arrows)*. Crossing of the midline is documented. Centrally necrotic parts of the tumor are visible

*Stage T3.* A tumor staged T3 is one over 4 cm in diameter that has not infiltrated structures beyond the tongue. In contrast-enhanced T1-weighted images, inhomogeneous enhancement pointing to a necrotic inner structure is quite common. Additional coronal images are very helpful in demonstrating the craniocaudal extent of the lesion. The mobility of the tongue is impaired because most of the intrinsic muscles are affected by the tumor, so swallowing difficulties are characteristic.

*Stage T4.* A tumor classified T4 has infiltrated structures beyond the oropharynx and the oral cavity. In tumors originating from the body of the tongue, the mandible, the hyoid bone, and the epiglottic and supraglottic laryngeal structures, such as the thyroid cartilage, are likely to be involved. The tumors mostly show a necrotic inner structure best visualized in contrast-enhanced T1-weighted sequences. The image quality of T2-weighted sequences is impaired by motion artifacts, because the patients suffer from dyspnea and pain during swallowing.

### 10.4.4 Vallecula and Base of Tongue

Squamous cell carcinomas of the vallecula show primary infiltration of the floor of the mouth (Fig. 10.5). Tumors of higher stage extend into the epiglottis, the supraglottic larynx, and the intrinsic muscles of the tongue (Fig. 10.6). A characteristic sign of low staged tumors in this area is the displacement of normal structures, causing evident asymmetry on MRI. The tumors are relatively large by the time they infiltrate surrounding structures. An important differential diagnosis of lesions in the vallecula is lymphatic hyperplasia (Fig. 10.7).
The longer T2 relaxation times of lymphatic tissue with similar signal intensity on T1-weighted images allow fairly reliable differentiation between tumor and lymphatic tissue. Both structures take up contrast medium equally, but lymphatic tissue shows no inhomogeneity of inner structure and no signs of infiltration. The contrast enhancement after

administration of Gd-DTPA reaches 100%, causing intermediate T1 and increased T2 relaxation times. The combination of T1-weighted sequences with Gd-DTPA and plain T2-weighted sequences is obligatory for examinations in this area. Axial slices are mandatory, and, especially in this topographic region, images in the sagittal plane prove very helpful. These images visualize the anterior-caudal to posterior-cranial extent of the epiglottis to best advantage, yielding information concerning infiltration of the epiglottis.

### 10.4.4.1 Characteristic Tumor Growth

*Stage T1.* Small tumors of the vallecula are a severe problem both for the clinician and for the radiologist. Due to the intricate anatomy tumors often "hide" in the mucosa between the glossoepiglottic folds or at the posterior-caudal part of the tongue. The resolution and the S/N of imaging techniques are not yet sufficient to discover such small tumors reliably. Only the of use Gd-DTPA improves the diagnostic value of MRI significantly, but overall the results of imaging techniques are unsatisfactory for small tumors.

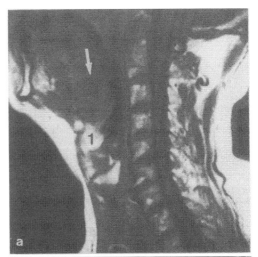

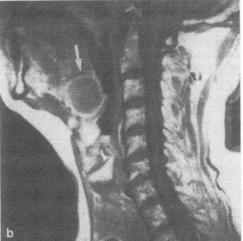

▷

**Fig. 10.5a–c.** Necrotic tongue base carcinoma, stage T3
**a** Plain sagittal MRI (SE, 500/17). Homogeneous lesion of low signal intensity in the tongue base (*arrow*). The preepiglottic fatty tissue appears with high signal intensity (*1*)
**b** Sagittal MRI (SE, 500/17) with Gd-DTPA. Halo-like contrast medium enhancement of the margins, infiltration of the dorsal tongue
**c** Subtraction image (**b** − **a**). The halo-like enhancement is also documented in this image (*arrow*). Displacement of the epiglottis without infiltration

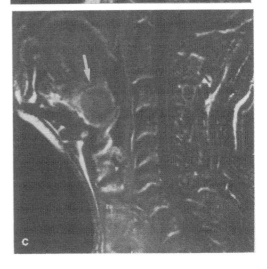

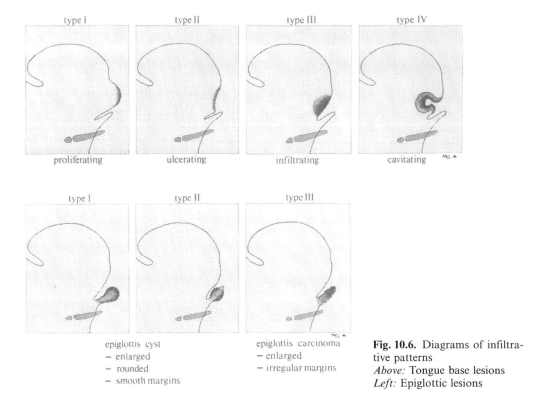

type I    type II    type III    type IV

proliferating    ulcerating    infiltrating    cavitating

type I    type II    type III

epiglottis cyst
– enlarged
– rounded
– smooth margins

epiglottis carcinoma
– enlarged
– irregular margins

**Fig. 10.6.** Diagrams of infiltrative patterns
*Above:* Tongue base lesions
*Left:* Epiglottic lesions

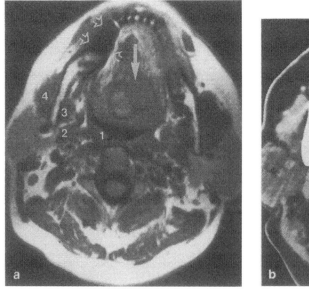

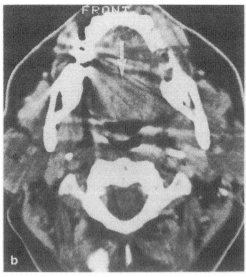

**Fig. 10.7 a, b.** Legend see p. 149

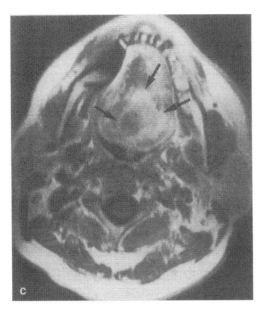

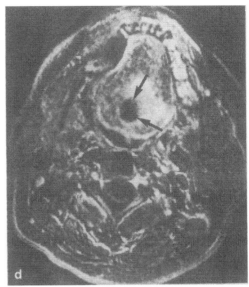

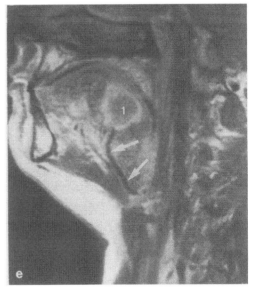

◁ **Fig. 10.7 a–e.** Tongue carcinoma with areas of necrosis

**a** Plain axial MRI (SE, 500/17). Inhomogeneous appearance of the tongue muscle (*solid arrow*). Beam-hardening artifact (*open arrows*). *1*, Longus colli muscle; *2*, medial pterygoid muscle; *3*, lateral pterygoid muscle; *4*, masseter muscle

**b** CT. The beam-hardening artifacts do not permit satisfactory information

**c** Axial MRI (SE, 500/17) with Gd-DTPA. Exact delineation of the lesion and enhancement at the margins (*arrows*). Necrotic internal pattern

**d** Subtraction image (**c** − **a**). Documentation of the enhancement of the lesion with central necrosis (*arrows*)

**e** Plain sagittal MRI (SE, 500/17) Demonstration of the halo-like tumor (*1*) and the supplying lingual artery (*arrows*)

*Stage T2.* Tumors staged T2, between 2 and 4 cm in size, are a clear indication for MRI. Plain T1-weighted images show anatomic details, and contrast enhancement of T1-weighted images optimizes the information by delineating the exact tumor margins. Additional T2-weighted sequences allow the differentiation of inflammatory or edematous tissue. Sagittal slices are important for the visualization of affected intrinsic muscles of the tongue and the epiglottis. The structures usually infiltrated by tumors in this area are the glossoepiglottic folds, the valleculae and the floor of the mouth (Fig. 10.8).

*Stage T3.* Tumors are staged T3 when reaching a diameter of over 4 cm without spreading beyond the oropharynx. Due to the enormous size of the tumor the patients often complain of the feeling of lump in their throat. The tumors show the same characteristic locations, but more and more intrinsic and extrinsic muscles are affected and infiltrated. The tumors show significant contrast medium enhancement in T1-weighted sequences, usually with an inhomogeneous inner structure pointing to central necrosis.

*Stage T4.* A tumor is classified T4 when reaching a diameter of over 4 cm and infiltrating neighboring structures such as the mandible, the soft tissues of the neck, the supraglottic larynx, or even the skin. The normal anatomy of the tongue is almost totally destroyed, and the pharyngeal cavity is narrowed. Clinical symptoms include pain during swallowing or even dyspnea. In these patients the quality of MR images is often reduced because of motion artifacts. If the diagnosis is evident from the first sequence, the further diagnostic procedure can be reduced to a second measurement.

---

MRI with Gd-DTPA is the method of choice for the diagnosis of tumors of stage T2 and above. Different planes and exact analysis of anatomic details, are important, especially in the mandible. If any doubt remains concerning osseous infiltration, additional CT can be very helpful.

---

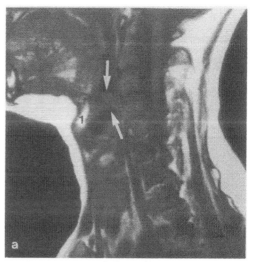

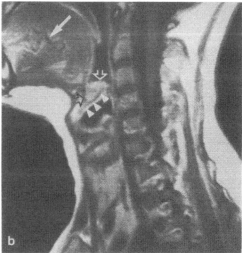

**Fig. 10.8a, b.** Carcinoma of the epiglottis, stage T2, without infiltration of the tongue base or the epiglottic cartilage
**a** Plain sagittal MRI (500/17). Lesion of low signal intensity in the cranial area of the epiglottis (*arrows*) *1*, Preepiglottic fatty tissue
**b** Sagittal MRI (SE, 500/17) with Gd-DTPA. Documentation of the squamous cell carcinoma of the epiglottis. Marked enhancement after Gd-DTPA (*open arrows*). The cartilage of the epiglottis and the tongue base are not infiltrated (*arrowheads*). Demonstration of the lingual artery within the normal tongue muscles (*white arrow*)

## 10.5 Other Lesions

### 10.5.1 Kaposi Sarcoma

Kaposi sarcoma is associated fairly closely with the acquired immune deficiency syndrome (AIDS) [6–8]. These semimalignant tumors demonstrate only a low rate of infiltration; primarily, they displace and narrow the pharyngeal cavity (Fig. 10.9). Characteristic morphologic criteria are the homogeneous inner structure and the smooth margins. The T1 and T2 relaxation times resemble those of squamous cell carcinoma, so certain differentiation based only on the optical impression of the MR image is not possible. The diagnosis is revealed by biopsy combined with serologic HIV antibody tests.

### 10.5.2 Glomus Tumor

A characteristic sign of glomus tumors is an immense increase in signal intensity (up to 250%) after administration of Gd-DTPA. This enhancement is caused by the very rich

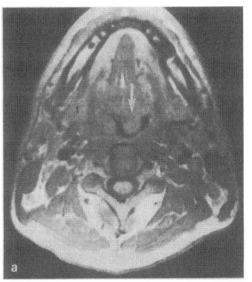

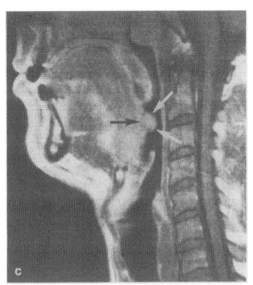

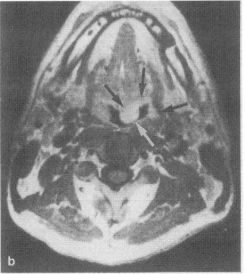

Fig. 10.9 a–c. Kaposi sarcoma in the dorsal third of the tongue in an HIV-positive patient
a Plain axial MRI (SE, 500/17). Tumor (*arrow*) filling the oropharynx. Isointense to tongue muscle and submandibular gland (*1*). No exact delineation possible
b Axial MRI (SE, 500/17) with Gd-DTPA. Medium enhancement of the lesion in the midline, precise differentiation from the tongue muscles (*arrows*). Enhancement is also seen in the mucosa of the pharynx
c Sagittal MRI (SE, 500/17) with Gd-DTPA. Documentation of the lesion without infiltration of tongue muscles (*arrows*). Histologic findings: clearly defined Kaposi sarcoma, resected completely

vascularization of these tumors. The tumors show a typical lobulated outline and preferential growth into the parapharyngeal space. On T1-weighted images they have the same intermediate signal intensity as muscles. However, their high T2, due to the rich vascularization, allows certain differentiation of glomus tumors from the other lesions that arise in the oropharynx.

### 10.5.3 Adenoma

The only common benign lesion of the oropharynx is pleomorphic adenoma, which typically exhibits distinct, regular tumor margins. Adenomas do not tend to infiltrate other structures, but the displacement and asymmetry of normal structures can narrow the pharyngeal cavity. Although the tumor is benign, large specimens show a necrotic inner structure, best seen on T1-weighted images after administration of Gd-DTPA. In plain T1-weighted sequences the tumor is isointense to muscles, whereas in T2-weighted sequences the tumors demonstrate higher signal intensity at the level of the salivary glands. The signal intensity after contrast medium administration increases by a factor of 110%.

### 10.5.4 Metastatic Lymph Nodes

The differentiation of inflammatory or metastatic lymph nodes is still difficult. Lymph nodes can be regarded as pathologic when they reach a diameter of 1.5 cm, when more than three nodes are fixed together, or when a necrotic inner structure is evident. The contrast medium enhancement reaches 100% in T1-weighted images. In T2-weighted images lymph nodes have a high signal intensity, comparable to that of the tonsils or other lymphatic tissue.

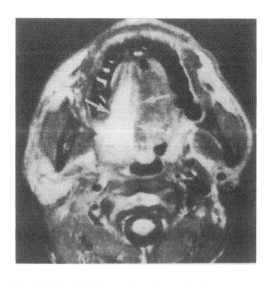

**Fig. 10.10.** Right hypoglossal paresis after trauma. Plain axial MRI (SE,1600/90). Area of high signal intensity in the right half of the tongue. Fatty replacement of tongue muscles. High signal intensity in T1- as well as T2-weighted sequences

### 10.5.5 Paresis of the Hypoglossal Nerve

One of the most important symptoms of tumors in the oropharynx is paresis of the hypoglossal nerve (Fig. 10.10). The typical signs include a strictly unilateral loss of tongue substance in the region of interest. The atrophy of the intrinsic muscle of the tongue gives rise to a prolonged T2 due to the fatty involution. Higher signal intensity of the affected side without contrast medium uptake are the corresponding characteristics in T1-weighted sequences. Thus, tumorous infiltration of the tongue can always be differentiated from hypoglossal paresis.

### 10.5.6 Hemangioma

Hemangiomas are benign lesions that can occur anywhere in the body, and their incidence in the oropharynx is more than negligible. They usually cause no clinical symptoms and are discovered by chance. On MRI hemangiomas can easily be differentiated from all other tumors by their extremely high signal intensity on T2-weighted images.

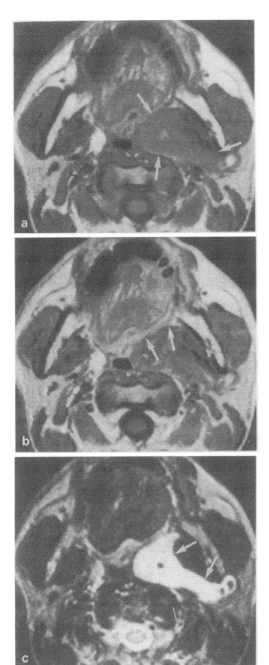

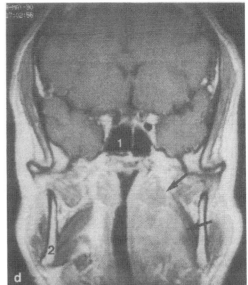

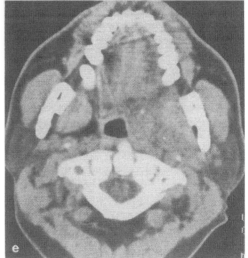

Displacement of tongue muscles ventrally. Good delineation due to the higher enhancement of superficial mucosa (*arrows*)

**c** Plain axial MRI (SE, 3000/90). In the T2-weighted image the lesion appears bright, representing acute bleeding. The pterygoid muscles are delineated laterally (*arrow*)

**d** Coronal MRI (SE, 500/25) with Gd-DTPA. In this plane the bleeding is documented from the naso- to the oropharynx. There is also evidence of bleeding within the pterygoid muscles. *1*, Sphenoid sinus; *2*, mandible

**e** Plain CT. The bleeding is seen in the region of the left parapharyngeal space with the same density as the tongue muscles

**Fig. 10.11 a–e.** Postoperative bleeding in the oropharynx

**a** Plain axial MRI (SE, 500/25). Extensive space-occupying lesion in the parapharyngeal space and tonsil region (*arrows*). Medium signal intensity somewhat resembling that of muscle tissue

**b** Axial MRI (SE, 500/25) with Gd-DTPA. Only low enhancement after Gd-DTPA administration.

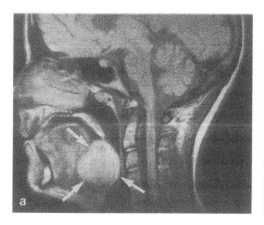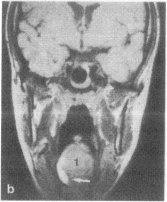

**Fig. 10.12a, b.** Thyroid tissue in the tongue base with a small hemorrhage
**a** Plain sagittal MRI (SE, 500/17). Homogeneous lesion with high signal intensity and distinct margins (*arrows*) in the tongue base. Displacement of surrounding tissues

**b** Plain coronal MRI (SE, 500/17). Documentation of a distinctly bordered lesion (*1*) in the tongue base. The area of higher signal intensity (*arrow*) represents bleeding

### 10.5.7 Plasmocytoma

Metastatic involvement of plasma cells in the oropharynx is extremely rare. On MRI, plasmocytoma appears as a tumor mass of intermediate signal intensity on plain T1-weighted images, with contrast medium enhancement of 100%. However, this appearance is similar to that of squamous cell carcinoma, so the diagnosis is revealed only by clinical biopsy.

### 10.5.8 Others

In rare cases other manifestations, such as bleeding or thyroid tissue, are found in this area (Figs. 10.11, 10.12).

## 10.6 Diagnostic Strategy

MRI is a highly sensitive and specific technique for the diagnosis of lesions in the oropharynx and the oral cavity because of its high soft tissue contrast and the multiplanar views. Although the oropharynx is relatively accessible for the examining clinician, the role of MRI is to define the extension of a tumor

into the surrounding deep soft tissues. Several points have to be clarified: the size and morphology of a tumor within the tongue, transgression of the midline, and infiltration of the tongue base or parapharyngeal space [2–5]. For visualizing normal anatomy, plain T1-weighted MRI is superior to any other imaging technique. The paramagnetic contrast medium Gd-DTPA is extremely valuable for assessment of tumorous involvement, particularly as T2-weighted sequences often lead to false tumor classification.

However, in view of the high costs and the invasivity of the technique, the use of Gd-DTPA must be considered carefully in every single case. Exact delineation of tumors classified T1 is extremely difficult; even after administration of Gd-DTPA these tumors "hide" in the mucosa. In general tumors of higher stages can be visualized at least adequately with the different MR sequences. Optimal results concerning the size and the character of the different lesions can be obtained using the combination of contrast medium, T2-weighted sequences and at least two planes.

In the primary diagnosis of oropharyngeal lesions clinical and endoscopic investigation is still obligatory because small and superficial

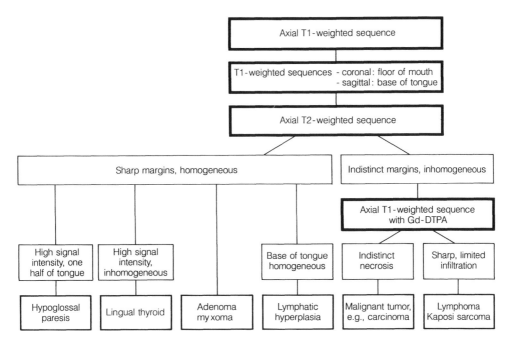

**Fig. 10.13.** Diagnostic strategy: oral cavity and oropharynx

stage T1 tumors can not be diagnosed by imaging techniques. For preoperative staging and assessment of deep infiltration, T1-weighted sequences with Gd-DTPA are of great value. Additional T2-weighted sequences help differentiate inflammatory and edematous reactions to the tumor. Therefore MRI is the method of choice for the diagnosis of high-grade tumors in the oropharynx and combines very well with the primary clinical examinations. The diagnostic strategy is outlined in Fig. 10.13.

---

In the primary diagnosis of oropharyngeal lesions clinical and endoscopic investigation remains mandatory. Preoperative staging and the visualization of deep infiltration can be improved using T1-weighted sequences and Gd-DTPA. T2-weighted sequences are still necessary to delineate inflammatory and edemous reactions to the tumor. MRI is the method of choice for primary diagnosis and for evaluating the efficacy of therapy in the oropharynx.

**References**

1. Hermanek P, Sohin LH (eds) TNM classification of malignant tumours, 4th ed. Springer, Berlin Heidelberg New York
2. Lenz M, Skalej M, Ozdoba C, Bongers H (1989) Kernspintomographie der Mundhöhle, des Oropharynx und des Mundbodens: Vergleich mit der CT. ROFO 150/4:425–433
3. Lufkin RB, Hanafee WN (1988) MRI of the head and neck. Magn Reson Imaging 6:69–88
4. Lufkin RB, Larsson SG, Hanafee WN (1983) Work in progress. NMR anatomy of the larynx and tongue base. Radiology 148:173–175
5. Lufkin RB, Hanafee WN (1985) Comparison of CT and MR of the head and neck. In: Carter BL (ed) Computed tomography of the head and neck. Churchill Livingstone, New York, p 303
6. Riederer A, Müller-Höcker J, Wilmes E, Vogl T (1988) Die aggressive Fibromatose im Kopf-Hals-Bereich. Arch Otorhinolaryngol 7:321
7. Riederer A, Vogl T, Wilmes E (1989) Kernspin-tomographische Befunde bei HIV-Manifestationen im Kopf-Hals-Bereich. Proceedings of 2nd German AIDS Congress, Berlin, p 315
8. Vogl T, Brüning R, Grevers G, Mees M, Bauer M, Lissner J (1988) MR imaging of the oropharynx and tongue: comparison of plain and Gd-DTPA studies. JCAT 12(3):427–433

# 11 Larynx and Hypopharynx

## 11.1 Clinical Findings

Disorders of the *larynx* can cause a variety of different symptoms, depending on the site of origin as well as the underlying disease.

In neonates, laryngeal abnormalities such as tracheomalacia, tracheoesophageal fistula, or branchiogenic cysts are the most common cause of congenital airway obstruction. Another frequent congenital laryngeal abnormality is vocal cord paralysis due to peripheral or central neurologic deficits.

Laryngeal infections are the most common diseases of the larynx, mostly preceded by an upper respiratory tract infection. Hoarseness is a major symptom in patients suffering from a variety of laryngeal diseases as well as laryngeal infection. For the clinician, knowledge of the rapidity of the progression of hoarseness and other associated symptoms, the duration of the infection, and the risk factors (e.g., nicotine abuse) are essential for an adequate diagnostic and therapeutic approach. Normally, an acute infection of the larynx should not last for more than 3–4 weeks. If a hoarseness of unclear origin lasts longer, the otorhinolaryngologist must exclude a malignancy. Tumors of the larynx can be of benign or malignant origin. Laryngeal cysts, e.g., saccular cysts, ductal cysts, and thyroid cartilage foraminal cysts, may range in diameter from a few millimeters to several centimeters. Another important benign lesion is the laryngocele, which has to be differentiated from saccular cyst. The latter does not communicate with the lumen of the larynx and is filled with mucus. Laryngoceles usually occur later in life and can be divided into three subtypes (internal, external, and combined). A laryngocele usually has to be regarded as a benign lesion; however, associations between laryn-goceles and laryngeal carcinomas have been described.

In addition to laryngeal cysts there is a wide variety of other benign tumors of the larynx; neoplasms of epithelial, cartilaginous, neural, glandular, vascular, adipose, muscular, and fibrous origin may be found at this site.

The most common malignant neoplasm of the larynx is squamous cell carcinoma. According to the National Cancer Institute of the United States, cancer of the larynx accounts for almost 1.3% of all new cancer diagnoses and 0.83% of all cancer deaths in that country. Several risk factors for the development of laryngeal cancer have been pointed out, including consumption of tobacco and alcohol, occupational hazards, and exposure to radiation. Carcinomas of the larynx may also develop in patients with a history of laryngeal papilloma. In many cases, laryngeal carcinoma can be detected in an early stage, because, at least in tumors originating at the glottic level, a voice change will be the first symptom. Other potential symptoms include dysphagia, throat pain, referred ear pain, and hemoptysis. Depending on the tumor stage, the prognosis of endolaryngeal cancer is usually better than in other regions of the upper aerodigestive tract.

The treatment of laryngeal cancer depends on the site and the extent of the tumor. Various surgical procedures such as chordectomy, partial or hemilaryngectomy, or even total laryngectomy may be necessary. Radiotherapy can also be useful under certain conditions.

The *hypopharynx* has a close relationship to the larynx and is divided into the postcricoid area, the piriform sinus, and the posterior pharyngeal wall.

Tumors of the hypopharynx occur less frequently than those of the larynx (less than

1/100000 newly diagnosed cancers). Most of the malignant neoplasms are squamous cell carcinomas. Swallowing disorders, throat pain, referred ear pain, and hemoptysis may occur in patients suffering from a hypopharyngeal carcinoma; as these symptoms are not specific they may be overlooked, and sometimes the appearance of a cervical lymph node metastasis will lead to the diagnosis. In many cases, parts of the larynx are already infiltrated by the time the diagnosis of hypopharyngeal cancer is established.

Depending on the site and extent of the tumor, it can be removed by either partial pharyngectomy or combined laryngectomy and partial pharyngectomy. In advanced stages, combined radiochemotherapy can be performed. The long-term prognosis of carcinoma of the hypopharynx, however, remains poor.

*Diagnostic Procedures.* Diseases of the larynx and hypopharynx require thorough physical examination. Mirror and fiberoptic laryngoscopy of these structures is mandatory.

If a tumor of the endolarynx is suspected, the patient must be examined under general anesthesia and a biopsy specimen taken endoscopically. During this procedure the extent of the tumor must be assessed carefully in order to determine the appropriate therapeutic approach. Sometimes binocular microscopy can help to determine the exact superficial borders of the lesion [4, 9].

Thorough palpation of the neck is obligatory for the detection of cervical lymph node metastases, which may be an early symptom of hypopharyngeal cancer or may appear in advanced laryngeal cancer.

*Demands on the Radiologist.* Some tumors of the larynx and/or hypopharynx do not show superficial tumor growth and will not be identified on endoscopy. These tumors tend to grow in the submucosal tissue layers, and biopsy of the suspicious area may not reveal any signs of malignancy. In these cases, neither the size nor the infiltration of the tumor can be ascertained by clinical or endoscopic evaluation alone.

In malignant tumors of supraglottic origin, and particularly in epiglottic cancer, the appropriate therapeutic procedure depends on the infiltration of surrounding structures, i.e., the vallecula and the base of the tongue. Endoscopic evaluation and palpation of this region will not always reveal the degree infiltrative tumor growth.

Although CT is superior to MRI in judging erosion of bone and cartilage it has the major disadvantages that multiplanar views can not be produced without changing the patient's position and that soft tissue contrast is poorer [7, 10, 12]. For these reasons MRI is of higher diagnostic value than CT in most cases.

## 11.2 Examination Technique

For the MR examination a special surface receiver coil, placed adjacent to the larynx, should be used. This coil, of the Helmholtz type, enables examination of the neck from the epiglottis to the supraclavicular region simultaneously without gaps. The examination should be started with a sagittal survey image for craniocaudal orientation followed by an axial T1-weighted sequence (500/17). Next another T1-weighted sequence should be obtained in a second plane depending on the location of the tumor as revealed by laryngoscopy. For hypopharyngeal lesions sagittal images are very helpful, whereas for tumors of the larynx coronal images are preferred. After intravenous administration of Gd-DTPA (0.1 mmol/l per kg body weight), another axial sequence follows. The whole examination lasts 18 min. If the first T1-weighted sequence is free of artifacts, a T2-weighted sequence (3000/25, 90) may be justified instead of using Gd-DTPA, especially if cartilage invasion is suspected. However, in many cases the diagnostic value of T2-weighted images is inferior to that of T1-weighted images with and without contrast medium. To achieve the best possible diagnostic information with respect to the extent and nature of the lesion, both T1-weighted sequences in combination with Gd-DTPA and T2-weighted sequences or images in three planes may be helpful in some cases. However, this enlarged strategy makes sense only when examining patients without dyspnea, otherwise the measurement time is too long for sufficient image quality.

> In most cases T1-weighted sequences with contrast medium are superior to T2-weighted sequences and shorten the examination time.

After measurement, special software allowing subtraction of corresponding T1-weighted images of the same slice before and after Gd-DTPA should be used [14, 15, 16].

## 11.3 Topographic Relations

The normal anatomy of the hypopharynx and the larynx is rather intricate and not easy to keep in mind in detail.

### 11.3.1 Hypopharynx

The hypopharynx extends from the oropharynx cranially to the supraglottic larynx caudally. Its cranial borders are the free margin of the epiglottis in the median line and, laterally, the pharyngoepiglottic folds forming the valleculae epiglotticae. The preepiglottic space lies ventral to the epiglottis and is filled with fatty tissue. The left and right piriform sinuses and the esophagus form the dorsal boundary of the hypopharynx.

### 11.3.2 Larynx

The larynx is subdivided into a supraglottic, a glottic, and a subglottic part. The supraglottic part reaches from the false vocal cords cranially to the true vocal cords caudally. Ventrally it is delineated by the thyroid laminae and the thyroid notch, laterally and dorsally by the aryepiglottic folds. The glottic part of the larynx contains the true cords with the vocal muscles and the laryngeal ventricle. The

ventral and dorsal regions of junction of the true cords are called the anterior and posterior commissures. The cords are moved by the intrinsic (e.g., cricoarytenoid and thyroarytenoid) laryngeal muscles, which are fixed on the arytenoid cartilages, and the extrinsic laryngeal muscles. The arytenoid cartilages are connected caudally with the cricoid cartilage, which forms the passage to the subglottic part of the larynx. The caudal notch of the cricoid cartilage forms the boundary between the larynx and the trachea (Fig. 11.1).

The main function of the larynx is to act as a sphincter rather than as an organ for producing sound. Keeping this in mind facilitates understanding of laryngeal anatomy and physiology. In addition to its role as a sphincter, the larynx is involved in respiratory, deglutition, and phonation.

### 11.3.2.1 Skeletal Structure

Several cartilages (cricoid, thyroid, epiglottic, arytenoid, corniculate, and cuneiform) and a single bone (hyoid) form the skeletal structure of the larynx. Numerous ligaments and folds (e.g., aryepiglottic and glossoepiglottic) attach to this skeleton.

### Cricoid Cartilage

The signet ring-shaped cricoid cartilage lies at the base of the larynx above the first tracheal ring. It is the only complete ring of cartilage encircling the airway. It has a narrow anterior arch and a wider, high posterior lamina. At the junction of the arch and the lamina on each side the cricoid cartilage articulates with the inferior cornu of the thyroid cartilage, forming the synovial cricothyroid joints. This level corresponds to the infraglottic or subglottic region. In older patients the cricoid, arytenoid, and thyroid cartilages have peripheral calcification, which appears as a zone of high density on CT and low signal intensity on MRI. The central area forms a cavity that contains fatty marrow and appears with low density on CT and high signal intensity on MRI.

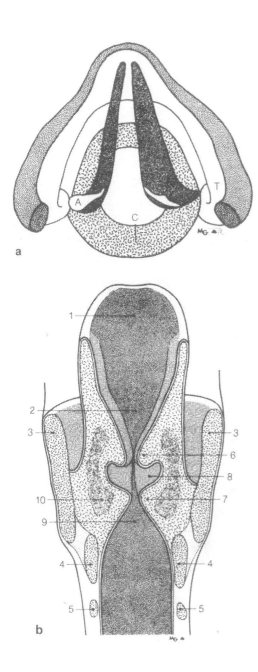

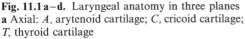

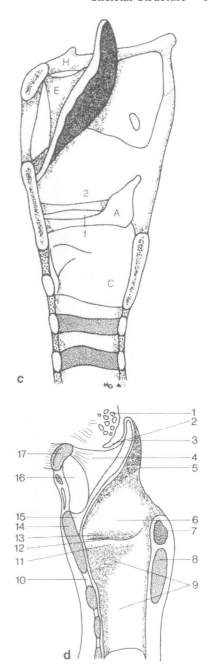

**Fig. 11.1 a–d.** Laryngeal anatomy in three planes
**a** Axial: *A*, arytenoid cartilage; *C*, cricoid cartilage; *T*, thyroid cartilage
**b** Coronal: *1*, Epiglottis; *2*, Supraglottic cavity; *3*, thyroid cartilage; *4*, cricoid cartilage; *5*, first tracheal cartilage; *6*, false vocal cord; *7*, true vocal cord; *8*, laryngeal ventricle; *9*, subglottic cavity; *10*, vocal muscle

**c** Sagittal: *A*, arytenoid cartilage; *C*, cricoid cartilage; *E*, epiglottis; *H*, hyoid bone; *1*, laryngeal ventricle; *2*, supraglottic cavity
**d** *1*, Tongue; *2*, vallecula; *3*, epiglottis; *4*, hyoepiglottic ligament; *5*, constrictor pharyngis muscle; *6*, supraglottic cavity; *7*, arytenoid cartilage; *8*, cricoid cartilage; *9*, subglottic cavity; *10*, cricothyroid ligament; *11*, true cord; *12*, laryngeal ventricle; *13*, false cord; *14*, thyroid cartilage; *15*, epiglottic petiolus; *16*, preepiglottic fat; *17*, hyoid bone

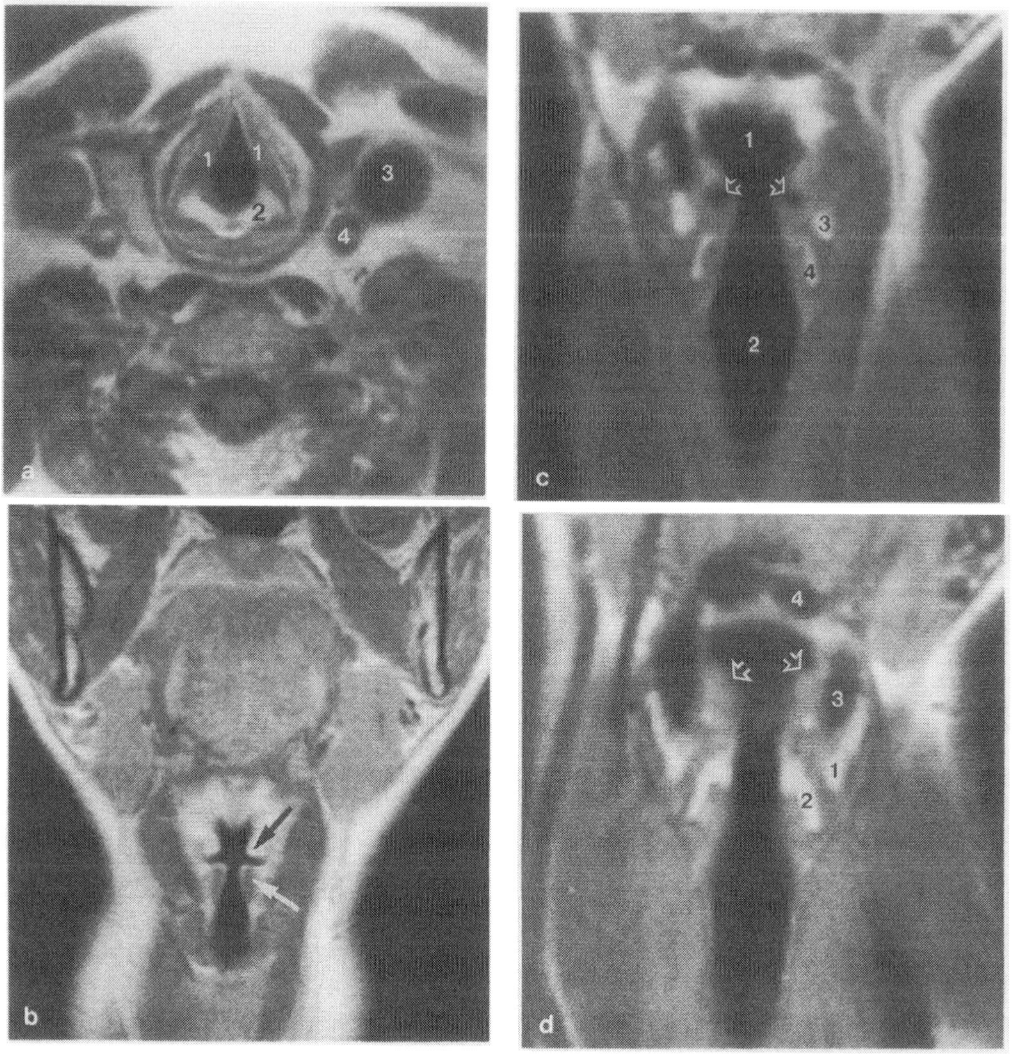

**Fig. 11.2a–d.** Normal topography of the larynx
**a** Plain axial MRI (SE, 500/17). Axial slice at the cricoid level showing the vocal cords (*1*), cricoid cartilage (*2*), internal jugular vein (*3*), and common carotid artery (*4*)
**b** Plain coronal MRI (SE, 500/17). The laryngeal ventricle is delineated by the caudal true vocal cords with low signal intensity (*white arrow*) and the cranial false cords with high signal intensity (*black arrow*)

**c** Plain coronal MRI (SE, 500/17). Visualization of supraglottic space (*1*), subglottic space (*2*), laryngeal ventricle (arrows), thyroid cartilage (*3*), and cricoid cartilage (*4*)
**d** Coronal MRI (SE, 500/17) with Gd-DTPA. Topographic relationship of the thyroid cartilage (*1*), cricoid cartilage (*2*), piriform sinus (*3*), epiglottic valleculae (*4*) and aryepiglottic folds (*arrows*)

In younger patients these cartilages are usually isointense with the surrounding fat. The mucosa of the subglottic larynx is less than 1 mm thick in the normal state. Any increase in thickness to more than 1 mm is abnormal and may represent subglottic extension of pathology. At the level of the highest portion of the posterior cricoid lamina, the true vocal cords constitute the glottis.

### Thyroid Cartilage

The shield-shaped thyroid cartilage is located above the cricoid cartilage and is attached anteriorly by the cricothyroid membrane. The midline fusion of two laminae gives the thyroid cartilage its characteristic appearance. It is the largest laryngeal cartilage and shields the vocal cords, which are attached to it at the anterior commissure. One centimeter above the anterior commissure is the thyroid notch, a narrow space between the laminae. Bilateral processes of the thyroid cartilage, known as the inferior cornua, extend downward to the level of the cricoid. Each thyroid lamina also has a superior cornu, which often extends to the level of the wings of the hyoid bone (Fig. 11.1 c).

### Hyoid Bone

The tripartite hyoid bone, consisting of a central body with two wings, is fixed caudally by the thyrohyoid membrane to the thyroid cartilage and is suspended cranially from the mandible and styloid process by the suprahyoid muscles. In patients of all ages, the cortex of the hyoid bone appears on MRI as an area of low signal surrounding a higher signal intensity marrow space.

### Epiglottis

The epiglottis consists of a elastic cartilage, pitted on the posterior aspect, that rarely calcifies and, on T1- and T2-weighted MRI, shows a signal intensity similar to fat. The epiglottis lies posterior to the thyroid cartilage and the hyoid bone. At its inferior tip (petiole) the epiglottis is connected to the thyroid cartilage by the thyroepiglottic ligament. The hyoepiglottic ligament links the body of the epiglottis to the hyoid bone and can be seen on MRI as a low-intensity structure dividing the high-intensity fat in the preepiglottic space. The free margin of the epiglottis lies above the hyoid bone and posterior to the valleculae. Here it is attached to the lateral hypopharynx and the tongue base by the paired pharyngoepiglottic folds and a single median glossoepiglottic fold respectively. The valleculae are paired air spaces anterior to the epiglottis, separated by the median glossoepiglottic fold (Fig. 11.1 b).

### Arytenoid, Corniculate, and Cuneiform Cartilages

The paired pyramid-shaped arytenoid cartilages rest on the posterior cricoid lamina. During respiration the arytenoids move laterally, closely approximating the thyroid laminae. During phonation they glide supramedially and rotate to adduct the vocal cords. An axial MR scan at the glottic level will visualize the arytenoids, the posterior lamina of the cricoid, and, of course, the true vocal cords. A scan through the superior processes of the arytenoids is at the level of the false vocal cords. At the apex of the arytenoids are the nodular paired corniculate cartilages. The paired cuneiform cartilages lie in the aryepiglottic folds (Fig. 11.1 a) slightly superior and anterior to the corniculate cartilages. The corniculate and cuneiform cartilages are not usually resolved with current MR imaging techniques.

### 11.3.2.2 Soft Tissues

MRI excels in delineation of the deep soft tissues of the larynx due to the presence of fatty tissue planes between the muscles of the preepiglottic, paralaryngeal, and deep subglottic spaces. The paired aryepiglottic folds extend from the corniculate cartilages, the cricoid lamina, and the adjacent triangular airway. The apex of the triangle represents the anterior commissure and the angles at the base of the triangle represent the paired posterior commissures. On MRI the true vocal cords are intermediate in signal intensity, due to the vocalis muscle, and can be distinguished from the high-intensity fat within the false vocal cords (Fig. 11.2 d). T1-weighted sequences after administration of contrast medium reveal the mucosal outline as structures of high signal intensity. The small vertical air column between the true cords is named the rima glottidis. At the anterior commissure of the true cords any more than 1 mm of soft tissue between the airway and inner surface of the thyroid cartilage is considered abnormal. Axial or sagittal images are best suited for examination of the anterior commissure. The false cords are cephalad to the true cords and are separated from them by the laryngeal ventricles. These ventricles are small, bilateral, air-filled outpouchings best seen on coronal scans.

## Preepiglottic, Paralaryngeal, and Infraglottic Spaces

The preepiglottic and paralaryngeal spaces are composed predominantly of fat and therefore are of low intensity on CT and give a high signal on MRI. The midline preepiglottic space extends downward from the hyoid bone to the anterior commissure; it can be traced as a continuum with the lateral paralaryngeal spaces, which are directly medial to the thyroid cartilage. The subglottic region normally contains no significant soft tissue between the airway and the cricoid cartilage. The conus elasticus is a fibrous sheath that originates from the cricoid cartilage and extends upward to the free margin of the true vocal cords, thereby forming the vocal ligaments. The conus elasticus is an important structure that limits lateral tumor extension and directs subglottic tumor spread inferiorly or superiorly along the airway.

## Intrinsic Laryngeal Muscles

Unlike CT, MR often allows visualization of the intrinsic musculature of the larynx. This can be attributed to increased tissue contrast and the ability to obtain direct coronal images. The muscles appear as vertical bands of moderate signal intensity surrounded by high-intensity fat. The paired intrinsic muscles act as a sphincter during swallowing. A superior group consisting of the aryepiglottic and thyroepiglottic muscles forms a protective cap over the aperture of the laryngeal airway by acting to invert the epiglottis during deglutition. The muscles of the vocal folds complete the sphincter inferiorly and can be subdivided into those muscles that open or close the sphincter and those that lengthen or shorten it. The posterior cricoarytenoid muscles act to open the vocal cords and are the only dilator muscles of this group. Their action is opposed by the lateral cricoarytenoid and transverse arytenoid muscles, which close the vocal folds. The vocal folds are lengthened by the action of the cricothyroid muscles and shortened by the thyrohyoid, arytenoid, and vocalis muscles (Fig. 11.2 b).

## Lymphatic Drainage

The lymphatic drainage of the larynx determines the spread of carcinoma. Embryologically, the larynx can be divided into superior and inferior portions at the level of the laryngeal ventricles, and lymphatic drainage reflects this division. Above the ventricles, the larynx is derived from branchial cleft anlage, and the lymphatics in this region drain over the top of the thyroid cartilage to submandibular nodes. Inferiorly, the larynx arises from tracheobronchial anlage, and the lymphatics of the true vocal cords and the subglottic region drain inferiorly, posteriorly, and occasionally anteriorly through the cricothyroid membrane to nodes in the lateral compartment (carotid sheath) and the lateral soft tissues of the neck and thoracic inlet.

## 11.4 Tumor Classification

A uniform classification of laryngeal and hypopharyngeal tumors is needed to enable clear description of tumor infiltration. Based on this information the appropriate therapy can be chosen. The most common classification of tumors is the TNM system proposed by the International Union Against Cancer (UICC) [5]. Tables 11.1–11.4 give the TNM classifications for tumors of the larynx and hypopharynx.

The TNM system defines *stage T1* as tumor extension limited to one part of this topographic region, not transgressing supraglottic, glottic, subglottic, or hypopharyngeal structures. Glottic tumors are subdivided into T1 a (confined to one vocal cord) and T1 b (affecting both vocal cords).

*Stage T2* tumors extend to adjoining parts of the laryngeal or hypopharyngeal region. Vocal cords show either normal or impaired mo-

bility. The hypopharynx is not fixed to the larynx.

*Stage T3* tumors invade, for example, the piriform sinus and the preepiglottic space in the case of supraglottic tumors. In glottic tumors one or both vocal cords are fixed.

*Stage T4* tumors invade structures beyond the larynx, such as the oropharynx or the soft tissues of the neck with the infrahyoid muscles. Glottic and supraglottic tumors invade the thyroid and/or cricoid cartilage, hypopharyngeal tumors the epiglottis.

The definitions of the N categories follow the same scheme (Table 11.3).

In our series, tumor masses pathologically classified T1 were seen on laryngoscopy in 100% of patients. Only limited information can be obtained in respect of the depth of infiltration. Laryngoscopy and pathology show equivalent results in 60% of T2 and T3 tumors and in 70% of T4 tumors. MRI often overestimates tumors of stage T1. Edematous

**Table 11.1.** Tumor classification of the larynx. (Modified from [5])

| TX | Minimum requirements to assess primary tumor not met | | |
|----|------|------|------|
| T0 | No evidence of primary tumor | | |

| | Supraglottis | Glottis | Subglottis |
|----|------|------|------|
| T | Carcinoma in situ | Carcinoma in situ | Carcinoma in situ |
| T1 | Tumor confined to the region with normal mobility | Tumor confined to the region with normal mobility | Tumor confined to the region |
| T1 a | Tumor confined to the laryngeal surface of the epiglottis or to an aryepiglottic fold or to a ventricular band | Tumor confined to one vocal cord | Tumor confined to one side of the region |
| T1 b | Tumor involving the epiglottis and extending to the ventricular bands or cavities | Tumor involving both vocal cords | Tumor with extension to both sides of the region |
| T2 | Tumor with extension to adjacent sites or to the glottis without fixation | Tumor extending to either the supraglottis or the subglottis with normal or impaired mobility | Tumor confined to the larynx impairing cord mobility |
| T3 | Tumor confined to the larynx with fixation and/or other evidence of deep invasion | Tumor confined to the larynx with fixation of one or both vocal cords | Tumor confined to larynx with fixation of vocal cords |
| T4 | Tumor with direct extension beyond the larynx | Tumor with direct extension beyond the larynx | Tumor with extension beyond the larynx |

**Table 11.2.** Tumor classification of the hypopharynx. (Modified from [5])

| | |
|---|---|
| TX | Minimum requirements to asses primary tumor not met |
| T0 | No evidence of primary tumor |
| Tis | Preinvasive carcinoma (carcinoma in situ) |
| T1 | Tumor confined to one site |
| T2 | Tumor with extension to adjacent site or region without fixation of hemilarynx |
| T3 | Tumor with extension to adjacent site or region with fixation of hemilarynx |
| T4 | Tumor with extension to bone, cartilage, or soft tissues |

**Table 11.3.** Classification of regional lymph node metastasis. (Modified from [5])

| | |
|---|---|
| NX | Regional lymph nodes cannot be assessed |
| N0 | No regional lymph node metastasis |
| N1 | Metastasis in a single ipsilateral lymph node, 3 cm or less in greatest dimension |
| N2a | Metastasis in a single ipsilateral lymph node, more than 3 cm but not more than 6 cm in greatest dimension |
| N2b | Metastases in multiple ipsilateral lymph nodes, none more than 6 cm in greatest dimension |
| N2c | Metastases in bilateral or contralateral lymph nodes, none more than 6 cm in greatest dimension |
| N3 | Metastasis in a lymph node more than 6 cm in greatest dimension |

Tumors in the entire head and neck region drain into the cervical lymph nodes. Their classification is thus uniform for all areas of origin except for the thyroid gland.

**Table 11.4.** Classification of distant metastasis (Modified from [5])

| | |
|---|---|
| Mx | Presence of distant metastasis cannot be assessed |
| M0 | No distant metastasis |
| M1 | Distant metastasis |

This classification is the same for all head and neck sites.

or inflammatory reactions of surrounding tissue may be impossible to distinguish from the primary tumor. T2 and T3 tumors are staged correctly in 80% of cases by MRI, using T1-weighted images with and without contrast medium and the subtraction technique. Tumors infiltrating neighboring structures, classified T4, can be diagnosed accurately in all cases (Table 11.5).

The primary tool for preoperative evaluation of the location and extent of laryngeal and hypopharyngeal tumors is clinical laryngoscopy. The choice of therapeutic procedure, e.g., surgery, radiotherapy, or chemotherapy, is based on the results. In the course of the past decade, imaging techniques such as CT, sonography, and MRI have become established in the diagnosis of primary tumors and lymph node involvement. Due to the excellent soft tissue contrast of MRI and its capacity for producing multiplanar views, certain clinical appearances have been established as indications for MRI [10, 11].

The improved information yielded by the paramagnetic contrast medium Gd-DTPA makes MRI the method of choice for the staging of laryngeal and hypopharyngeal tumors staged higher then T1 [9].

Clinical laryngoscopy and MRI combine very well and together represent the first choice of therapeutic procedure.

## 11.5 Differential Diagnosis

In contrast to other regions, tumors of the larynx and hypopharynx are of almost uniform histology: in almost every case they are squamous cell carcinomas. Other malignancies occasionally found in the larynx and hypopharynx include pseudosarcoma, adenocarcinoma, spindle cell carcinoma, and basal cell carcinoma. Laryngeal cancers of connective tissue and hematopoietic elements include comedocarcinoma, fibrocarcinoma, and lymphoma. Precise histologic classification is the domain of the pathologist and can not be

**Table 11.5.** Comparison of the results of MRI and laryngoscopy (L) with pathological staging (P)

| Stage | MRI = P | MRI > P | MRI < P | L = P | L > P | L < P |
|---|---|---|---|---|---|---|
| pT1 | 2 | 2 | – | 4 | – | – |
| pT2 | 4 | 1 | – | 3 | 2 | – |
| pT3 | 4 | – | 1 | 3 | – | 2 |
| pT4 | 14 | – | – | 10 | – | 4 |
| | Correlation: 85.7% | | | Correlation: 71.4% | | |

achieved by MRI. Benign lesions such as fibroma or amyloid tissue are also extremely rare in the larynx. Therefore the problem of diagnosis is often reduced to assigning the tumor to the correct TNM category (Table 11.6).

> Most tumors of the larynx and hypopharynx are squamous cell carcinomas – exact TNM classification is important. To facilitate exact description of the extent of tumors we have developed a checklist of anatomic structures that may be seen on the MR image.

## 11.6 Characteristic Diagnostic Findings

### 11.6.1 Principles of MRI

MRI is a highly sensitive and specific means of staging laryngeal and hypopharyngeal tumors. It improves the imaging of this area substantially by permitting high soft tissue contrast and by its capacity for producing multiplanar views. Fatty, cystic, and muscular structures can be precisely differentiated on the basis of their different T1 and T2 relaxation times.

Plain T1-weighted sequences alone visualize tumor margins less than perfectly in glottic and hypopharyngeal lesions, but are very useful in differentiating tumor from fatty tissue in the supraglottic area. Optimal image quality can be achieved with T1-weighted sequences after administration of Gd-DTPA; in particular, the interface between muscles (e.g., the transverse arytenoid muscle) and the tu-

**Table 11.6.** Checklist: larynx und hypopharynx

| | Normal | Abnormal |
|---|---|---|
| *Skeleton:* | | |
| Cricoid cartilage | | |
| Thyroid cartilage | | |
| Hyoid bone | | |
| Arytenoid cartilage | | |
| *Folds:* | | |
| Thyrohyoid fold | | |
| Cricohyoid fold | | |
| Thyroepiglottic fold | | |
| Hyoepiglottic fold | | |
| *Muscles:* | | |
| Suprahyoid muscles | | |
| Superior group | | |
| True cord level, vocal muscle | | |
| True cord level, thyroarytenoid muscle | | |
| Anterior commissure | | |
| Posterior commissure | | |
| Conus elasticus | | |
| Medial pharyngo-epiglottic fold | | |
| Lateral pharyngo-epiglottic fold | | |
| Vallecula | | |
| Extralaryngeal soft tissues | | |
| Soft tissues of the neck | | |

mor mass is seen more clearly. T2-weighted and spin density images are advantageous in judging cartilage invasion when they are of good quality; however, the long scan time means that delineation of the airway is often adversely affected by respiratory motion or coughing, especially in patients suffering from dyspnea and sore throat.

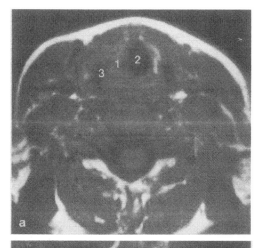

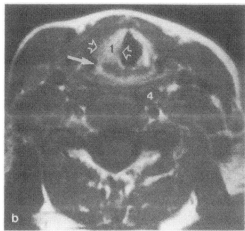

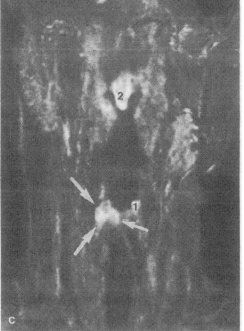

**Fig. 11.3a–c.** Supraglottic carcinoma pT2, pN0
**a** Plain axial MRI (SE, 500/17). Tumor (*1*) of intermediate signal intensity between airway (*2*) and piriform sinus (*3*) at the supraglottic level on the right side
**b** Axial MRI (SE, 500/17) with Gd-DTPA. The tumor (*arrows*) shows inhomogeneous contrast medium enhancement (*1*). The medial wall of the right piriform sinus is formed by tumor (arrow). Longus colli muscle (*4*)
**c** Coronal subtraction image. This image shows the longitudinal extent of the tumor and its exact medial delineation (*arrows*). Inflammatory lesion on the opposite side (*1*) and uvula (*2*) with high signal intensity

After the injection of contrast medium, all tumors show significant enhancement (by a factor of 1.8–2.3), due to the richer vascularization of the tumor than of the surrounding tissue. However, the normal mucosa coating the complete larynx and hypopharynx also takes up contrast medium (Fig. 11.4b). Therefore in some cases surrounding inflammatory tissue may lead to overstaging of the tumor. Central necrosis shows up as areas of intermediate signal intensity in T1-weighted sequences; after administration of Gd-DTPA enhancement can be documented in neighboring vascularized structures. T2-weighted sequences allow the diagnosis of necrotic or liquid-filled structures (Fig. 11.10c).

High-quality T2-weighted sequences yield the best visualization of cartilage, but many severe artifacts often restrict image quality and thus render exact diagnosis difficult. Accurate plain T1-weighted images, contrast-enhanced images and the subtraction technique allow good or at least sufficient judgement of cartilage invasion in all cases. The subtraction technique improves visualization of tumor spread beyond the larynx and hypopharynx, classified T4 (Table 11.7).

Axial images are mandatory for the staging of laryngeal and hypopharyngeal tumors. For accurate preoperative depiction of topographic detail, such as the distinction of vocal and vestibular folds, images in a second plane are helpful (Fig. 11.3c). In hypopharyngeal lesions, sagittal images are indispensable for clear visualization of the dorsal and cranial aspects of the epiglottis and for detection of infiltration of the preepiglottic space and tongue. In laryngeal lesions coronal images show the best diagnostic results.

Lymph node metastasis may be diagnosed if MRI shows a node more than 1.2 cm in greatest dimension or more than three nodes combined. Indistinct outline and inhomogeneous contrast medium enhancement with decreased central vascularization are additional criteria. Whereas patients with laryngeal tumors mainly show a lymph node involvement stage N0 or N1, in hypopharyngeal tumors stages N1 and N2 prevail. Following this scheme, MRI sensitivity and specificity of more than 80% can be reached.

### 11.6.2 Tumors

#### 11.6.2.1 Carcinoma

High-resolution MRI with multiplanar surface coil techniques have improved spatial resolution and S/N; however, resolution is not sufficient for demonstration of mucosal abnormalities. Therefore, endoscopy and MRI will remain complementary, the former used for diagnosing mucosal lesions and the latter for staging deep extension. Although laryngoscopy can show mucosal surfaces and masses within the lumen, submucosal extension cannot be evaluated. This information has profound implications on the management of disease, since planning for conservative laryngeal surgery depends on accurate knowledge of the extent of disease within the

**Table 11.7.** The Value of the different MRI sequences

|  | T1 weighted, plain | T1 weighted GD-DTPA | T2 | Spin density |
|---|---|---|---|---|
| Larynx |  |  |  |  |
| supraglottic | 2 | 3 | 2 | 1–2 |
| glottic | 3 | 3 | 2 | 1–2 |
| subglottic | 2 | 3 | 3 | 1 |
| Hypopharynx | 2 | 3 | 2 | 1–2 |

Grading of visualization: 1, satisfactory; 2, good; 3, optimal.

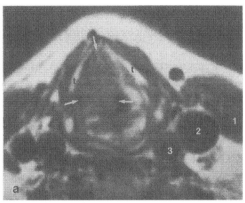

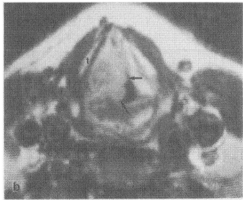

**Fig. 11.4a, b.** Supraglottic carcinoma of the larynx pT3
**a** Plain axial MRI (SE, 500/17). A tumor with low signal intensity is infiltrating the right vestibular fold (*arrows*). No exact visualization of the posterior tumor margins. *1*, sternocleidomastoid muscle; *2* internal jugular vein; *3*, common carotic artery; *t*, thyroid cartilage
**b** Axial MRI (SE, 500/17) with Gd-DTPA. Significant enhancement of tumor (*arrow*), borders precisely visualized. No infiltration of thyroid cartilage (*t*)

larynx. MRI provides vital information on laryngeal and hypopharyngeal anatomy in the following specific areas, which should be identified and evaluated for tumor extension:

1. Anterior and posterior commissures
2. Supraglottic extension (preepiglottic space, paralaryngeal space, piriform sinuses, valleculae)
3. Subglottic extension
4. Vocal cord fixation
5. Extralaryngeal spread (soft tissues of neck and tongue base)
6. Cartilage invasion
7. Carotid artery involvement
8. Cervical adenopathy

Laryngeal cancer may be divided into three groups based on location: supraglottic, glottic (true vocal cords), and subglottic. Each tumor has a characteristic pattern of spread. For instance, metastasis to lymph nodes is more common in supraglottic and subglottic tumors than in glottic lesions. This reflects the relatively poor lymphatic drainage of the vocal cords. Tumors of the piriform sinus, while actually of hypopharyngeal origin, will be included in this discussion because of their close relationship to supraglottic lesions.

In the various types of laryngeal cancers, the laryngeal cartilages may be distorted by tumor. Distortion can range from mild displacement to frank destruction. When marked, these changes are easy to recognize on CT or MRI. However, slight asymmetrical deformity and focal infiltrative destruction may be difficult to assess. Normal variations in patterns of cartilage calcification can simulate destruction on MRI as well as on CT. Neither CT nor MRI can detect microscopic cartilage invasion.

### Supraglottic Carcinoma

Supraglottic tumors, arising anywhere from the false vocal cords to the epiglottis, comprise 20% to 35% of laryngeal cancers. They tend to spread to lymph nodes high in the neck, involving the internal jugular chain and often the jugular digastric nodes, because of the abundant lymphatics in this region. Con-

sequently, supraglottic cancers often present at a more advanced stage than glottic lesions. Thyroid cartilage invasion is not a common finding unless the tumor extends to the anterior commissure. The hyoid bone is usually displaced rather than destroyed by tumor.

Carcinomas of the supraglottic region can be subdivided into two groups: anterior tumors, arising in the epiglottis or preepiglottic space, and posterolateral tumors, found in the aryepiglottic folds and the paralaryngeal spaces. The former have a better prognosis than the latter. Suprahyoid epiglottic cancers may initially present as thickening of the free margin and can be treated by surgery or radiotherapy. More advanced lesions may spread to the pharyngoepiglottic folds, lateral pharyngeal walls, valleculae, or base of tongue. Infrahyoid epiglottic cancers often extend into the preepiglottic space, which then loses its normal fatty appearance. Preepiglottic space abnormalities may also result from edema, hemorrhage, or inflammation. Posterolateral supraglottic tumors appear as thickening of the aryepiglottic folds or as a mass in the paralaryngeal space. Their natural tendency is to grow posteriorly and inferiorly to the arytenoids, rather than anteriorly to the preepiglottic space. Advanced piriform sinus carcinomas often resemble lateral supraglottic (marginal) lesions.

*Stage T1*. Supraglottic tumors staged T1 are usually too small to be detected prospectively by MRI, despite its high resolution and high soft tissue contrast. T1 tumors are limited to mucosal structures of the supraglottic region, e.g. the aryepiglottic fold or the false cord, on either the left or the right side. The motion of the hemilarynx is not yet impaired.

*Stage T2*. Stage T2 tumors of the supraglottic larynx are the smallest tumors that should be diagnosed routinely by MRI, assuming excellent image quality and the use of the paramagnetic contrast medium Gd-DTPA. The tumor enhances by a factor of 1.8−2.3. The normal mucosa also takes up the contrast medium, but to a lesser degree than the tumor. In difficult cases of similar enhancement the subtraction technique may enable accurate differentiation of tumor masses and normal or inflamed mucosa. The tumor tends to spread either cranially, infiltrating the hypopharyngeal region with the epiglottis or the pharyngoepiglottic folds, or caudally, into the glottic region and the lateral pharyngeal walls. The false cords may be partially fixed, but the mobility of the true vocal cords is not impaired (Fig. 11.3).

*Stage T3.* Tumors of stage T3 are a clear indication for MRI, which provides a detailed assessment of deep infiltration and gives important information on which to base the decision on subsequent surgical therapy. Exact delineation of tumors should be possible using contrast medium, and the subtraction technique can be employed if necessary. If infiltration of the thyroid cartilage or the epiglottis remains uncertain a T2-weighted and a spin density sequence may be helpful. Stage T3 tumors often erode the thyroid cartilage or even the arytenoid cartilages. An overlapping of the tumor to the pre-epiglottic space, the valleculae epiglotticae, or the vocal cords, even with fixation of the cords, is quite common (Fig. 11.4).

*Stage T4.* Stage T4 tumors infiltrate structures beyond the larynx and hypopharynx. Starting from the supraglottic larynx, the base of the tongue and the mylohyoid and geniohyoid muscles are frequently involved. In the dorsal direction the piriform sinus and esophagus may be infiltrated. As patients with advanced tumors often suffer from dyspnea, shortness of breath, and sore throat, the MR images tend to be of a lower quality. In particular, the long measurements like T2-weighted and spin density sequences often do not make any useful contribution to diagnosis because of severe motion artifacts. On the other hand, tumors of this size can be visualized with sufficient clarity by CT in most cases. Therefore CT may obviate MRI and is less burdensome for the patient (Fig. 11.5).

> Extensive laryngeal tumors can be seen on CT as well as on MRI, and CT is less troublesome for the patient.

### Glottic Carcinoma

Glottic tumors, arising from the true vocal cords, are the most common laryngeal cancers. They comprise 50%–70% of laryngeal malignancies and are usually well-differentiated, slow-growing lesions. Some 75% of these tumors arise from the anterior half of the true vocal cord. Because of their early presentation and the ease of clinical examination, most glottic carcinomas do not require investigation by imaging techniques [3]. Nodal spread is uncommon because there is an absence of lymphatics along the free margin of the vocal cords. However, advanced lesions associated with cord fixation have a higher incidence of lymphatic involvement. Glottic tumors may extend to the anterior commissure and into the subglottic or supraglottic region, the contralateral vocal cord, or the thyroid cartilage and cricothyroid membrane. Alternatively, they may grow posteriorly to the ipsilateral posterior commissure, the arytenoid cartilages, and the cricoarytenoid joints. From the posterior commissure, tumors may extend further into the contralateral cord or into the soft tissues of the neck. Early glottic lesions have an excellent prognosis: the 5-year survival rate approaches 95% with surgery or radio-therapy. MRI adds valuable staging information to laryngoscopy by revealing or excluding deep tumor extension and lymphadenopathy. Unfortunately, some positive MRI and CT findings are nonspecific; for example, thickening of a cord may be secondary to tumor, fibrosis, edema, inflammation, or hemorrhage.

Anterior commissure involvement necessitates extended hemilaryngectomy. Occasionally, an abundance of tissue displaying the typical MRI signal of soft tissue at the anterior commissure, despite the symmetric appearance of the vocal cords, is the major clue to extension of tumor. In general, early mucosal

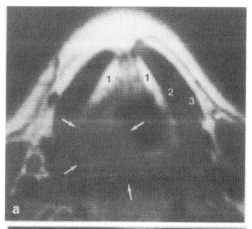

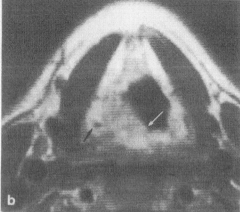

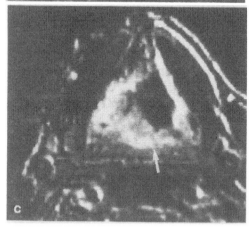

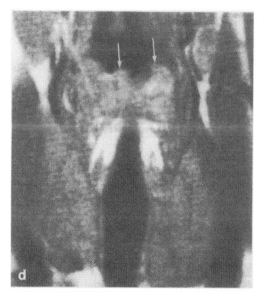

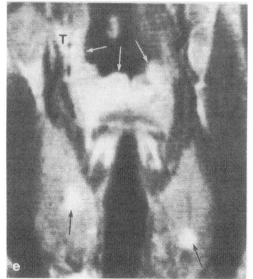

**Fig. 11.5a–e.** Supraglottic carcinoma pT4, pN1
**a** Plain axial MRI (SE, 500/17). Tumor of intermediate signal intensity at the false cord level (*arrows*).
*1*, Thyroid cartilage; *2*, thyrohyoid muscle; *3*, sternohyoid muscle
**b** Axial MRI (SE, 500/17) with Gd-DTPA. Significant enhancement of the tumor, which reaches the
midline at the posterior commissure (*white arrow*).

Right piriform sinus is surrounded by tumor (*black
arrow*)
**c** Axial subtraction image. Infiltration of the thyroid cartilage and the inferior constrictor pharyngis
muscle (*arrow*)
**d** Plain coronal MRI (SE, 500/17). The coronal
image shows the supraglottic growth of the tumor
(*arrows*). No exact delineation of tumor and infrahyoid muscles
**e** Coronal MRI (SE, 500/17) with Gd-DTPA.
Marked, enhancement of the tumor (*white arrows*).
Infiltration of the thyrohyoid muscle up to the tonsil level (*T*). Note the thyroid adenoma on both
sides (*black arrows*)

disease is best evaluated with laryngoscopy. Vocal cord fixation can also be diagnosed by MRI when an arytenoid cartilage is shown in the median or paramedian position. Cord fixation may be the result of several mechanisms. Tumor may infiltrate the intrinsic laryngeal musculature and fix the cord to the thyroid cartilage, bulky tumor may limit cord mobility by the mass effect, tumor may involve the cricoarytenoid joint, or vocal cord fixation may be due to invasion and paralysis of the laryngeal nerve.

*Stage T1.* Tumors of this low stage can not normally be depicted with MRI. The vocal cords are visualized as normal or can not be differentiated from inflammatory or edematous lesions prospectively. Clinical symptoms like hoarseness are suspicious of a tumor of the glottis and must be investigated by clinical laryngoscopy. The tumor stage is designated T1 a if the tumor involves only one cord and T1 b if both cords are involved. Both vocal cords remain fully mobile.

*Stage T2.* Glottic tumors of stage T2 should normally be detected by MRI, assuming excellent image quality and the use of Gd-DTPA and the subtraction technique. Glottic tumors can spread in any direction, most frequently the thyroid and arytenoid cartilages are involved. Infiltration of the false vocal cords and of the aryepiglottic folds is also very common. Another typical route of infiltration is dorsal, involving the cricoid cartilage and the dorsal parts of the piriform sinus. Even caudal growth into the subglottic area is possible. The vocal cords are still fully or almost fully mobile (Fig. 11.6).

*Stage T3.* Tumors of stage T3 show more advanced growth than those of stage T2, but still are restricted to the larynx. The combination of the different MRI techniques is very helpful in giving a detailed description of the tumor with respect to the following therapy. The criterion for classifying a tumor as stage T3 rather than stage T2 is fixation of the vocal cords. Therefore, knowledge of the clinical symptoms and the progress of the patient's complaints is of great importance for tumor classification (Fig. 11.7).

*Stage T4.* Tumors staged T4 have already infiltrated anatomic structures beyond the larynx. The most common routes of infiltration are dorsally, involving the esophagus and ventrally, to the hyoid bone and the base of the

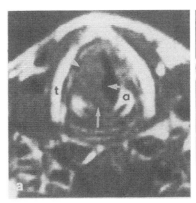 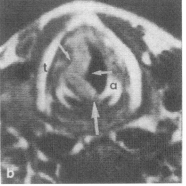

**Fig. 11.6a, b.** Glottic carcinoma pT2, pN0
**a** Plain axial MRI (SE, 500/17). Tumor (*arrows*) with low signal intensity infiltrating the vocal muscle on the right side. Normal thyroid (*t*) and arytenoid (*a*) cartilage. The lateral and dorsal extension of the tumor are depicted exactly. On laryngoscopy the right vocal fold showed impaired mobility
**b** Axial MRI (SE, 500/17) with Gd-DTPA. Marked enhancement of the tumor (*small arrows*). The tumor crosses the midline at the posterior commissure (*large arrow*)

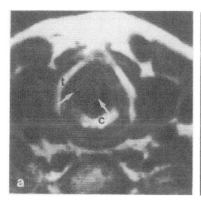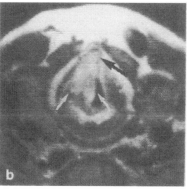

**Fig. 11.7a, b.** Glottic carcinoma pT3, pN0
**a** Plain axial MRI (SE, 500/17). Tumor of the right vocal cord narrowing the airway (*arrows*). No infiltration of the thyroid cartilage (*t*). The posterior tumor margins are not visualized exactly. Clinically, the right vocal cord was fixed. *c,* Cricoid cartilage

**b** Axial MRI (SE, 500/17) with Gd-DTPA. The laryngeal tumor (*white arrows*) and the normal mucosa at the left side show increased signal intensity. The tumor crosses the midline at the anterior commissure (*black arrow*). The aryepiglottic folds are not infiltrated

tongue. Due to the severe motion artifacts that may occur with long scan times, CT instead of MRI may be considered for patients with advanced clinical symptoms such as dyspnea.

> Glottic tumors generally have a good prognosis because clinical symptoms arise at a lower tumor stage.

### Subglottic Carcinoma

Subglottic tumors arising between the true vocal cords and the inferior border of the cricoid cartilage comprise 2%–6% of laryngeal cancers. True subglottic primary malignancies are rare. Tumors arising from this area spread easily to the trachea, thyroid, hypopharynx, and lateral compartment lymph nodes. Subglottic tumors most often represent inferior extensions of glottic and, occasionally, supraglottic cancers. On scans below the level of the true vocal cords any soft tissue between the cricoid cartilage and the airway is abnormal and may represent subglottic extension. The conus elasticus is an anatomic barrier to tumor spread. Tumors infiltrating deep to the conus elasticus (e.g., transglottic) tend to re-

main on its deep surface (paralaryngeal surface), while those beginning on its mucosal side tend to remain mucosal.

Generally, if a subglottic tumor extends more than 1 cm caudal to the true vocal cords, total laryngectomy is indicated because it is necessary to remove the cricoid cartilage to obtain a clear margin of excision. With more aggressive voice-conservation techniques, parts of the superior rim of the cricoid lamina may be excised, leaving the cricoid ring intact to preserve laryngeal function. In advanced lesions the cricoid cartilage may be eroded and total laryngectomy is then necessary. Transglottic tumors are defined as those involving the true cords and subglottic space or those that cross the laryngeal ventricles. Involvement of the true and false vocal cords may cause vocal cord fixation. A few transglottic tumors begin in the laryngeal ventricle: many more originate from the true vocal cords with laryngeal spread. Transglottic tumors are characterized by higher rate of thyroid cartilage invasion and extension through the cricothyroid membrane. Treatment is usually total laryngectomy with or without radiotherapy (Fig. 11.8).

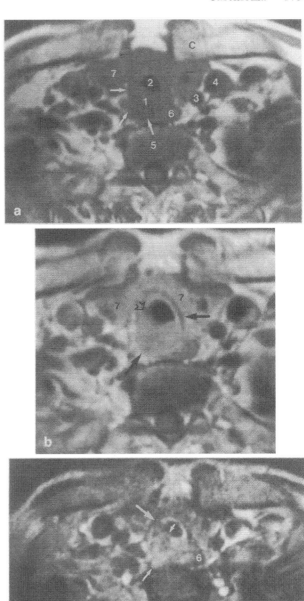

**Fig. 11.8 a–c.** Subglottic tumor pT3, pN1

**a** Plain axial MRI (SE, 500/17) Homogeneous tumor (*1* and *arrows*) lying between the trachea (*2*) and the spine. Exact delineation of the tumor margins is not possible. *3*, Common carotid artery; *4*, internal jugular vein; *5*, second thoracic vertebral; *6*, esophagus; *7*, thyroid gland; *C*, clavicle

**b** Axial MRI (SE, 500/17) with Gd-DTPA. Enhancement of tumor solid (*solid arrows*) and thyroid gland (*7*) is evident. The right tracheal cartilage is infiltrated by tumor (*open arrow*)

**c** Plain axial MRI (SE, 3000/90). In the T2-weighted sequence the infiltrative character of the tumor (*large arrow*) and its inhomogeneous inner structure (*small arrows*) are demonstrated

### Hypopharyngeal Carcinoma

Piriform sinus tumors behave more aggressively than endolaryngeal lesions and comprise 10%–20% of "laryngeal" cancers. They are usually squamous cell cancers of inferior hypopharyngeal origin. Early nodal involvement occurs because of the rich lymphatics anterior to the piriform sinuses. Piriform sinus tumors grow in two major patterns: Lateral wall lesions invade the thyroid cartilage and soft tissues of the neck, forming bulky masses about the piriform sinus. Medial wall lesions extend into the paralaryngeal space and vocal muscle, resembling marginal supraglottic lesions. Less commonly, piriform sinus cancers invade the preepiglottic space and extend across the midline. Tumors of either wall of the piriform sinus may spread supramedially to the aryepiglottic fold, again simulating marginal supraglottic lesions.

Despite the aforementioned similarities, piriform sinus tumors have several characteristics that distinguish them from marginal supraglottic lesions. They frequently invade the thyroid cartilage, usually at its posterolateral margins. Also, piriform sinus lesions tend to be unilateral and submucosal. If extensive, these tumors may widen the space between the thyroid and cricoid cartilages. When this occurs, the conus elasticus tends to direct the tumor posterolaterally and inferiorly.

There is no clear dividing line between supraglottic laryngeal carcinomas and hypopharyngeal carcinomas. In most cases it is difficult or even impossible to be sure of the site of origin of the tumor. The cranial hypopharyngeal carcinomas have a strong tendency to infiltrate the floor of the mouth with the mylohyoid and geniohyoid muscles and the epiglottis, while supraglottic laryngeal carcinomas tend to erode laryngeal structures like the true and false vocal cords.

*Stage T1.* Hypopharyngeal tumors of stage T1 often escape clinical detection. On MRI, too, the tumors are too small to be diagnosed with sufficient confidence, because they conceal themselves in the mucosa coating the complete hypopharynx. Even clinical laryn-goscopy does not achieve 100% detection of T1 tumors, as the intricate anatomy of this area often obstructs the laryngoscopic view into the complete hypopharynx.

> Hypopharyngeal tumors of stage T1 can not be visualized by MRI and may even escape detection by clinical laryngoscopy.

*Stage T2.* T2 tumors of the hpopharynx can be diagnosed accurately with MRI. Short T1-weighted sequences and the paramagnetic contrast medium Gd-DTPA yield detailed description of the tumor margins and permit classification. The contrast medium enhancement (by a factor of 1.8–2.3) in combination with the subtraction technique enables the observer to distinguish tumors from surrounding mucosa. The most common sites of tumor growth are the piriform sinus on both sides, the pharyngoepiglottic fold, and the posterior wall of the hypopharynx. In stage T2 the tumor infiltrates one or several of these structures, often erodes the epiglottis, but is not yet fixed to the hemilarynx.

*Stage T3.* In tumors of stage T3 MRI is the method of choice for exact visualization of deep infiltration. Again, Gd-DTPA and the subtraction technique generally delineate the tumor margins in detail. Additional images in the sagittal plane are particularly helpful in visualizing the epiglottis in its characteristic position extending from anterior caudal to posterior cranial. T3 tumors are characterized by greater size and more extensive infiltration. Posteriorly growing tumors have infiltrated the piriform sinus and the posterior pharyngeal wall, while cranially spreading tumors may have reached the epiglottis, the pharyngoepiglottic folds, and the valleculae epiglotticae. If the tumor reaches the larynx it tends to infiltrate the postcricoid area, the false vocal cords, and the arytenoid cartilage and is fixed to the hemilarynx (Fig. 11.9).

*Stage T4.* A tumor of stage T4 infiltrates anatomic structures beyond the hypopharynx. Most frequently the base of the tongue

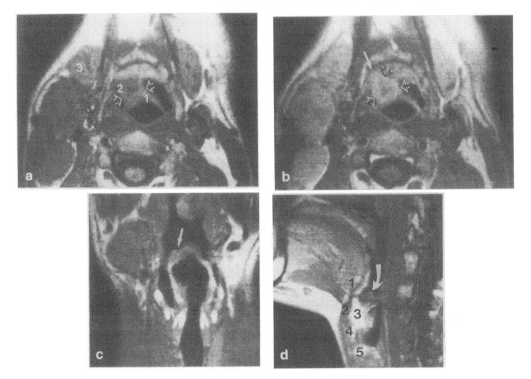

**Fig. 11.9 a–d.** Hypopharyngeal carcinoma pT3, pN1

**a** Plain axial MRI (SE, 500/17). Tumor of the right vallecula (*open arrows*) displacing the medial (*1*) and lateral (*2*) glossoepiglottic folds and the submandibular gland (*3*)

**b** Axial MRI (SE, 500/17) with Gd-DTPA. Inhomogeneous enhancement of the tumor (*open arrows*). Erosion of the lateral glossoepiglottic fold (*solid arrow*) is evident

**c** Coronal MRI (SE, 500/17) with Gd-DTPA. The tumor shows its ulcerating morphologic structure. No infiltration at the true cord level with cricoid cartilage (arrow)

**d** Plain median sagittal MRI (SE, 500/17). Topographic relations of the tumor (arrow) to the base of the tongue (*1*) hyoid bone (*2*), preepiglottic space (*3*), thyroid cartilage (*4*), and cricoid cartilage (*5*)

and the mylohyoid and geniohyoid muscles are reached first. The hyoid bone is often affected, and erosions of the thyroid area may be found. Infiltration of the cricoid cartilage or soft tissues of the neck are further criteria for staging a hypopharyngeal tumor T4. On MRI, large tumors of the hypopharynx, in particular, show a characteristic necrotic inner structure. The necrotic tissue is visualized best using contrast medium, when circular enhancement surrounding an area of extremely low signal intensity is obvious.

A necrotic inner structure is a characteristic for a hypopharyngeal tumor stage T4.

### 11.6.2.2 Other Malignant Neoplasms and Benign Lesions

An increasing number of HIV-positive patients are suffering from Kaposi sarcoma in the pharynx and neck. MRI is helpful in the diagnosis of these patients due to the characteristic findings. Plain MRI in different planes accurately localizes the tumor. In our series all sarcomas showed an enormous uptake of Gd-DTPA, which resulted in high signal intensity in T1-weighted sequences (Fig. 11.10).

Papillomas are the only benign neoplasms to occur more than rarely in the larynx. They are found more commonly in children than adults and are in fact the most common laryngeal

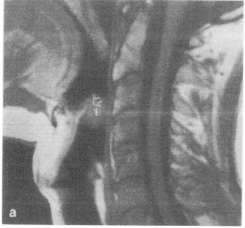

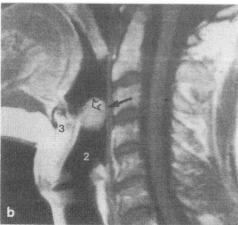

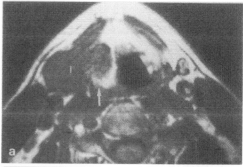

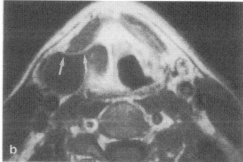

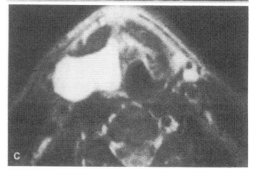

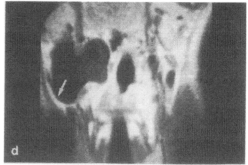

**Fig. 11.10a, b.** Kaposi sarcoma of the epiglottis
**a** Plain median sagittal MRI (SE, 500/17). Sagittal images are very helpful in the diagnosis of epiglottic tumors (*1*). The epiglottic cartilage is infiltrated by the tumor (*arrow*)
**b** Median sagittal MRI (SE, 500/17) with Gd-DTPA. The tumor shows an immense increase of signal intensity. Infiltration of the inferior constrictor pharyngis muscle can be excluded (*black arrow*). The preepiglottic space (*3*) and supraglottic cavity (*2*) are not infiltrated

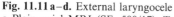

▷

**Fig. 11.11a–d.** External laryngocele
**a** Plain axial MRI (SE, 500/17). Tumor with low signal intensity on the right side (*1*) displacing the pharyngeal airway (*arrows*). No exact delineation of the lesion possible
**b** Axial MRI (S, 500/17) with Gd-DTPA. Circular enhancement of the tumor (*arrows*) with no change in central signal intensity

**c** Plain axial MRI (SE, 3000/90). In the T2-weighted sequence the lesion shows extremely high signal intensity, pointing to a liquid-filled structure
**d** Coronal MRI (SE, 500/17) with Gd-DTPA. Again, the mucosa (arrow) shows high contrast medium uptake, so the lesion is delineated clearly. The contrast medium technique enables exact diagnosis of this laryngocele

tumors in the pediatric age group. Children usually have multiple lesions, whereas in adults a single lesion is more common. A characteristic juvenile papilloma originates in the anterior larynx on the true or false vocal cords and extends subglottically. Extension throughout the tracheobronchial tree may follow incomplete removal.

A laryngocele is a dilation of the saccule (appendix) of the laryngeal ventricle. Sometimes this appendix extends superiorly in the paralaryngeal space, medial to the thyroid cartilage, where it is known as an internal laryngocele and can present as a submucosal supraglottic mass [2, 6–8, 13]. Lateral displacement of the thyroid lamina can occur. If the dilated saccule extends through the thyrohyoid membrane, it is an external laryngocele. The most common type, mixed laryngoceles, combine components of both internal and external laryngoceles.

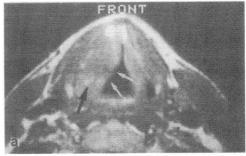

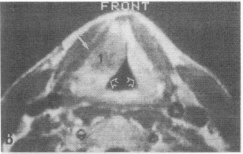

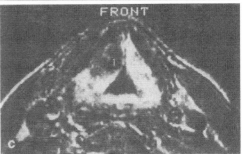

▷

**Fig. 11.12 a–d.** Amyloid tissue in the supraglottic larynx

**a** A supraglottic lesion with intermediate signal intensity is shown (*arrows*). Delineation of thyroid cartilage and infrahyoid muscles is not possible

**b** TR/TE = 500/17, transverse, Gd-DTPA. A certain part (*1*) of the enlarged mucosa shows no contrast medium uptake, in contrast to the highly vascularized mucosa at the false cord level. Additional contrast medium uptake by the enlarged mucosa due to an inflammatory reaction (*open arrows*). Exact delineation from the thyroid cartilage (*white arrow*)

**c** Subtraction image. Clear delineation of amyloid tissue (*1*) and homogeneously enhanced false cords. Increased enhancement of the enlarged mucosa due to inflammatory reaction

**d** Coronal MRI (SE, 500,17) with Gd-DTPA. Topographic relations of the tumor (*arrows*) to the supraglottic space (*1*), piriform sinus (*2*), and floor of the mouth (*3*)

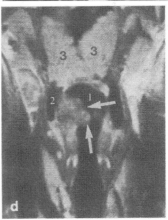

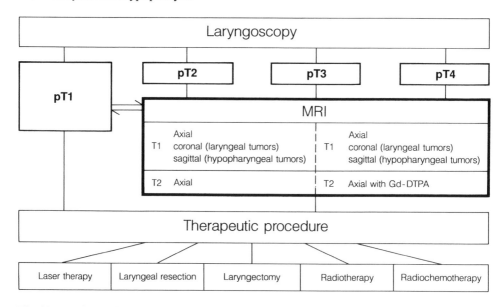

**Fig. 11.13.** Diagnostic strategy: larynx

Laryngoceles are unilateral in around 75% of cases. Presumably, they arise from increased intralaryngeal pressure, as in glass-blowing or playing wind instruments. Laryngoceles commonly present in adulthood; many are asymptomatic. An unobstructed laryngocele is filled with air [1]. With obstruction, fluid accumulates within the dilated appendix. Sometimes a small cancer near the neck of the saccule causes the obstruction and subsequent laryngocele. Laryngoceles are also associated with chronic granulomatous disease, such as tuberculosis. On MRI a laryngocele is a well-circumscribed mass extending superiorly from the laryngeal ventricle and false cord into the paralaryngeal space (internal laryngocele) or lateral to the thyrohyoid membrane (external laryngocele). In mixed laryngoceles the internal and external features can be identified (Fig. 11.11).

Rare benign laryngeal neoplasms include adenoma, chondroma, hemangioma, neurofibroma, and plasmacytoma. Except for chondroma, the MRI appearance is not specific. Chondromas arise most frequently from the cricoid cartilage and show matrix calcification. Generally, benign lesions are distinguished from malignant tumors by biopsy.

Amyloidosis may also involve the larynx, and displays nonspecific MRI tissue characteristics (Fig. 11.12).

### 11.6.3 Trauma

Occasionally, posttraumatic changes mimic cancerous masses in the laryngeal cartilages. Most commonly, thyroid cartilage fractures heal in a distorted position, giving rise to the appearance of supraglottic masses. Vocal cord paralysis after trauma may be incorrectly attributed to malignancy. MRI is useful in the study of laryngeal trauma. Significant acute injuries should be identified and repaired within 7–10 days. Delay in the treatment of fractured laryngeal cartilages may lead to posttraumatic laryngeal stenosis. Chronic posttraumatic abnormalities such as laryngeal stenosis are also easily studied by these techniques.

The direct sagittal scanning capability of MRI is particularly useful for demonstrating the extent of airway lesions and is of value in planning laryngeal reconstruction. Unsuspected or forgotten old laryngeal trauma simulating a laryngeal mass may be recognized for what it is by the posttraumatic deformity of the laryngeal cartilages.

## 11.6.4 Diagnostic Strategy

The following diagnostic strategy is recommended for MRI of the larynx and hypopharynx (Fig. 11.13).

## *References*

1. Becker H, Naumann H, Pfalz C (1982) HNO-Heilkunde. Thieme, Stuttgart
2. Fenzl G, Heywang S, Vogl T, Obermüller J, Einhäupl K, Clados D, Steinhoff H (1986) Die Kernspintomographie der Wirbelsäule und des Rückenmarks im Vergleich zu Computertomographie und Myelographie. ROFO 144(6):636–643
3. Gademann G, Semmler G, Bachert-Baumann P, Zabel H-J, van Kaick G, Lorenz W-J (1987) 31P-spectroscopy follow up studies of human tumor after chemotherapy. Society of Magnetic Resonance in Medicine, 6th Annual Meeting and Exhibition. Book of abstracts, p 506
4. Giovaniello J, Grieco RV (1970) Laryngocele. AJR Radium Ther Nucl Med 9:108
5. Hermanek P, Sobin LH (eds) (1987) TNM classification of malignant tumors. Springer, Berlin Heidelberg New York
6. Hippel RV (1910) Über Kehlsackbildungen beim Menschen (Laryngozele ventricularis). Dtsch Z Chir 107:477
7. Hofmann U, Hofmann D, Vogl T, Wiesinger H, Coerdt J (1990) Rezidivierende Atemnotattacken bei Neugeborenen mit gestieltem nasopharyngealen Hamartom. Pädiatr Praxis 39:55–59
8. Jensen AM, Samulsen U (1963) On laryngocele. Acta Otolaryngol (Stockh) 57:475
9. Lufkin RB, Hanafee WN (1986) MR reveals subtleties of head and neck pathology. Diagn Imaging 8:98–104
10. Lufkin RB, Hanafee WN (1988) MRI of the head and neck. Magn Reson Imaging 6:69–88
11. Lufkin RB, Wortham DG, Dietrich RB, Hoover LA, Larson SG (1986) Tongue and oropharynx: findings on MR imaging. Radiology 161:69–75
12. Requard H, Sauter R, Bayerl J, Weber H (1987) Helmholtzspulen in der Kernspintomographie. Electromedia 55/2:61–67
13. Schätzle W, Baumert U (1962) Über die Laryngozele. Laryngologie 4:270
14. Vogl T (1989) Erkrankungen des Aerodigestivtraktes und der Halsweichteile: Vergleich MRI und CT. Röntgenblätter 42:199–209
15. Vogl T, Schuler M, Hahn D, Funk W, Mees K (1986) Vergleichende Darstellung einer Laryngozele im MR, CT und konventioneller Röntgendiagnostik. Digitale Bilddiagn 6:64–66
16. Vogl T, Steger W, Grevers G, Schreiner M, Dresel S, Lissner J (1991) MRI with Gd-DTPA in tumors of larynx and hypopharynx. European Radiology 1:58–64

# 12 Neck

## 12.1 Clinical Findings

Many pathologic conditions of the neck are manifested by cervical swelling, depending on the extent of the lesion. Only in the deeper layers, such as the parapharyngeal region, do space-occupying diseases sometimes present as pharyngeal tumors.

In children the most common cause of a cervical mass, after nonspecific lymphadenopathy, is a congenital neck tumor. These abnormalities can originate from the muscles, the skin, the blood vessels, the lymphatic vessels, or the branchial apparatus. Not all congenital neck masses are present at birth. Malignant tumors are relatively rare in children but must be considered in the differential diagnosis of cervical masses.

In adults, a wide variety of different causes must be considered in the case of a cervical swelling. In addition to nonspecific or specific lymphadenopathies, possible benign causes include lateral and median cervical cysts, tumors of vascular and neural origin, lipomas, and hypertrophy of the thyroid gland. Symptomatic lymphadenopathy preceded by an acute viral or bacterial infection of the upper aerodigestive tract commonly causes a cervical swelling. In most cases, these lymphadenopathies can be effectively treated with antibiotics. An abscess occasionally develops, requiring drainage of the infected area. In the case of recurrent lymphadenopathy of unknown origin HIV must be excluded. Specific lymphadenopathies that may be manifested by cervical masses include those caused by tuberculosis, sarcoidosis, toxoplasmosis, and actinomycosis.

Lateral cervical cysts can produce a swelling located mainly anterior to the sternocleidomastoid muscle. This common entity is supposed to be of branchiogenic origin. The therapy of choice is surgical removal.

Median cervical cysts are believed to be remnants of the embryologic thyroglossal duct. They are found submentally in the midline of the neck superior to the hyoid bone. When removing the cyst, the medial parts of the hyoid bone have to be resected concomitantly to prevent recurrence.

Vascular tumors can also present as cervical swellings. Still, in this group aneurysms of the supraaortic branches have to be distinguished from glomus tumors and hemangiomas.

Aneurysms of the extracranial parts of the carotid artery are quite rare. An important symptom is pulsation of the tumor, which can easily be detected by palpation.

Glomus tumors manifesting as cervical swellings mainly originate from the glomus caroticum. This tumor is the most common paraganglioma in the neck. The therapy of choice is surgical resection, provided the other arteries can maintain a sufficient cerebral blood supply. Glomus tumors are benign in most cases, but metastatic spread has been described.

Hemangiomas are vascular tumors which usually appear shortly after birth. The majority shows a spontaneous remission within the first 6 or 7 years of life. The tumors are usually located in the subcutaneous tissue layers and can be diagnosed easily by inspection. Occasionally, however, they occur in deeper tissue layers. The treatment of choice is either surgical removal or laser therapy.

Malignant vascular tumors (angiosarcomas, hemangiopericytomas) are very rare. The best treatment is a combination of surgery, radiotherapy, and chemotherapy. The prognosis, however, is poor.

Lymphangiomas are benign tumors originating from the lymphatics. The etiology of these lesions is unclear. Almost 90% of lymphangiomas appear by the age of 2 years. The therapy of choice is surgical resection.

Neurogenic tumors can also cause cervical swellings. They can originate from the autonomic nervous system, from the cranial nerves (with the exception of the optic and oculomotor nerves), or from the peripheral nerves.

Neurinomas (schwannomas) originate from Schwann cells. Usually, they do not show any specific symptoms, at least in an earlier stage. Depending on the size of the tumor, however, they may produce symptoms like dysphagia and hoarseness. Almost 25% of schwannomas are located in the head and neck. The vagus nerve and the cervical sympathetic chain are most commonly involved.

Neurofibromas occurring in patients suffering from neurofibromatosis have to be distinguished from schwannomas. These patients usually show additional, cutaneous lesions such as café au lait spots or peripheral neurofibromas.

Lipomas are benign tumors, mainly located subcutaneously. Rare cases of malignant transformation have been described. The therapy of choice is surgical resection.

Finally, lymph node metastases of malignomas of the head and neck, as well as lymph nodes in Hodgkin's disease and non-Hodgkin's lymphomas, may present as cervical swellings. Particularly in patients exhibiting risk factors such as chronic alcohol and nicotine abuse, metastatic lymph nodes in the neck might represent an early manifestation of a cancerous lesion in the nasopharynx, the oral cavity, the oropharynx, the hypopharynx, or the larynx.

*Diagnostic Procedures.* In the diagnostic evaluation of cervical swellings, thorough physical examination, including inspection and palpation, is mandatory. In many cases, physical examination and the patient's history will establish the diagnosis. Ultrasound can be useful as a screening method in cervical tumors. If a patient with a cervical mass has a history of alcohol and nicotine abuse, the lesion must be biopsied. In addition, the upper aerodigestive tract must be checked carefully. Even if the patient does not complain of any other symptoms, endoscopic evaluation of the nose, nasopharynx, oropharynx, oral cavity, hypopharynx, larynx, trachea, and esophagus must be undertaken to exclude primary cancer that might be responsible for a metastatic lymph node.

The diagnostic approach to the parapharyngeal space tends to be difficult. Many diseases of this space first become apparent in an advanced stage, due to its inaccessibility. If a tumor of the parapharyngeal space is suspected, careful clinical investigation including inspection of the pharynx and palpation of the neck is obligatory.

*Demands on the Radiologist.* As in many other diseases, the main purpose of the diagnostic evaluation in cervical swellings is to establish whether the process is benign or malignant. Additionally, the topographic relation of the tumor to the surrounding tissue is important, especially if surgical intervention is planned. Possible involvement of the carotid sheath must also be considered; the major vessels in the neck can either be displaced by a benign cervical mass or infiltrated by a malignant process, usually a cervical lymph node metastasis of a carcinoma of the head or neck. In addition, vascular lesions such as glomus caroticum tumors and aneurysms have to be considered. In these cases thorough investigation of the vascular supply is mandatory to enable informed planning of treatment.

## 12.2 Examination Technique

The examination technique for the neck corresponds to that for the larynx and hypopharynx (Chap. 11).

## 12.3 Topographic Relations

### 12.3.1 Neck Compartments

The neck is defined as the anatomic region between a plane defined by the lower margin of the mandible and the superior nuchal line of the occipital bone and an imaginary line joining the suprasternal notch and the top of the seventh cervical vertebra (Fig. 12.1 e). Fascial planes divide the neck into multiple compartments. For the interpretation of axial images it is useful to define four anatomic compartments: the visceral, the posterior, and the two lateral compartments.

The *visceral compartment* is the most anterior and contains structures of the aerodigestive tract, including the larynx, trachea, and esophagus. The thyroid and parathyroid glands also lie within this compartment. The sternocleidomastoid and pharyngeal constrictor muscles form the lateral and posterior boundaries, respectively, of the visceral compartment.

The *posterior compartment* includes the cervical vertebrae, posterior extensor muscles, and anterior flexor muscles, including the scalene, longus capiti, and longus colli muscles (Fig. 12.1 a, b). These muscle groups have the same intermediate signal intensity as muscles in the tongue and paralaryngeal structures, due to their similar MRI tissue characteristics (long T1, short T2). The fibrous tissue of the nuchal ligament has a low intensity, similar to that of dense cortical bone in the vertebral bodies and ribs. Hematopoietic and fatty marrow within cancellous bone has a high signal intensity on most T1- and T2-weighted pulse sequences. On administration of Gd-DTPA only richly vascularized structures enhance, such as the mucosa lining the pharynx and lymphoid tissue. Vessels, fascial planes

**Table 12.1.** Checklist: compartments of the neck

|  | Normal | Abnormal |
|---|---|---|
| *Visceral compartment* |  |  |
| Larynx |  |  |
| Hypopharynx |  |  |
| Trachea |  |  |
| Esophagus |  |  |
| Thyroid gland |  |  |
| *Posterior compartment* |  |  |
| Cervical spine |  |  |
| Scalene muscles |  |  |
| Longus colli muscle |  |  |
| Longus capitis muscle |  |  |
| *Lateral compartment* |  |  |
| Common carotid artery |  |  |
| Jugular vein |  |  |
| Lymph nodes |  |  |

and muscles typically do not show significant enhancement.

The *lateral compartments* contain the carotid sheaths. The carotid arteries and jugular veins are easily distinguished from adjacent fat, muscle, and lymph nodes because of the low signal intensity of flowing blood, which shows up black on the MR image. Because of the inherently superior contrast of blood vessels and absence of streak artifacts, MRI is better than CT for delineation of vessels at the thoracic inlet. Small branches of major cervical vessels can easily be traced from section to section on axial images. Images obtained in the coronal or coronal oblique planes may be useful for delineation of cervical vessels and vascular relations near the aortic arch. Lymph nodes are best seen with T1 weighted sequences. Normal lymph nodes resemble thyroid and thymic tissue in having relatively long T1 and T2, allowing discrimination from fatty tissues on T1-weighted images and from muscle on T2-weighted images.

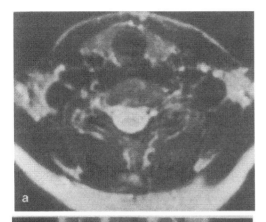

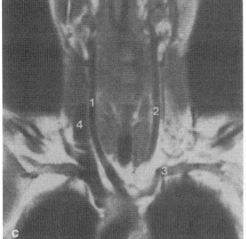

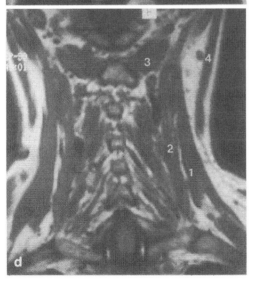

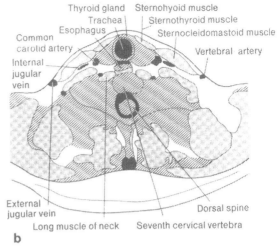

Thyroid gland   Sternohyoid muscle
Trachea         Sternothyroid muscle
Esophagus       Sternocleidomastoid muscle
Common
carotid artery                  Vertebral artery
Internal
jugular
vein
External
jugular vein                    Dorsal spine
Long muscle of neck   Seventh cervical vertebra

**b**

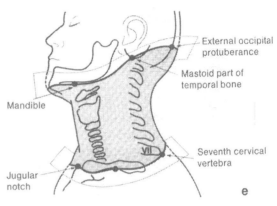

External occipital
protuberance

Mastoid part of
temporal bone

Mandible

Seventh cervical
vertebra

Jugular
notch

**e**

**Fig. 12.1 a–e.** Topography of the neck
**a** Plain axial MRI (SE, 2000/60)
**b** Schematic representation of **a**
**c** Plain coronal MRI (SE, 500/17). Visualization of
soft tissues, vessels, and musculature. *1*, Right common carotid artery; *2*, left common carotid artery;
*3*, left subclavian artery; *4*, right jugular vein
**d** Plain coronal MRI (SE, 500/17). *1*, Splenius capitis muscle; *2*, semispinalis capitis muscle; *3*, inferior
oblique muscle; *4*, sternocleidomastoid muscle
**e** Schematic representation of the boundaries of the
neck

### 12.3.2 Thyroid Gland

The thyroid gland develops as a tubular invagination from the root of the tongue called the foramen cecum. The thyroglossal duct grows downward, in front of the hyoid bone and thyroid cartilage, to the trachea. At birth the thyroid gland is located inferior to the thyroid cartilage and in adults extends over a craniocaudal distance of 3–5 cm as a symmetric, homogeneous, wege-shaped structure on either side of the trachea. The average weight of the gland in adults is 25 g. The thyroid isthmus crosses anterior to the second and third tracheal rings to connect the inferior portions of the right and left thyroid lobes. The thyroid gland capsule is fixed to the pretracheal fascia, causing the gland to move upward on deglutition.

Axial images alone are often sufficient in examination of the thyroid gland. When craniocaudal relations have to be delineated, the coronal plane is favored because of the symmetry of the thyroid gland in this plane. The normal thyroid gland is readily distinguished from the sternothyroid and sternocleidomastoid muscles because its long T2 relaxation time results in greater signal intensity on T2-weighted images.

### 12.3.3 Parathyroid Glands

Four parathyroid glands normally exist as upper and lower bilateral pairs posterior to the thyroid lobes in the tracheoesophageal groove. The upper pair, along with the thyroid, arises from the fourth branchial cleft, while the lower pair, along with the thymus, arises from the third branchial cleft. The position of the upper pair of glands is relatively constant, near the level of the cricoid cartilage in 95% of cases. The position of the inferior pair is more variable; in 40% of cases they are located within the thymic tongue, a distinct bilateral structure at the thoracic inlet extending from the lower thyroid pole to the mediastinal thymus. Some 5%–10% of the population have more than four parathyroids, with a fifth gland most commonly located in the thymic remnant. Normal parathyroid glands measure 4–6 mm in their largest (craniocaudal) dimension, 2–4 mm in width, and weigh an average of 20 mg, and are not routinely imaged by ultrasound, CT, or MRI.

### 12.3.4 Lymph Nodes

In looking for abnormalities in the neck, knowledge of the normal appearance and distribution of the lymph nodes is important (Fig. 12.2). Axial MR slices enable the radiologist to survey all groups of lymph nodes in the neck. For diagnostic purposes it is essential to distinguish between the submental, submandibular, and deep cervical groups of lymph nodes. The deep cervical nodes are divided into three levels by the thyroid and the cricoid cartilage and the digastric muscle. The most cranial of these levels is known as the jugulo-digastric area and is delineated by the posterior belly of the digastric muscle and the hyoid bone. At the caudalmost level is found the important jugulo-omohyoid node [11] (Table 12.2).

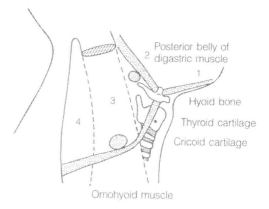

**Fig. 12.2.** Topographical relations of lymph nodes in the neck. *1*, Submental; *2*, submandibular; *3*, deep cervical; *4*, posterior neck triangle

**Table 12.2.** Checklist: lymph nodes of the neck

| Lymph nodes | Number | Central necrosis | Greatest diameter | Infiltration of adjacent structures |
|---|---|---|---|---|
| 1. Submental | | | | |
| 2. Submandibular | | | | |
| 3. Deep cervical<br>3a. Upper level:<br>    posterior digastric muscle | | | | |
| 3b. Middle level:<br>    hyoid bone to cricoid | | | | |
| 3c. Lower level:<br>    cricoid to supraclavicular | | | | |
| 4. Retropharyngeal | | | | |
| 5. Deep visceral<br>Paratracheal | | | | |
| Paraesophageal | | | | |
| Scalene gap | | | | |

## 12.4 Thyroid Gland

### 12.4.1 Diagnostic Concept

MRI of the neck combines the advantages of CT and ultrasound.

In evaluating tumors of the thyroid and parathyroid glands, neither MRI nor CT can match the low cost, availability, ease of use, and overall effectiveness of ultrasound. When nodal metastases are suspected, the full cross-sectional field of view of MRI has advantages similar to those established for CT. Intrathoracic extension of thyroid goiters or ectopic parathyroid glands can be evaluated better by MRI due to the good delineation of blood vessels and the excellent tumor/fat contrast. Suspected adenopathy or vascular pathology in the thoracic inlet is also well delineated by MRI [3].

The advantage of MRI over CT, then, is the exact differentiation of soft tissue lesions and lymphadenopathies with the possibility of obtaining images in various planes during one examination.

In many cases, however, the MR diagnosis is restricted to an exact delineation of tumors; histologic information has to be obtained via biopsy. New technical developments such as gradient echo sequences and FLASH sequences with a flip angle of 40° yield improved distinction of tumors.

### 12.4.2 Anatomic Abnormalities

Some characteristic anatomic abnormalities arise from disturbances in the development of the thyroid gland.

Persistence of the embryonal thyroglossal duct results in formation of an anterior midline cyst. Duct remnants can extend from the foramen cecum of the dorsal tongue to the level of the thyroid isthmus. Although the diagnosis is often clinically apparent, imaging is helpful to delineate extensions above the hyoid bone that must be removed to prevent recurrence [3].

Lingual thyroid is the term used for a functioning midline mass of thyroid tissue in the posterior third of the tongue. The normal thyroid is usually absent in these patients. An ectopic maldescended thyroid is a functioning midline nodule; the normal thyroid may be present or absent.

### 12.4.3 Goiter

Enlargement of the thyroid gland, whether diffuse and symmetrical or irregular and focal, is known as goiter. Goiter is due to diffuse hyperplasia (Graves' disease) in 25% of cases; nodular thyroid disease accounts for the remaining 75%. Scintigraphy with pertechnetate $^{99m}TcO_4^-$, $^{123}I$, or $^{131}I$ can be used to assess function of thyroid tissue and plan therapy of Graves' disease or hyperfunctioning (hot) nodules. MRI cannot determine thyroid function by means of signal intensity or T1 or T2 measurements. Although permanganate ($MnO_4^-$) is selectively accumulated by functioning thyroid tissue, manganese in this form is not paramagnetic. Nonspecific extracellular agents such as Gd-DTPA are not likely to show tissue-specific patterns of enhancement. In the absence of a functional contrast agent MRI provides only anatomic informa-tion. Thus, in simple goiter with diffuse normal uptake of tracer on scintigraphy, MRI shows a diffuse homogeneous enlargement of the thyroid gland. In diffuse toxic goiters (Graves' disease) with higher tracer uptake, the MRI findings are characterized by prolonged T2 values, with homogeneous high signal intensity (Fig. 12.3). In all other thyroid disease with diffuse high or low uptake of tracer, the MRI findings are nonspecific.

### 12.4.4 Nodular Disease

The major clinical value of MRI in evaluating nodular thyroid disease lies in morphologic assessment of the extent of disease in patients with cancer or benign goiters that require surgical excision to relieve symptoms caused by the mass effect. The value of CT is often limited by streak artifacts caused by swallowing or respiratory motion and beam hardening. Furthermore, large amounts of iodinated contrast material must be injected to identify the complex vascular structures of the neck and thoracic inlet. Ultrasound is superior to CT and MR for visualization of the cervical thyroid gland; however, the lower pole of the thyroid gland often lies within the thoracic inlet where bone and air hamper transmission of sound waves. MR combines the advantages of CT and ultrasound in that both the neck and the thoracic inlet can be examined without streak artifacts and vascular structures can be separated from soft tissue masses without intravenous contrast material. As the vast majority of hot nodules are benign, there is no role for cross-sectional imaging in their clinical management. Thyroid disease presents with symptoms of hyperfunction in one third of patients; the other two thirds have nontoxic nodular goiters. The rare nontoxic goiters that display some evidence of function on scintigraphy ("warm" nodules) may in fact be nonfunctioning ("cold") nodules overlain by functioning thyroid tissue. Cold nodules require biopsy and/or endocrine therapy with careful imaging follow-up to exclude cancer. Approximately 10% of cold nodules are malignant and 85% represent benign colloid ade-

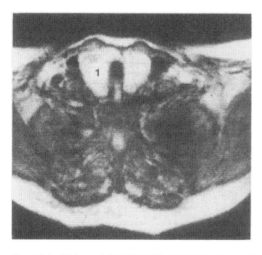

**Fig. 12.3.** Plain axial MRI (SE, 2000/60) Graves' disease. The thyroid gland (*1*) is visualized with high signal intensity and distinct margins

nomas; cysts and focal thyroiditis constitute fewer than 5% of benign lesions.

### 12.4.5 Adenoma

Thyroid adenomas show prolonged T2 relaxation times and are best distinguished from normal thyroid tissue using T2-weighted SE images. Although the mean T1 of adenomas is longer than that of normal thyroid tissue, values frequently overlap and adenomas are commonly isointense on T1-weighted images (Fig. 12.4). Adenomas may also appear brighter than normal thyroid tissue on T1-weighted images, an inconsistent finding possibly associated with hemorrhagic degenera-

tion. Hemorrhagic changes have not been observed in thyroid cancer. As for diffuse thyroid disease, an overall increased in signal intensity in T2-weighted sequences may be observed in some cases of thyroiditis and hyperfunction. Thyroid carcinoma shows T1 and T2 prolongation that is nonspecific and indistinguishable from the majority of benign lesions (Fig. 12.5). Tissue characterization by MRI is most useful in distinguishing posttreatment fibrosis, which has a low signal intensity due to short T2, from recurrent cancer.

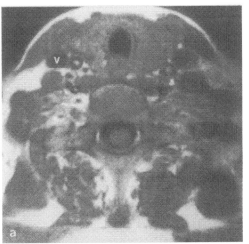

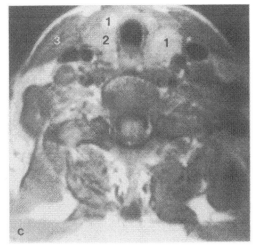

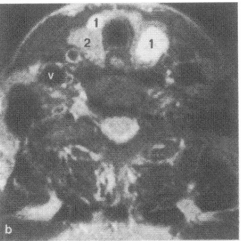

Fig. 12.4a–c. Bilateral multifocal thyroid adenoma
a Plain axial MRI (SE, 500/15). The thyroid gland is slightly enlarged, no exact delineation from the sternohyoid muscles is possible. *V*, jugular vein
b Plain axial MRI (SE, 3000/90). Due to prolonged T2 values, the adenomas (*1*) show higher signal intensity than normal thyroid tissue (*2*)
c Axial MRI (SE, 500/17) with Gd-DTPA. After Gd-DTPA administration the adenomas (*1*) can be differentiated from the normal thyroid gland (*2*) and the sternocleidomastoid muscle (*3*)

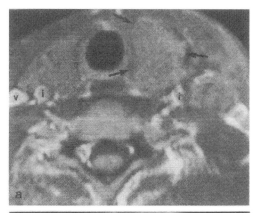

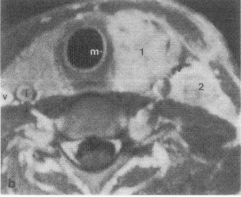

**Fig. 12.5 a, b.** C-cell carcinoma pT3, pN2
**a** Plain axial MRI (SE, 550/17). In the T1-weighted image a homogeneous tumor of the left lobe of the thyroid gland is evident (*arrows*). Its signal intensity is equal to that of the normal thyroid gland, so the tumor margins can not be depicted exactly. *i*, common carotid artery; *v* jugular vein
**b** Axial MRI (SE, 550/17) with Gd-DTPA. The tumor (*1*) shows inhomogeneous enhancement with diffuse infiltration. The tracheal cartilage is free of tumor, but at the left side a large lymph node is demonstrated (*2*). *m*, Tracheal mucosa; *i*, common carotid artery; *v*, jugular vein

### 12.4.6 Conclusions

There are some specific indications for the use of MRI in thyroid imaging:
MR determines well the extent of large goiters and their relationship to the cervicothoracic vessels.
MRI is very sensitive in the detection of muscle.
In medullary carcinoma, which cannot be detected by the uptake of radioactive iodine, MRI can differentiate between nonfibrous tumor and fibrous tissue.
MRI does not require the administration of iodinated contrast medium, thereby avoiding unwanted iodine loading in patients with thyroid disease [25, 28].

---

There are currently few indications for the primary use of MRI in the diagnosis of thyroid lesions:
1. MRI is superior to CT with iodinated contrast medium for investigation of suspected neoplasia
2. Recurrent carcinoma
3. Before surgery of a large thoracic goiter

---

## 12.5 Parathyroid Glands

### 12.5.1 Diagnostic Concept

A dramatic increase in the clinically apparent incidence of primary hyperparathyroidism has occurred with the introduction of automated methods for routine measurement of serum calcium. In the United States, it is estimated that one in 700 persons over the age of 60 develops hyperparathyroidism each year, and overall a total of 50000 new cases are diagnosed annually. A surgeon experienced in parathyroid surgery can treat 90%–95% of patients without any preoperative localization procedure. Nevertheless, recurrent or persistent hyperparathyroidism is common, and the most frequent cause is incomplete exploration of the neck. Extensive neck dissection and biopsy of all four glands may also result in

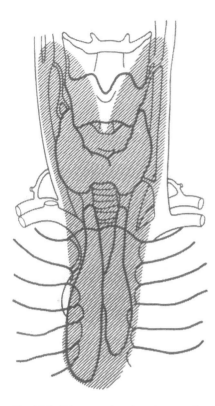

**Fig. 12.6.** Diagram showing the area in which the parathyroid glands may be located

**Table 12.3.** Sensitivity and specificity of MRI, CT and ultrasound (US) for the diagnostic of primary hyperparathyroidism

|  | Sensitivity (%) | Specificity (%) |
|---|---|---|
| MRI: Primary surgery | 79 | 98 |
|       Secondary surgery | 67 | 88 |
| CT | 56 | 95 |
| US | 56 | 91 |
| MRI + CT + US | 93 | 96 |

laryngeal nerve trauma or postoperative complications such as tetany. Surgery is prolonged, and complication rates are highest in patients who have scarring from previous neck operations. Due to the variability in location of the parathyroids the neck must be examined craniocaudally from the hyoid bone to the aortic arch and ventrodorsally from the thyroid gland to the esophagus (Fig. 12.6). Slightly abnormal position of the parathyroids is found in 20% of cases, but in 10% of cases the glands are situated in the mediastinum.

Due to their small volume (2–3 mm × 1 mm) and low weight (25–40 mg), normal parathyroids are not easily differentiated from surrounding structures. With increasing enlargement of the glands in older patients and in pathologic changes, MRI reveals the parathyroids as areas of high signal intensity, especially in T2-weighted images. On CT too the fat content facilitates the recognition of the parathyroids. On ultrasound the fibrous capsule and the mixed fatty and fibrous internal pattern result in a weaker echo than from thyroid tissue. These features become more pronounced in pathologic changes such as adenoma and hyperplasia. Ultrasound is the procedure of choice for imaging the thyroid and parathyroid glands because of its superior spatial resolution, multiplanar capabilities, and ability to distinguish solid masses from blood vessels. Unfortunately, acoustic transmission is blocked by air or bone, and therefore retrotracheal or mediastinal tumors are not detected. CT has proven to be advantageous in patients with ectopic parathyroid tumors due to its larger field of view and ability to image all areas of the neck and mediastinum. Unfortunately, CT is limited by the numerous tortuous blood vessels at the thoracic inlet that are poorly opacified even with large doses of contrast medium. Furthermore, beam-hardening artifacts from the shoulders often obscure anatomic detail (Table 12.3). Parathyroid scintigraphy using a double-tracer ($^{201}$Tl, $^{99m}$Tc) subtraction technique is effective for localizing parathyroid tumors in the neck and mediastinum. Since the basis for differential $^{201}$Tl uptake by parathyroid adenomas is poorly understood, no rationale exists for the observed accuracy rates.

On MRI the differentiation of the parathyroid adenomas and hyperplasia by MR-specific parameters such as proton density and T1 and T2 relaxation times require discrimination between cystic and noncystic le-

**Table 12.4.** T1 and T2 of parathyroid adenomas and of normal muscle relative to normal thyroid tissue

|  | Parathyroid adenoma | | Normal muscle |
|---|---|---|---|
|  | Cystic | Non cystic |  |
| T1 ratio | 1.59 | 2.01 | 1.07 |
| T2 ratio | 8.64 | 1.37 | 2.01 |

sions. For non-cystic lesions the small difference in T2 between parathyroid and thyroid lesions is not useful in individual cases. Using T1, both cystic and noncystic adenomas are clearly differentiated from fatty tissues. Discrimination between adenomas and hyperplasia is not possible. The diagnostic value of MRI can be improved further with the paramagnetic contrast medium Gd-DTPA. Due to the enhancement of parathyroid adenomas and hyperplasia the administration of Gd-DTPA helps to reveal small lesions. There are significant differences in T1 and T2 between parathyroid adenomas and thyroid tissue and between muscle and thyroid tissue (Table 12.4).

### 12.5.2 Nodular Disease

As in the thyroid gland, parathyroid carcinoma shows no significant difference in relaxation times from the much more common parathyroid adenomas. Parathyroid adenomas tend to have longer T2 relaxation times than thyroid adenomas; however, the difference is too small to be useful in individual cases. Posterior thyroid adenomas and lymph nodes are the most common causes of false positives on MRI. Axial slices are preferred at the thoracic inlet to minimize volume averaging of structures that are predominantly oriented perpendicular to this plane (Fig. 12.7). Left-right symmetry is also valuable in identifying normal muscles and vessels. Planar surface coils are ideal for this region, and anterior positioning of the coil will significantly improve the S/N for the region of interest (Fig. 12.8). With improved S/N

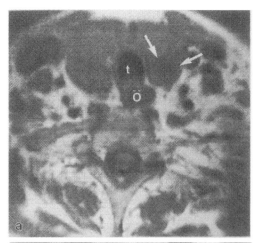

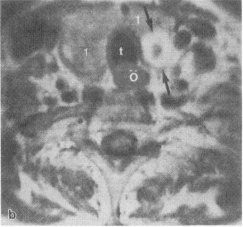

**Fig. 12.7 a, b.** Left parathyroid adenoma in primary hyperparathyroidism
**a** Plain axial MRI (SE, 500/25). An area of lower signal intensity (*arrows*) is evident at the left posterior pole of the thyroid gland. There is no displacement or infiltration of surrounding tissues. *ö*, Esophagus; *t* trachea
**b** Axial MRI (SE, 500/25) with Gd-DTPA. The thyroid gland (*1*) shows moderate enhancement whereas the adenoma (*arrows*) enhances markedly. The lesion is distinctly bordered and shows a central area of lower enhancement representing necrosis

the achievable spatial resolution of MRI ($0.5 \times 1 \times 5$ mm voxel size) nearly matches that of CT. Surface coil techniques can now detect more than 85% of parathyroid adenomas in extracervical locations. A rare finding is recurrent adenoma of a parathyroid gland transplantated to the soft tissues of the forearm. The signal intensity and contrast medium uptake of such an adenoma are analogous to those of cervical parathyroid adenomas.

### 12.5.3 Conclusions

The value of MRI, CT, and ultrasound for the diagnosis of parathyroid lesions must be judged in the light of operative findings. Gd-DTPA-enhanced MRI has better sensitivity (86%) than CT (66%) or sonography (69%). All three modalities have similarly high specificity, ranging from 94% to 96%. Their diagnostic accuracy is also similar, between 88% and 91%. Combining all three methods, the sensitivity can be increased to 93%.
MRI may be particularly valuable in cases of recurrent or persistent hyperparathyroidism where tissue planes are obscured by previous surgery. Surgical clips interfere with ultrasound and CT, and fibrous tissue can mask or mimic tumors. MRI offers superior contrast, freedom from artifacts, and can distinguish fibrous tissue (short T2) from tumor (long T2) [26, 27].

## 12.6 Lymph Nodes

### 12.6.1 Diagnostic Concept

Diseases of the lymphatics in the neck can be divided into primary (Hodgkin's, non-Hodgkin's lymphoma) and secondary tumors and inflammatory lesions. The grading of lymphomas follows the Ann Arbor classification. The lymph node groups of the neck have very intricate drainage paths which follow the venous system. Hence the most important guiding structure in the neck is the internal jugular vein. Lymphadenopathy appears above all with lesions in the oropharynx, hypopharynx, and supraglottic larynx. Typical for systemic diseases is infiltration of the supraglottic lymph nodes, which form the connection between the jugular and the cervicoposterior lymph nodes.

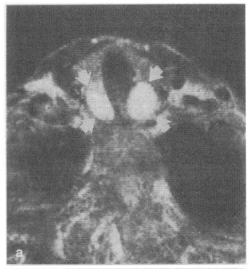

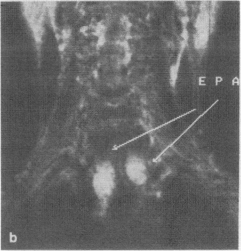

**Fig. 12.8 a, b.** Parathyroid adenomas
**a** Plain axial MRI (SE, 3000/90)
**b** Plain coronal MRI (SE, 3000/90). In the T2-weighted sequence the adenomas display distinct margins and high signal intensity (*arrows*). The signal intensity of the thyroid gland lies between that of adenoma and that of normal muscles. *EPA,* epithelial parathyroid adenoma

For MRI of the lymph nodes the SE mode can be used with long and short TR. After a sagittal survey with short TR, imaging should proceed with continuous axial slices with a thickness of 5–10 mm, using a long (3000/25, 90) and a short (600/25) sequence. Depending on the examination, a short sequence should then be performed in either the sagittal or the coronal plane. Better information about the inner structure and the degree of infiltration of diseased lymph nodes can be obtained using Gd-DTPA-enhanced T1-weighted sequences. Further improvement in the MRI diagnosis of lymph node disease is to be expected from the use of fast imaging techniques.

Normal lymph nodes in the neck measure about 3–10 mm in diameter and have a homogeneous structure on MRI. They can be detected from a diameter of approximately 3–8 mm. As they are often surrounded by fatty tissue rather than compact connective tissue, distinction from blood vessels is possible after contrast medium administration, especially in T1-weighted images.

The advantage of MR over CT and ultrasound is the optimal, exact differentiation of involved from uninvolved lymph nodes and the infiltration of adjoining structures, especially in the retropharyngeal space, where a combination of T1- and T2-weighted sequences is obligatory. Outstanding results are obtained using a mixed T1/T2 sequence, which also allows an interpretation of the internal structure of sized lymph nodes. T1-weighted images permit the distinction of normal and pathological lymph nodes from fatty tissue, but are not as useful for distinguishing nodes from muscle. In T2-weighted sequences, lymph nodes can be distinguished from adjoining muscles by their higher signal intensity.

### 12.6.2 Inflammatory Lesions

Acute inflammations of the lymphatic system (tuberculosis, fever of unknown origin) show increased T1 and T2 on plain images, in contrast to chronic inflammatory processes. Liquefaction and central necrosis of lymph nodes has an MRI appearance resembling that of cystic processes. After administration of Gd-DTPA all inflamed lymph nodes show a significant increase in signal intensity on T1-weighted images (Fig. 12.9). In all patients suffering from viral lymphadenitis the GE technique reveals homogeneous enlarged

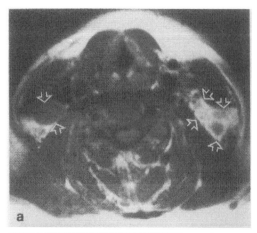

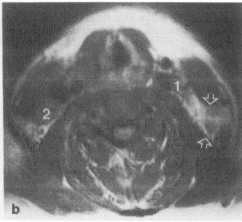

**Fig. 12.9a, b.** Bilateral tuberculous infiltration of the cervical lymph nodes
**a** Plain axial MRI (SE, 500/17). A T1-weighted sequence shows areas of low signal intensity in the neurovascular sheaths (*arrows*). Note the excellent contrast between enlarged lymph nodes and fatty tissue
**b** Axial MRI (SE, 500/17) with Gd-DTPA. After Gd-DTPA administration the tuberculous lymph nodes show homogeneous enhancement. Better delineation of the mass on the right side (2). Tumor/fat contrast is poorer on the left side (1)

lymph nodes of high signal intensity with distinct margins.

### 12.6.3 Malignant Lymphoma

Lymphomas occur preferentially in the lymphatic tissue of the deep neurovascular sheath of the neck and are predominantly bi-

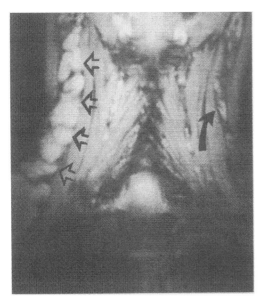

**Fig. 12. 10.** Non-Hodgkin's lymphoma on the right side. Plain coronal MRI (FLASH, 500/17, flip angle 40°). A FLASH sequence shows a chain of enlarged lymph nodes in the right posterior neck (*open arrows*). The nodes increase in size caudally. Note the homogeneity and the distinct margins. On the left, small nonpathologic lymph nodes (*black arrow*)

**Table 12.5.** Classification of regional lymph node metastasis in the neck (all sites except thyroid gland). [From: Hermanek P, Sobin LH (eds) (1987) TNM classification of malignant tumours. Springer-Verlag, Berlin Heidelberg New York]

NX  Regional lymph nodes cannot be assessed

N0  No regional lymph node metastasis

N1  Metastasis in a single ipsilateral lymph node, 3 cm or less in greatest dimension

N2  Metastasis in a single ipsilateral lymph node, more than 3 cm but not more than 6 cm in greatest dimension, or in multiple ipsilateral lymph nodes, none more than 6 cm in greatest dimension, or in bilateral or contralateral lymph nodes, none more than 6 cm in greatest dimension

  N2a Metastasis in a single ipsilateral lymph node, more than 3 cm but not more than 6 cm in greatest dimension

  N2b Metastasis in multiple ipsilateral lymph nodes, none more than 6 cm in greatest dimension

  N2c Metastasis in bilateral or contralateral lymph nodes, none more than 6 cm in greatest dimension

N3  Metastasis in a lymph node more than 6 cm in greatest dimension

Midline nodes are considered ipsilateral nodes.

lateral. In plain T1-weighted sequences they give a low signal, allowing distinction of tumor from fatty tissue, while in T2-weighted sequences tumor can be differentiated from muscle on the basis of its increased T2 (Figs. 12.10, 12.11). After therapy, decreased signal intensity in T1- and T2-weighted sequences indicates response to treatment. After administration of contrast medium there is homogeneous enhancement of the lymphoma.

### 12.6.4 Metastatic Cancer

Most lymph nodes metastases in the neck are from squamous cell carcinoma. The nodes most often involved are those of the jugular and cervicoposterior groups. Both MRI and CT reliably demonstrate pathologic lymph nodes from a diameter of 5–8 mm (Table 12.5). The T1 and T2 relaxation times resemble those of normal lymph nodes, with long T1 and intermediate T2. The S/N is better in T2-weighted sequences. Increases in TR and TE reduce the signal intensity of fatty tissue and increase that of the metastasis, decreasing the contrast and marking the tumor. Metastases that are surrounded by little or no fatty tissue (e.g., those in retrolaryngeal lymph nodes), are distinguished best with a T2 sequence or a mixed T1/T2 sequence. After administration of contrast medium metastatic lymph nodes show an enhancement and an increase of signal intensity in T1-weighted images that may allow even heterogeneous structures to be discerned. A central hypodensity with ring-shaped enhancement on MRI and CT after contrast medium administration may correspond to metastasis of squamous cell carcinoma.

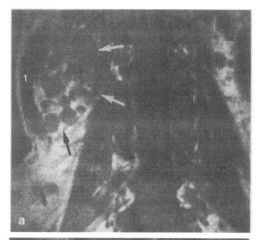

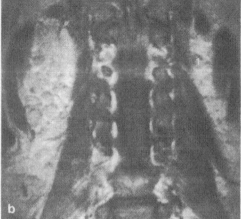

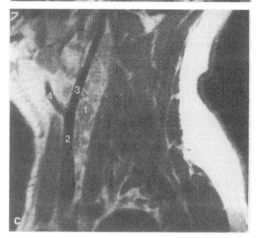

## 12.6.5 Conclusions

The advantage of MRI over CT is the exact differentiation of lymphadenopathies with the possibility of obtaining images in various planes during one examination. New technical developments, such as the GE sequence and the FLASH sequence with a flip angle of 40°, improve visualization. Measurements of T1 and T2 are not sufficient, in themselves, to distinguish between various types of tumors; this can be achieved only on the basis of characteristics known from CT. Signs of lymph node involvement on MR images are (1) central necrosis and (2) transgression of the capsule and infiltration of adjoining structures [4, 5, 6–9, 15, 18, 19, 21–24].

---

MRI diagnosis of lymph nodes offers high sensitivity but only intermediate specifity. The criteria for pathologic lymph nodes are:
1. Diameter exceeding 15 mm
2. Central hypointensity
3. Indistinct margins, infiltration of neighboring structures
4. Fixation and loss of normal anatomic structures
5. More than three lymph nodes in a group

---

◁
**Fig. 12.11 a–c.** Hodgkin's lymphoma stage II in a 35-year-old patient
**a** Coronal MRI (SE, 500/17). A plain T1-weighted sequence shows multiple enlarged lymph nodes in the right posterior area of the neck (*arrows*). Additionally single nodes are detected on the left side. *1*, Sternocleidomastoid muscle
**b** Coronal MRI (SE, 500/17) with Gd-DTPA. After Gd-DTPA administration there is homogeneous enhancement of the involved lymph nodes. Note the lower tumor/fat contrast. Lymph nodes on the opposite side also show high signal intensity (*1*)
**c** Sagittal MRI (SE, 500/17) with Gd-DTPA. In the sagittal plane the relationship of the involved lymph nodes to the carotid artery is exactly demonstrated. *1*, Lymph nodes; *2*, common carotid artery; *3*, internal carotid artery; *4*, external carotid artery

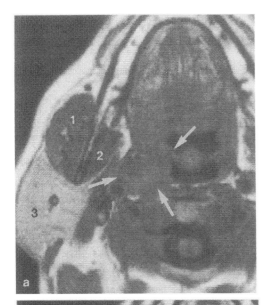

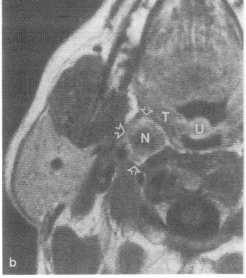

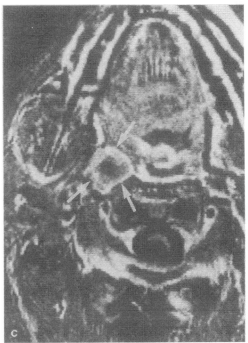

**Fig. 12.12a–c.** Tonsillar tumor with retropharyngeal lymph node involvement

**a** Plain axial MRI (SE, 500/17). A tumor in the tonsillar area narrows the pharyngeal cavity (*arrows*). Normal anatomy of masseter muscle (*1*), pterygoid muscle (*2*), and parotid gland (*3*)

**b** Axial MRI (SE, 500/17) with Gd-DTPA. After the administration of Gd-DTPA a retropharyngeal lymph node (*N, arrows*) can be delineated from the tumor (*T*). The normal uvula (*U*) also shows high signal intensity due to its vascularization

**c** Axial subtraction image. The lymph node (*arrows*) can be exactly delineated from the surrounding tissue and shows central necrosis

## 12.7 Soft Tissue Masses

### 12.7.1 Inflammation, Abscess

In patients suspected of having inflammatory masses in the neck, the main possibilities are abscess, inflammatory or malignant lymphadenopathy, jugular thrombophlebitis, and an infected branchial cyst. It is of great impor-

tance to distinguish abscess, in particular, from any kind of cellulitis, because the treatment is different. The most common site of abscesses is peritonsillar, followed by subcutaneous, submandibular, retropharyngeal, and parapharyngeal locations. An abscess usually appears as a well-defined low-attenuation mass that may contain gas bubbles. The wall is thick and shows enhancement after

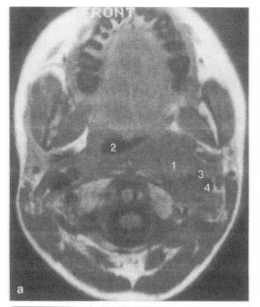

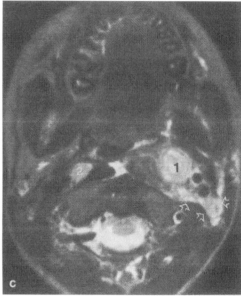

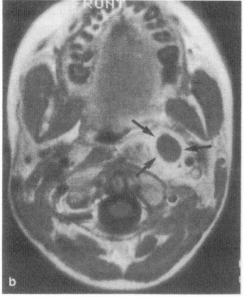

**Fig. 12.13a–c.** Parapharyngeal abscess
**a** Plain axial MRI (SE, 600/17). In the left parapharyngeal space a tumor (*1*), isointense to the muscles of the tongue, displaces the pharyngeal cavity (*2*), internal carotid artery (*3*), and internal jugular vein (*4*)
**b** Axial MRI (SE, 600/17) with Gd-DTPA. An oval inner area shows no contrast medium enhancement (*arrows*), whereas the surrounding tissue shows considerable increase in signal intensity
**c** Plain axial MRI (SE, 3000/90). In the T2-weighted image the abscess shows high signal intensity (*1*) with inflammatory and edematous surrounding (*arrows*). On the opposite side a reactive lymph node (*2*) can be identified

intravenous injection of contrast medium. This finding, however, is nonspecific, and can also be seen with neoplasms and tuberculous adenitis. The MRI appearance of an abscess also depends on its contents: it may exhibit high signal intensity in T2-weighted sequences due to liquid structures, or a shortened T1 relaxation time if fatty tissue prevails. Gas bubbles show no signal at all. Typical signs of an abscess include a medially displaced tonsil and displacement of the uvula toward the opposite side (Fig. 12.13).

### 12.7.2 Cysts

Cysts of the neck can be divided into median or lateral cysts.

The most common median cyst, the thyroglossal duct cyst, can occur anywhere along this duct from the foramen cecum of the tongue to the pyramidal lobe of the thyroid gland. Some 65% of these cysts present as masses in the infrahyoid region, and only 12% occur in the suprasternal area. Thyroglossal duct cysts are typically in the midline with a history of gradually increasing size, often associated with infection.

Lateral cysts typically arise from the second branchial cleft. Because the sternocleidomastoid muscle develops from mesoderm, which is posterior to the last branchial cleft, the external sinuses or fistulas that may be associated with these cysts open anterior to or along this muscle's anterior border.

Many other cystlike lesions, such as cervical thymic cysts, thyroid cysts, hygromas, teratomas, and tracheo-esophageal cysts, may be found in the neck.

On MRI, cysts present high T1 (low signal intensity) and high T2 (high signal intensity) due to a lymphatic or liquid inner structure respectively (Fig. 12.14). MRI with contrast medium proves to be helpful in delineating the exact borders with the surrounding tissue. Images in the coronal plane, to ascertain the extent of the cyst, are obligatory.

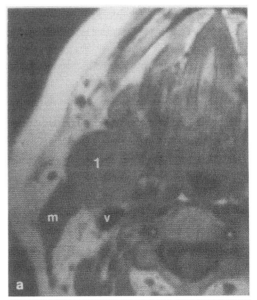
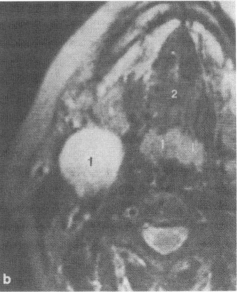

**Fig. 12.14 a, b.** Neck cyst
**a** Plain axial MRI (SE, 550/17). The T1-weighted sequence shows a tumor in the right parapharyngeal space (*1*). It is isointense to the surrounding muscles; thus, no clear delineation is possible. *v* Jugular vein; *m* sternocleidomastoid muscle
**b** Plain axial MRI (SE, 3000/90). The tumor proves to be a liquid-filled cyst showing high signal intensity. Its margins are depicted. The signal intensity of lymphatic tissue (*1*) is higher than that of the normal muscles of the tongue (*2*)

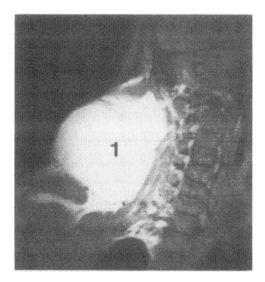

**Fig. 12.15.** Lipoma. Plain coronal MRI (SE, 500/17). A large benign lipoma is visualized in the lateral neck (*1*). The muscles are displaced without signs of infiltration

### 12.7.3 Lipoma

Lipomas are benign tumors of the neck ranging in size from very small to enormous. MRI is helpful in gaining information on the exact extent and morphology.

The tumor is homogeneous and can be delineated clearly from the surrounding structures. In most cases internal septae can be seen (Fig. 12.15). Fatty tissue shows the highest signal intensity in axial T1-weighted images and enables the best visualization of anatomic structures (Fig. 12.16). Another advantage of T1 weighting is the short scan time, an important issue in patients suffering from dyspnea or hoarseness. Additional information on the morphology of the lipoma can be acquired with T2-weighted images by virtue of the high signal intensity of liquid-filled cysts or lymphatic tissue. Images in the coronal plane prove to be very helpful for visualizing the craniocaudal extent of the tumor.

### 12.7.4 Neural Tumors

Neural tumors can occur anywhere along the course of the cranial or cervical nerve roots. Benign neurinomas of the neck arise from the trigeminal, vagus, and hypoglossal nerves (Fig. 12.17). Smooth expansion of a vertebral foramen may be seen secondary to a tumor arising from a cervical nerve root. The morphology of a neural tumor depends on the relative proportions of neural tissue and fibrous elements and on the degree of cystic degeneration.

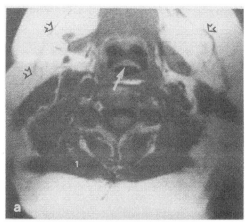

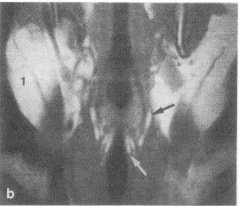

◁
**Fig. 12.16a, b.** Madelung's disease
**a** Plain axial MRI (SE, 550/17). Enlarged fatty tissue at the anterior and posterior parts of the neck. Normal epiglottis (*white arrow*) and paravertebral muscles (*1*). Normal platysma (*open arrows*)
**b** Plain coronal MRI (SE, 550/17). Normal topography of the larynx showing the enlarged neck (*1*), the thyroid cartilage (*black arrow*), and the cricoid cartilage (*white arrow*)

Schwannomas are of epithelial origin and are often malignant (Fig. 12.18). The clinical symptoms of neural tumors vary greatly. Trigeminal neuromas may affect the sensitivity of facial skin and cause pain all over the face, while hypoglossal neurinomas lead to paralysis and atrophy of the tongue. Dysphagia, hoarseness, and headache are very common, but are nonspecific symptoms. A characteristic sign for neuromas on MRI is enormous enhancement after administration of Gd-DTPA. Although malignant nerve sheath tumors like schwannoma are usually infiltrative and heterogeneous in appearance, it is not always possible to distinguish reliably between benign and malignant processes. MRI is very helpful in showing the intraspinal extension of paraspinal neurogenic tumors. Central areas of decreased signal intensity, possibly representing fibrous tissue, have been described in some neurofibromas. Contrast medium increases the sensitivity and specificity of MRI in neural tumors.

Neuroblastoma is a frequent tumor in infants but remains rare in absolute terms and seldom occurs primarily in the neck. The tumor can reach from the skull base and preauricular region to the clavicle and supraclavicular fossa. On MRI the tumor is seen with high signal intensity on T2-weighted and proton density images, and vascular structures, even vascular bifurcations, can be demonstrated. The lesion is isointense with the cervical cord in all sequences, probably because the tumor is composed predominantly of neural tissue. The differential diagnosis is limited to tumors of the carotid or of the poststyloid parapharyngeal space, such as nodal tumors (lymphoma, metastasis), and neurogenic tumors (schwannomas, neurofibromas, and paragangliomas). Although MRI shows the exact relation of the tumor to the surrounding vessels, depicts the vascular structures inside the tumor, and yields exact information on the extent of the lesion, diagnosis must be confirmed by biopsy and measurement of urinary 3-methoxy-4-hydroxymandelic acid or homovanillic acid.

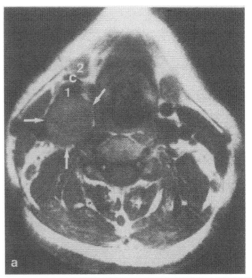

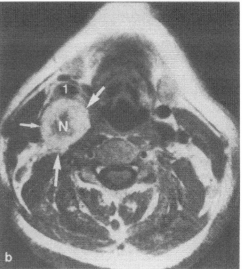

**Fig. 12.17 a, b.** Neurinoma of the vagus nerve
**a** Plain axial MRI (SE, 550/17). In the right parapharyngeal space a large tumor (*arrows*) displaces the internal jugular vein (*1*), submandibular gland (*2*), and internal carotid artery (*C*)
**b** Axial MRI (SE, 550/17) with Gd-DTPA. The tumor shows circular enhancement with a necrotic inner structure (*N*) and clearly defined margins, pointing to a benign lesion. The retropharyngeal topography and the characteristic contrast medium enhancement prove that the lesion is a neurinoma

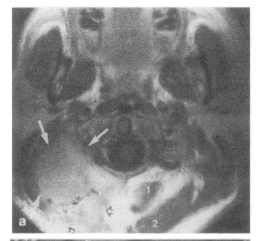

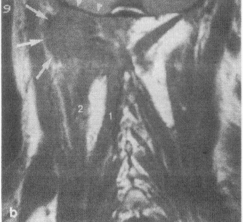

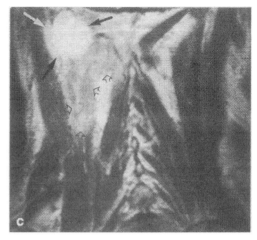

**Fig. 12.18a–c.** Malignant Schwannoma
**a** Axial MRI (SE, 550/17) with Gd-DTPA. Tumor of intermediate signal intensity displacing the posterior muscles of the neck (*white arrows*). Medially an area of high contrast medium enhancement because of lymphangiosis and edema is visualized (*open arrows*) *1*, Posterior rectus capitis muscle; *2*, semispinalis capitis muscle (2)
**b** Plain coronal MRI (SE, 550/17). In a T1-weighted sequence the tumor is isointense to the surrounding muscles and the evaluation of infiltration is not possible. The occipital bone is not eroded (*arrowheads*)
**c** Coronal MRI (SE, 550/17) with Gd-DTPA. After Gd-DTPA administration differentiation of a solid tumor (*solid arrows*) and infiltrations reaching from the skull base to the supraclavicular muscles (*open arrows*) is possible

## 12.7.5 Rhabdomyoma, Rhabdomyosarcoma

Rhabdomyoma is one of the rarest types of tumor known in humans. The majority of these tumors are of cardiac origin, but the next most common site is the head and neck. Clinical symptoms are respiratory distress, dysphagia, the feeling of a lump in the throat and hoarseness, while fever, detectable cervical lymph nodes, and weight loss are often absent. Adult rhabdomyomas probably arise from the musculature of the third and fourth branchial arches. They are found most commonly in middle age, with a male to female ratio of 4:1. On MRI a solid structure with distinct margins and relatively high contrast medium enhancement is evident; however, the histologic diagnosis is only revealed by biopsy.

Malignant rhabdomyosarcoma is more common than its benign counterpart. In most cases it does not originate in malignant transformation of a rhabdomyoma, but arises primarily. On MRI the malignancy of the tumor can be recognized by its spreading and asymmetric margins with inhomogeneous contrast medium enhancement, but of course biopsy is needed for histologic verification.

### 12.7.6 Chordoma

Although some 85% of chordomas occur in the skull base and sacrococcygeal area, primary cervical chordomas are sometimes found. MRI reveals vertebral body destruction along with an associated soft tissue mass, the predominant part of which is located anterior or lateral to the spinal column. Some chordomas contain solitary or multiple septated areas of low attenuation. The soft tissue component is commonly contained within a fibrous pseudocapsule, which contributes to the MRI finding of a distinct margin. Areas of amorphous calcification, scattered sparsely and randomly within the tumor, are noted in some cases. The clinical symptoms are variable and nonspecific. On MRI, chordomas have lower signal intensity than gray matter on T1-weighted images and display the same intensity as cerebrospinal fluid on T2-weighted images. They show a certain, but not characteristic, contrast medium uptake.

### 12.7.7 Others

Lymphoceles show high signal intensity in T2-weighted sequences due to their liquid or lymphatic contents. Therefore, it is sometimes difficult to distinguish a lymphocele from a laryngocele or liquid-filled cyst. Chondroma of the cricoid, arytenoid, or cricoid cartilage, hamartoma, and teratoma may be found, but have no characteristic appearance on MRI.

### 12.7.8 Conclusions

For all soft tissue lesions MRI is the imaging modality that yields the best information with respect to the extent and infiltrative nature of the tumor due to its excellent soft tissue contrast (Table 12.6). For precise histologic diagnosis biopsy is often mandatory.

**Table 12.6.** Comparison of plain and contrast-enhanced MRI and value of MRI relative to CT in the diagnosis of lesions of lymph nodes, blood vessels and soft tissues

|  | Plain MRI | MRI with Gd-DTPA | MRI vs CT |
|---|---|---|---|
| *Lymph nodes* | | | |
| Primary lymphoma | 2 | 3 | + |
| Secondary infiltration | 2 | 3 | + |
| Inflammatory lesions | 2 | 3 | = |
| *Soft tissues* | | | |
| Cyst | 2 | 3 | + |
| Lipoma | 3 | 3 | = |
| Neurinoma | 2 | 3 | + |
| Mesenchymal lesions | 2 | 3 | + |
| *Vessels* | | | |
| Glomus caroticum tumor | 2 | 3 | + |
| Angioma | 3 | 3 | + |
| Hemangioma | 3 | 3 | + |
| Arteriovenous shunt | 2 | 3 | + |
| Aberrant vessels | 2 | 3 | + |

Visualization: *1*, adequate; *2*, good; *3*, optimal.

Follow-up
*T1-weighted sequence*
Scar, tumor, and muscle isointense

*T2-weighted sequence*
Scar and tumor show higher signal intensity than muscle

*T1-weighted sequence with Gd-DTPA*
Scar: no significant enhancement
Tumor: considerable enhancement

---

*Cervical soft tissue lesions*
Abscesses have a typical MRI appearance but differential diagnosis of other inflammatory lesions is more difficult. Median and lateral neck cysts can be identified on the basis of their prolonged T1 and T2 relaxation times. The combination of short T1 and long T2 is a sure sign of a lipoma. The topography and internal structure of the mass are decisive in the diagnosis of neural lesions. Careful analysis of the MRI appearance and the clinical findings should point to other rare lesions of the neck.
A major application of MRI is checking the response to surgery, radiotherapy, or chemotherapy. The most important criterion is the uptake of contrast medium by neighboring structures.

## 12.8 Vascular Lesions

### 12.8.1 Glomus Tumor

Glomus tumors arise from paraganglia, which are found at various sites in the human body. Precapillary arteriovenous shunts and nonchromaffin cells are characteristic histologic features of these tumors. Although glomus tissue is found at different locations, its histology and functions are always the same. In the literatur glomus tumors are also referred to as chemodectomas and paragangliomas. They are characterized by their slow progression and their mostly benign, nonmetastatic growth.

We have found no instances of metastatic spread in our patients, but it has been described in the literature. CT with thin slices and contrast enhancement has hitherto been the method of choice for diagnosis of glomus tumors and their growth in the skull base and neck. Before the introduction of CT the preoperative diagnosis of glomus tumors had been based on selective angiography. However, the diagnosis of small tumors, especially at the glomus caroticum, proves difficult with CT, especially regarding differentiation from lymph nodes and other lesions.

The two principal advantages of MRI over CT for the diagnosis of lesions in the neck and adjacent structures are its superb soft tissue contrast and the flow phenomenon [1, 2]. Generally, in the conventional SE techniques flowing blood has a low signal intensity; therefore, the lumina of vessels are easily distinguished from surrounding tissue. By using thin slices and individually adapted head or surface coils with high S/N, the carotid artery, the superior and inferior jugular bulb, and the jugular vein are easily identified on nonenhanced MRI. MRI enables demonstration of smaller vessels within the tumor.

The advantages of noninvasive investigation are forfeited when the contrast medium Gd-DTPA is used; however, MRI with Gd-DTPA is considerably less invasive than angiography. The paramagnetic contrast medium helps to differentiate inflammatory lesions from tumors (Figs. 12.19, 12.20). In our series, inflammatory lesions showed significantly lower enhancement by Gd-DTPA than did tumors. Gd-DTPA is even more important in detecting tumors of the glomus with a diameter of 5 mm or less.

As in dynamic CT, it is possible to evaluate the pattern of enhancement over time with the fast imaging technique, using short exposure sequences (GE sequences) repeated in a standardized pattern. Typically, paragangliomas show uptake starting immediately after injection of the paramagnetic contrast medium and decreasing gradually until the end of measurement at 7 min. Peak enhancement is reached after approximately 150 s. This enhancement/time pattern with the washout

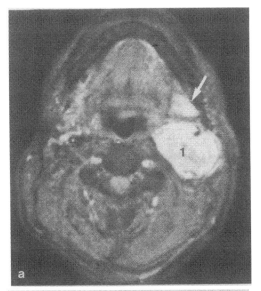

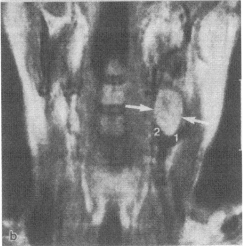

effect helps to differentiate paragangliomas from meningiomas and neurinomas (Fig. 12.21).

MRI of the glomus caroticum offers the same advantages described for glomus tumors of the skull base. Because glomus caroticum lesions may be difficult to detect clinically, an imaging study takes on particular importance. MRI is able to define the position of the common, external, and internal carotid arteries, especially when the MR angiography technique is used. Glomus caroticum tumors 5 mm in diameter can be identified by MRI, while CT with iodinated contrast medium only allows detection of glomus tumors greater than 8 mm in diameter.

Additionally, the new 3D reconstruction technique accurately demonstrates vascular lesions of the neck in various projections. The lower image quality compared with the SE technique yields no additional radiologic information, but by virtue of acquiring thin slices and offering the possibility of transforming the examination data into any required plane, this technique has important advantages for the planning of surgery.

**Fig. 12.19 a, b.** Glomus caroticum tumor
**a** Axial MRI (FLASH, 30/12, flip angle 40°) with Gd-DTPA. The tumor (*1*) is located around the left carotid artery and shows marked, inhomogeneous contrast-medium enhancement. The submandibular gland (*arrow*) can be differentiated from the solid tumor
**b** Coronal MRI (SE, 1600/30). Exact visualization of the tumor (*arrows*) in the bifurcation of the external (*1*) and the internal (*2*) carotid artery

▷

**Fig. 12.20.** Glomus caroticum tumor. Plain coronal MRI (SE, 1600/28). The craniocaudal extension of the tumor is shown. The common carotid artery (*c*) flowing into the tumor (*1*) is visualized

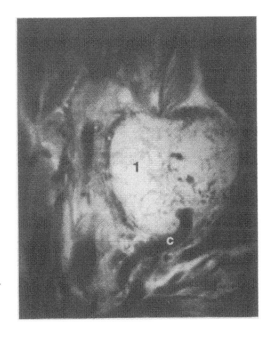

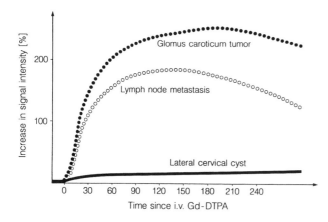

**Fig. 12.21.** MR contrast medium enhancement of different lesions in the neck

In conclusion, our experience has shown the advantages of MRI in patients with suspected carotid and jugular paragangliomas. For the detection of glomus tumors in the head and neck, the use of contrast-enhanced MRI including short sequences and a dynamic technique is recommended.

### 12.8.2 Hemangioma

Hemangiomas of the neck have an MRI appearance similar to that of hemangiomas in other parts of the body. On T2-weighted images, they have very high signal intensity. Areas of low signal intensity may be seen secondary to phleboliths or fibrosis, and feeding or draining vessels may also be seen as serpiginous areas of low intensity. In comparison, neck cysts show lower signal intensity in T1-weighted sequences reflecting the long T1 of fluids. In some circumstances complicated neck cysts may mimic hemangiomas due to varying appearance in different sequences.

## 12.9 Value of MRI and Diagnostic Strategy

Magnetic resonance imaging of the neck combines the advantages of CT and ultrasound. In aerodigestive tract tumors, MRI can take the place of CT in assessing the deep extension of mucosal lesions [10, 16, 17, 20, 23].

In evaluating tumors of the thyroid and parathyroid glands, neither MRI nor CT can match the low cost, availability, ease of use, and overall effectiveness of ultrasound. When nodal metastases are suspected, the full cross-sectional field of view of MRI has advantages similar to those established for CT [12–14]. Intrathoracic extension of goiters or ectopic parathyroid glands can be evaluated better by MR due to its superior delineation of blood vessels and excellent tumor/fat contrast. Suspected adenopathy or vascular pathology in the thoracic inlet is also well delineated by MRI.

Due to the number of different soft tissue lesions in this area, the clinical symptoms are not characteristic. However, in every case diagnostic investigation should ensue. The most common complaints are dysphagia, dyspnea, sore throat, and the feeling of a lump in the neck. Careful history taking, palpation, and endoscopy seem to be the most important steps in arriving at an exact diagnosis. Additional information is conveyed by imaging techniques, above all ultrasound, and by endoscopy. Often the symptoms can be explained by neural or vascular problems and MRI reveals no further information. For tumors, MRI is a very helpful diagnostic tool by virtue of its high soft tissue contrast and its capacity to produce multiplanar images. However, in many cases MRI can merely describe the morphology of a process, and only pathologic examination reveals the precise diagnosis (Fig. 12.22).

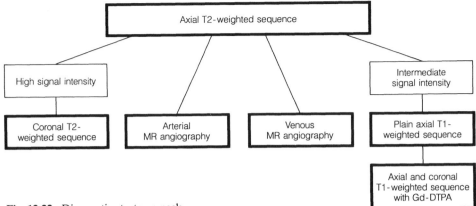

**Fig. 12.22.** Diagnostic strategy: neck

With reduction of motion artifacts, faster scan times, and the introduction of MR spectroscopy, MRI has now partially replaced CT as the imaging modality of choice in the neck.

## References

1. Ackermann JJH, Grove TH, Wong GG, Gadian DG, Radda GK (1980) Mapping of metabolites in whole animals by 31P-NMR using surface coils. Nature 283:167–170
2. Bauer M, Obermüller H, Vogl T, Lissner T (1984) MR bei zerebraler alveolärer Echinokokkose. Digitale Bilddiagn 4:S 129–131
3. Bauer WM, Baierl P, Vogl T, Obermüller H (1985) Contrast-enhancement in intercranial tumors – a comparison of CT and MR. Radiology 157 (P):126
4. Beimert U, Grevers G, Vogl T (1991) Differentialdiagnostische Kriterien bei der Dignitätsbeurteilung zervikaler Schwellungen. Otorhinolaryngol (in press)
5. Beimert U, Grevers G, Vogl T (1989) Differentialdiagnose zervikaler Schwellungen: Thrombose der Vena subclavia. HNO-Information 1:98
6. Bruneton JN, Normand F, Balu-Maestro C, Kerboul P, Santini N, Thyss A, Schneider M (1987) Lymphomatous superficial lymph nodes. US-detection. Radiology 165:233
7. Dillon WP (1986) Applications of magnetic resonance imaging to the head and neck. Semin US CT MR 7:202
8. Dillon WP (1986) Magnetic resonance imaging of head and neck tumors. Cardiovasc Intervent Radiol 8:275
9. Dooms GC, Hricak H, Moseley ME, Bottles K, Fisher MR, Higgins CB (1985) Characterization of lymphadenopathy by magnetic resonance relaxation times: preliminary results. Radiology 155:691
10. Friedmann M, Shelton VK, Mafee MF, Bellity P, Grybauskas V, Skolnik E (1985) Metastatic neck disease, evaluation by computed tomography. Radiology 155:555
11. Glazer HS, Niemeyer JH, Balfe DM et al. (1986) Neck neoplasms: MR imaging part 2. Radiology 160:349–354
12. Grodd W, Schmitt WGH (1983) Protonenrelaxaionsverhalten menschlicher und tierischer Gewebe Invitro, Änderungen bei Autolyse und Fixierung. ROFO 139/9:233–240
13. Haels J, Lenarz T, Gademann G, Kober B, Mende U (1986) Kernspintomographie in der Diagnostik von Kopf- und Halstumoren. Laryngol Rhinol Otol (Stuttg) 65:180–186
14. Hagemann J, Witt CP, Jend-Rossmann R, Hörmann L, Jend HH, Bücheler E (1983) Wertigkeit der Computertomographie bei Tumoren des Epi- und Oropharynx. ROFO 139:373–378
15. Hajek PC, Salomonowitz E, Türk R, Tscholakoff D, Kumpan W, Czernbirch H (1986) Lymph nodes of the neck, evaluation with US. Radiology 158:739–742
16. Jinkins JR (1987) Computed tomography of the cranio-cervical lymphatic system: anatomical and functional considerations. Neuroradiology 29:317
17. Lee YY, Van Tassel P, Nauert C, North LB, Jing BS (1987) Lymphomas of head and neck. CT findings at initial presentation. AJR 149:575
18. Lufkin RB, Hanafee WN (1985) Application of surface coils to MR anatomy of the larynx. AJR 145(9):483–485
19. McCunniff AJ, Raben M (1986) Metastatic carcinoma of the neck from an unknown primary. Int J Radiat Oncol Biol Phys 12:1849
20. Reede DL, Bergeron RT (1985) Cervical tuberculous adenoids: CT manifestations. Radiology 154:701

21. Schedel H, Vogl T, Hahn D, Mees K, Peer F, Lissner J (1988) Erkrankungen des lymphatischen Systems im Kopf-Hals-Bereich. Vergleichsstudie KST und CT. Digitale Bilddiagn 8:158–167

22. Som PM (1987) Lymph nodes of the neck. Radiology 165:593

23. Stark DD, Moss AA, Gamsu G, Clark OH, Gooding GA, Webb WR (1983) Magnetic resonance imaging of the neck II. Pathological findings. Radiology 150:455–461

24. Steinbrich W, Beyer D, Mödder U (1985) Möglichkeiten der Lymphomdiagnostik mit der MR-Tomographie. Ein Vergleich mit anderen bildgebenden Verfahren. Radiology 25:199

25. Vogl T (1989) Erkrankungen des Aerodigestivtraktes und der Halsweichteile: Vergleich MRI und CT. Röntgenblätter 42:199–209

26. Vogl T, Mees K (1989) Bildgebende Verfahren: Computertomographie und Kernspintomographie des Gesichtsschädels und des Halses. Otorhinolaryngology [Suppl]:1–40

27. Vogl T, Hefele B, Hahn D, zur Nieden J, Mühlig H-P (1986) Ergebnisse einer Vergleichsstudie von MR, CT und Sonographie bei Patienten mit primärem Hyperparathyreoidismus. ROFO 145(2):39–44

28. Vogl T, Mühlig H-P, zur Nieden J, Moser E, Spelsberg F (1986) KST zur Diagnostik von Erkrankungen der Schilddrüse und der Nebenschilddrüsen. Therapiewoche 46:4740–4744

29. Vogl T (1992) Hypopharynx, larynx, parathyroid and neck. Eds. Stark/Bradley. Mosby, St. Louis/MO, pp 1318–1358

# 13 Temporomandibular Joint

A dense fibrocartilaginous structure, the articular disk, separates the mandibular condyle from the mandibular fossa of the temporal bone. The disk is fixed to the medial and lateral aspect of the mandibular condyle. Because some fibers of the lateral pterygoid muscle insert into the anterior margin of the disk, it moves anteriorly during opening of the mouth. Several stabilizing structures exist, such as the lateral temporomandibular ligament, which prevents subluxation of the joint during extreme opening.

MRI as screening for diseases of the temporomandibular joint (TMJ) has to be accompanied by exhaustive clinical examination in order to exploit the excellent diagnostic potential of the method [5, 7, 26].

## 13.1 Clinical Approach

A major part of the population (particularly women) suffers from craniomandibular pain and dysfunction. Often there is a classical triad of symptoms: pain and tenderness in the joint and the muscles of mastication, joint noise, and changed mobility of the mandible. These problems may occur for a variety of reasons, but commonly TMJ disorders are to blame. Etiologic factors are trauma, bruxism, stress, and occlusal abnormalities.

The different parts of the stomatognathic system, particularly the occlusion of teeth, the muscles of mastication, and the TMJ, interact closely with each other and with the psyche of the patient. This complicates the diagnosis and leeds to a wide range of problems. Clinical methods are used in combination with diagnostic tools such as imaging techniques to discover what structures are involved.

Adaptive structural changes of the TMJ are a common finding and not necessarily connected with pain. This process, called remodeling, may, however, develop into a degenerative disease. In its transitional stage no differentiation is possible.

The aim of the clinical examination is the distinction of articular from muscular disorders. MRI of the TMJ should be carried out if structural changes (especially internal derangement) are suspected. Acute disorders as well as chronic, unsuccessfully treated problems may indicate MRI. Within the framework of therapy planning the major indication for MRI is verification of the diagnosis to prevent iatrogenic lesions of the TMJ. During therapy MRI may be necessary to check treatment, to depict causes of complications, and to find out the reasons for any failure of treatment.

Because of the structural diversity of the TMJ the effective application of imaging procedures requires specific analysis of the problem. The observed changes of the joint can be judged only with regard to the clinical findings. Exact elucidation of the history of the presenting illness is important in order to reveal any existing pathologic changes in the neighborhood of the joint that might give rise to similar symptoms. The causes for craniomandibular pain embrace a variety of conditions, such as central nervous system disease and tumors, intracranial vascular disorders, and cervical neuritis. It is particularly important that all observations on the part of the patient regarding pain, joint noise, and changes of mobility of the lower jaw are recorded.

The joint itself, the masticatory muscles, and the occlusal situation are the major points of interest during clinical examination. The range and disturbance of mandibular mobility are established. The regularity of condyle movement is checked by the ensuing palpation and auscultation of the joint area. Clicking and crepitus may be symptoms of internal derangement and degenerative changes, but are not necessarily idiopathic. Lateral joint tenderness is a sign of a capsular affliction, dorsal tenderness a sign of retrodiskal tissue inflammation. Manual manipulation of the lower jaw may reveal joint surface irregularities.

Tenderness of masticatory muscles and cervical muscle pain are of importance.

The occlusal surfaces have to be checked for indications of bruxism and other irregularities. Discrepancies in occlusion lead to pathologic movement patterns, which result in muscle pain and joint overload.

There are several methods for the therapy of TMJ problems. The most common are intraoral splint therapy, medical management, and surgery. Splint therapy aims to change the position of the mandible. An acutely displaced articular disk may be repositioned with the help of a protrusive splint. Flat splints serve to relieve a damaged condyle in chronic disorders. There are various methods of surgery to replace and fix a displaced meniscus (disc plication), remove damaged tissue, and replace joint structures with alloplastic implants. Late results lead to a restrictive use of these methods [5, 7, 10, 11, 16].

## 13.2 Examination Technique

Modern MRI of the temporomandibular joint has developed from static joint imaging with the mouth closed and open to dynamic functional analysis. Cine techniques and threedimensional imaging methods improve the diagnostic possibilities to better understand TMJ-disease.

The use of specially designed surface coils is essential for exact imaging of the TMJ. Depending on the type of MR scanner, different surface coil techniques are in use. In our experience the best diagnostic information is obtained with a laterally placed surface coil in a supine patient. Further improvement is achieved via the use of a double TMJ coil which allows the simultaneous imaging of both sides.

T1-weighted SE sequences are routinely recommended for the interpretation of intraarticular relations and disk morphology. This high-resolution technique (600/15) is especially useful for the diagnosis of diskopathy with disk perforation or degenerative changes (Table 13.1) [3, 4, 12, 14, 21, 26].

T2-weighted SE sequences are used for the diagnosis of fluid in the joint space of either

**Table 13.1.** The applications of MRI techniques in diagnostic examination of the TMJ

| SE technique | T1 weighted | Visualization of intraarticular situation | – Diskopathy (perforation, displacement)<br>– Degenerative changes of smooth tissues (bilaminar zone)<br>– Pre-/postoperative status |
|---|---|---|---|
| | T2 weighted | Visualization of fluid in joint space (serous/hematogeneous) | – Arthritis |
| Cine technique | 2D FISP | Functional analysis of coordinated lower joint motion | – Analysis of motion<br>– Control of splint therapy<br>– Arthrosis<br>– Protrusive movement of lower joint<br>– Handicapped patient<br>– Extreme mouth opening |
| 3D technique | 3D FISP, MPRAGE | Topographic visualization of TMJ correlated with other structures of head | – Cystic and tumorous process<br>– Dislocated fractures of the mandible (collum, intracapsular)<br>– Pre-/postoperative status |

posttraumatic or inflammatory origin [13, 15, 24, 25].

Cine techniques with GE sequences (300/15) allow the visualization of the disk-condyle complex in relation to the surrounding structures during each phase of mouth opening. Due to the very short examination time (1 min 19 s) the patient can tolerate extreme positions of the lower jaw such as maximum opening, protruding mandible, or posterior positions of the condyle. These techniques are extremely useful for the examination of handicapped or old patients or patients with very intense pain [1, 4, 18, 24, 27]. The indications for cine techniques are the clinical interpretation of coordinated mandibular movements, the functional diagnosis of torn disk, arthrosis with remodeling effects, and checking the results of treatment using stabilizing or repositioning splints. Three-dimensional MRI techniques (3D FISP, MPRAGE) are used in the diagnosis of tumorous or cystic processes, the assessment of pre- and postoperative status, and the examination of dislocated fractures of the mandible [6, 29] (see Fig. 13.1).

The principal movement of the lower jaw is in the sagittal plane, so this is the most important plane for MRI of the TMJ. For interpretation of asymmetric changes of the TMJ, both joints have to be examined. In order to diagnose lateroposition of the disk or partial disk displacement, coronal images of the TMJ have to be obtained.

## 13.3  Topographic Relations

The TMJ is a synovial (diarthrodial) articulation. It consists of three articulating components: the mandibular condyle, the articulating portion of the squamous part of the temporal bone, and, between them, the articular disk. Its unique features include the fibrocartilaginous articulating surfaces, the exclusively bilateral action, the complexity of the joint, and the definite end point of closure [19]. The crucial importance of the condition of the articular disk for TMJ disorders, in combination with the concealed location of the joint at

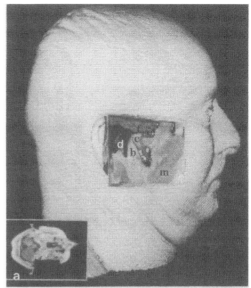

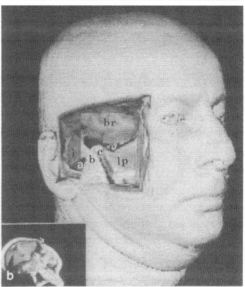

Fig. 13.1 a, b. Topographic relations of TMJ and surrounding structures in a 49-year-old man: joint compression, no visible joint space and disk
a Lateral view, 3D MPRAGE
b Frontolateral view, 3D MPRAGE. *a*, External auditory canal; *b*, retromandibular space; *br*, cerebrum; *c*, condyle; *d*, mastoid; *e*, articular eminence (tubercle); *f*, mandibular fossa; *i*, cerebellum; *lp*, lateral pterygoid muscle; *m*, medial pterygoid muscle

the base of the skull, makes MRI the procedure of choice for visualization of TMJ structures (Table 13.2).

### 13.3.1 Mandibular Condyle

The condyle is oriented perpendicular to the ramus of the mandible (Fig. 13.2). Since the rami diverge posteriorly, the longitudinal axes of the condyles form an angle of about 150° in the horizontal plane. For radiographic examinations it is important to measure this value in each individual patient in order to be sure of obtaining true sagittal and coronal images. There is wide interindividual variation in length (13–25 mm) and breadth (5.5–16 mm) of the condyle. The average length is about 20 mm in the mediolateral and 10 mm in the anteroposterior direction [20]. The upper outline of the condyle is convex in two thirds of cases and flat in a further one fourth [2]. White fibrocartilage lines the articular surfaces of the condyle and the temporal bone.

### 13.3.2 Mandibular Fossa

The anterior part of the mandibular fossa and the articular tubercle form the articulating surface of the temporal bone, the second component of the joint (Fig. 13.2). The posterior part of the mandibular fossa is extracapsular. The articulating surface of the temporal bone is about 3 times bigger in the anteroposterior direction and slightly wider mediolaterally than that of the condyle. At birth the articular surface is almost flat, but in the course of postnatal development the articular slope of the condyle becomes steeper, creating a definitely S-shaped profile in the sagittal plane. In the coronal plane, the articular fossa and the articular tubercle – the latter due to adaptive processes of remodelling – are concave. As an adaption to articular function, the articular tissue is approximately 6 times thicker at the crest of the articular tubercle than in the roof of the fossa [2, 11, 30].

**Table 13.2.** Checklist: temporomandibular joint

| | |
|---|---|
| *Condyle-disk complex* | |
| Mouth closed: | Normal position |
| | Anterior displacement of disk |
| | – partial |
| | – complete |
| | With/without posterior dislocation of condyle |
| Mouth open: | Normal position with both rotation and translation of condyle |
| | Reduction or not of disk displacement |
| | Posterior or eccentric displacement of disk |
| | Restricted translation of disk but translation of condyle |
| | Restricted translation of disk and condyle |
| | Hypermobility of condyle |

| | |
|---|---|
| *Enlarged upper or lower compartment of joint space caused by fluid* | |
| *Disk* | Signal intensity |
| | Shape/dimensions |
| | Comparison of shape with mouth closed/open |
| *Retrodiskal tissue* | Signal intensity (inflammatory disease) |
| | Perforation |
| *Condyle* | Shape |
| | Surface |
| | Signal intensity (avascular necrosis) |
| *Temporal bone* | Steepness of articular tubercle |
| | Attached tissue (gap between disk and bone) |
| | Degenerative lesions |
| *Other structures* | Lateral pterygoid muscle |
| | Tumors |

### 13.3.3 Articular Disk

The third component of the TMJ is the articular disk, a connective tissue sheet which compensates the incongruities of the condyle and the mandibular fossa or articular tubercle. It is an oval plate of dense fibrous tissue (like the other articulating surfaces in this joint) which divides the joint cavity completely into an upper and a lower compartment. The articular disk is usually neither vascularized nor inner-

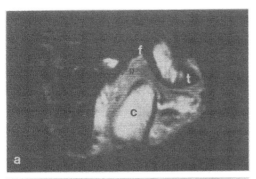

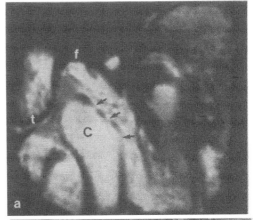

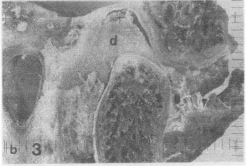

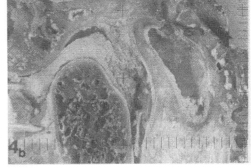

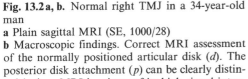

**Fig. 13.2a, b.** Normal right TMJ in a 34-year-old man
**a** Plain sagittal MRI (SE, 1000/28)
**b** Macroscopic findings. Correct MRI assessment of the normally positioned articular disk (*d*). The posterior disk attachment (*p*) can be clearly distinguished on MRI by virtue of its high signal intensity. The cortical bone of the condyle (*c*), the articular tubercle (*t*), and the mandibular fossa (*f*) is delineated by the surrounding tissue

**Fig. 13.3a, b.** Left TMJ of the same patient
**a** Plain sagittal MRI (SE, 1000/28)
**b** Macroscopic findings. Correct demarcation of the soft tissue similar to imaging of right joint. Cortical bone may be misinterpreted due to partial volume artifacts (*arrows*). The condyle (*C*), articular tubercle (*t*), and mandibular fossa (*f*) are indicated

vated. Two thick zones, the posterior and the anterior band, and an intervening thinner zone can be distinguished. The posterior band, with a maximum thickness of about 3 mm, is generally larger than the anterior band. Because of the resulting double convex profile the condyle keeps the disk in the physiologically correct position. The disk, covering the condyle like a tight-fitting cap [11], is fixed rigidly to the condylar neck in the mediolateral direction and is attached to the joint capsule anteriorly, contiguous with the superior head of the lateral pterygoid muscle.

On MRI, the meniscus usually can be distinguished clearly from the surrounding tissue by virtue of its low signal intensity (Figs. 13.2, 13.3). A highly vascularized and well-innervated tissue called the bilaminar zone (or retrodiskal pad) builds the posterior attachment of the disk (Fig. 13.4). The upper part is attached to the posterior portion of the mandibular fossa, the lower part to the condyle. Sometimes small linear structures of low signal intensity, representing elastic tissue fibers, are visible within the posterior attachment. The disk forms a movable socket, which allows the different forms of condyle motion,

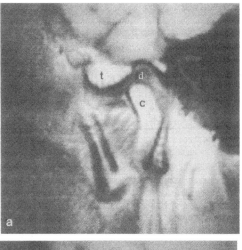

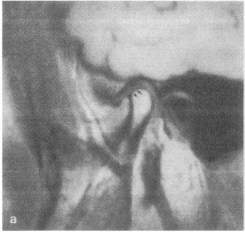

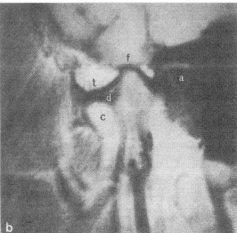

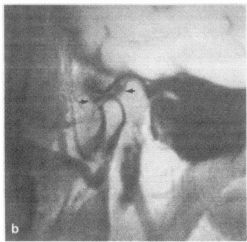

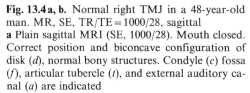

**Fig. 13.4 a, b.** Normal right TMJ in a 48-year-old man. MR, SE, TR/TE = 1000/28, sagittal
**a** Plain sagittal MRI (SE, 1000/28). Mouth closed. Correct position and biconcave configuration of disk (*d*), normal bony structures. Condyle (*c*) fossa (*f*), articular tubercle (*t*), and external auditory canal (*a*) are indicated
**b** Plain sagittal MRI (SE, 1000/28). Mouth open (interincisal distance 25 mm). Physiological translation of disk (*d*) and condyle (*c*) to apex of articular tubercle (*t*)

**Fig. 13.5 a, b.** Right TMJ in a 30-year-old woman: restricted movement of articular disk
**a** Plain sagittal MRI (SE, 1000/28). Mouth closed. Slightly flattened surface (*arrows*) and slightly dorsal position of the condyle, normal biconcave configuration and position of the disk
**b** Plain sagittal MRI (SE, 1000/28). Mouth open (interincisal distance 25 mm). Restricted anterior movement of the disk (*arrows*) with normal anterior mobility of the flattened condyle. The high mobility in the lower joint space is an adaptive functional alteration resulting from adhesions between the disk and the temporal bone

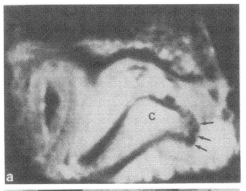

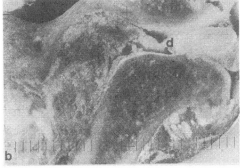

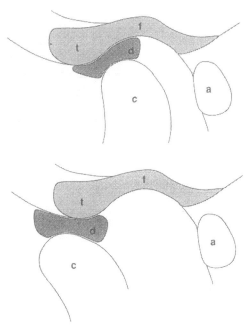

**Fig. 13.6 a, b.** Right TMJ in a 50-year-old man
**a** Plain sagittal MRI (SE, 1000/28)
**b** Macroscopic findings. Correct demarcation of bony changes. The prominent exostosis (*arrows*) of the condyle (*C*) is shown clearly on MRI. Disk (*d*)

**Fig. 13.7 a, b.** Diagram showing the normal topographic relations of the TMJ structures with the mouth closed (**a**) and open (**b**). *c,* condyle; *d,* disk, *t,* tubercle; *f,* mandibular fossa; *a,* auditory canal

such as gliding, spinning, rolling, and angulation.

The fibrous capsule encloses the joint like a downward-directed cone. It is attached anteriorly in front of the highest prominence of the articular tubercle, posteriorly to the tip and the anterior surface of the postglenoid process, and mediolaterally to the rim of the mandibular fossa. It reaches down to the mandibular neck.

In addition to the postnatal development there are substantial structural changes of fully developed joints in adult life (Fig. 13.5 a, b). In autopsy studies, 40% of the joints in the 20–39 age group and about 60% of the joints in the group aged 40 years and over showed remarkable changes in shape (Fig. 13.6). This "remodeling," defined as an adaptive, proliferative process of the subarticular tissue layers can be regarded as normal. In contrast,

"arthrosis" is defined as destruction of the articular surface layer [2, 9, 20].

### 13.3.4 Mandibular Movement

There are four main possibilities for mandibular movement with reference to the position of centric occlusion of the teeth: retrusion, 0–2 mm; protrusion, 7–10 mm; opening, 40–60 mm; and laterotrusion, 10–15 mm [7]. When the mouth is being opened, both mandibular condyles rotate below the disk and also move anteriorly with the disk. The superior and inferior heads of the lateral pterygoid muscle are active (Fig. 13.7 a, b). This muscle, which is depicted clearly in sagittal MRI, plays an important role in many theories on the pathogenesis of TMJ dysfunction [7]. The lateral pterygoid muscle has an upper and a lower belly, separated by fat planes with high signal intensity surrounding their fascial coverings [12, 14].

At maximum opening the condyle is slightly anterior to the crest of the tubercle. When the mouth closes, the retraction of the disk is achieved by the elastic tissue fibers in the bilaminar zone and the congruence in shape of condyle and disk. The masseter, temporal, and medial pterygoid muscles produce the elevation of the mandible.

Protrusion of the mandible is a result of contraction of the lateral and medial pterygoid muscles. Retraction of the condyle is effected by activation of the posterior fibers of the temporal muscle, assisted by middle and deep parts of the masseter, digastric, and geniohyoid muscles.

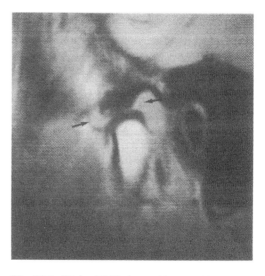

**Fig. 13.8.** Right TMJ in a 42-year-old woman: acute hemarthrosis. Plain sagittal MRI (SE, 1000/ 27). The disk is pressed tightly against the surface of the condyle because of liquid in the upper joint space (*arrows*). During puncture 5 ml of blood could be aspirated. Clinical findings were malocclusion (anterior position of the condyle) and suspected posterior disk displacement

## 13.4 MRI and Clinical Findings

### 13.4.1 Traumatic Injuries

Traumatic injuries can result from external trauma (e.g., a blow) and from excessive or prolonged opening of the mouth (e.g., in the course of dental treatment). They include fractures, dislocation of the condyle, soft tissue damage, hemarthrosis, serous joint effusion, perforation of the disk, and lesions of the joint surfaces. During the healing process, proliferative or regressive remodeling of the joint surfaces may occur and lead to adhesions and exostoses. These joint surface changes lead to TMJ dysfunction.

MRI is of minor importance in the diagnosis of TMJ trauma; however, soft tissue damage and joint effusion may be detected by this method (Fig. 13.8). Joint function and avascular necrosis of bone can be visualized [2, 9, 12, 27].

Ankylosis is most often found following traumatic injuries, but may occur subsequent to inflammatory joint disease (especially infectious arthritis) or after surgery. Ankylosis is classified according to extracapsular or intracapsular location and osseous or fibrous origin. The most important clinical finding is restricted joint mobility. On MRI fibrous anky-

losis is depicted by an obliterated joint space of low signal intensity. Therapy is primarily surgery to mobilize the condyle [23, 25, 26].

Acute TMJ dislocation may occur as a result of trauma. Loose capsular ligaments, muscular incoordination, and emotional disturbances may result in recurrent dislocation of the condyle [5]. The patient is not able to reduce the mandible by himself; an "open lock" is the clinical finding. Acute and chronic condylar dislocation are treated by sedation and manipulation of the jaw inferiorly and posteriorly. Recurrent dislocation may require myofunctional training, injection of sclerosing solution, or surgery (Table 13.3).

Table 13.3. MRI findings in 80 patients suspected to have disorders of the TMJ. (Prospective study)

| | |
|---|---|
| *Changes in disk position* | 11 |
| a) With reduction | |
| – posterior luxation | 4 |
| – anterior luxation | 19 |
| b) Without reduction | |
| – anterior luxation (adhesion of disk) | 12 |
| – disk rupture | 12 |
| *Changes in disk shape* | |
| a) Deformation | 4 |
| b) Compression | 7 |
| c) Perforation | 2 |
| *Changes in shape and position of condyle* | |
| a) Subluxation | 8 |
| b) Deformation of head | 14 |
| c) Malposition | |
| – compression | 7 |
| – distraction | 5 |
| – anterior malposition | 6 |
| – posterior malposition | 8 |
| d) Fracture | 3 |
| *Others* | |
| a) Fibrous ankylosis | 5 |
| b) Aggressive fibromatosis | 1 |
| c) Hematoma | 1 |
| d) Arthritis with effusion | 4 |
| *Normal TMJ* | 6 |

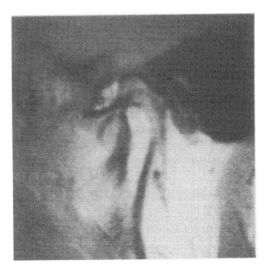

Fig. 13.9. Right TMJ in a 50-year-old man: TMJ effusion in arthritis. Plain sagittal MRI (SE, 1000/28). Mouth closed. Expanded superior and inferior joint space with degenerative thinned disk and anteriorly dislocated condyle. Bloody, serous, or proteinaceous fluid can not be distinguished by MRI. These slight degenerative findings are not typical for psoriatic arthritis, which was diagnosed in other joints of this patient

## 13.4.2 Arthritis

Degenerative arthritis is a common finding following joint overload and internal derangement (see Fig. 13.8). Other forms of arthritis may also affect the TMJ.

The incidence of TMJ involvement in patients with rheumatoid arthritis (RA) reported in the literature varies greatly, from 5% to 86%. Clinical findings include pain, swelling, crepitus, stiffness on opening the mouth and limitation of movement; progressively anterior open bite because of the resorption of the condyle is reported as a typical sign [5]. Ankylosis following RA is relatively rare. The diagnosis of RA by imaging techniques is difficult because of the primarily nonspecific nature of the joint changes; on MRI too, only severe changes may be identified as RA. The condyle may display degenerative changes, including signs of avascular necrosis of bone or osteo-chondritis dissecans, which is identified on MRI by changes of shape and marrow signal characteristics [24]. Degenerative lesions of the articular disk and joint effusion with or without synovial thickening may be observed (Fig. 13.9). These alterations are detected on T2-weighted images and, less sensitively, by T1-weighted or fast imaging. The therapy is similar to the medical management of RA of other joints.

The findings following psoriatic arthritis are similar, but bony changes and osseous resorption may develop more rapidly than in RA.

Infectious arthritis may develop after hematogenous spread of tuberculosis, syphilis, or other diseases, or after perforating external trauma, or the infection may spread directly from adjoining processes (e.g., otitis media) [13, 15, 21, 24, 25].

### 13.4.3 Internal Derangement

Internal derangement of the TMJ is defined by changes of the physiologic relations of the anatomic structures associated with the condyle as well as changes in their form and structure. Degenerative processes in the TMJ are complex and dynamic and are divided into characteristic stages according to their intensity. Internal derangement of TMJ is characterized by disk luxation and deformation, abnormal position of the condyle, and, as a result, increasing deformation of osseous structures.

Occlusal instability and functional disorders of the stomatognathic system of arthral or muscular origin lead to abnormal and excessive strains on the TMJ. The results are diskopathy and arthrosis of the glenoid surfaces caused by excessive remodeling or adaption. Arthrosis is recognized at an early stage by changes of the articular cartilage of the condyle and the temporal fossa and changes of the fibrous components of the disk and bilaminar zone. These processes of modification and shape change cause mechanical detrition and disturb the normal joint function, increasing the functional strain on tissues. The continuity of the smooth articular surfaces is interrupted, and consequently degeneration and destruction of the cartilaginous components of the TMJ increases and osseous arthrosis develops. The pathogenesis of this progressive process can be examined using MRI techniques (Table 13.4).

The MRI findings regarding tissue changes enable diagnosis, and thus initiation of treatment, at an early stage of internal derangement. Visualization of the articular disk, the bilaminar zone, and the osseous portions of the joint permits a functional analysis of the intraarticular situation. This enables prophylaxis and early treatment of this disorder. The MRI stages of internal derangement of the TMJ are divided into an early phase of reducible displacement (stages I and II), an intermediate phase of irreducible displacement (stage III), and a late phase with arthrosis (stages IV–VI).

The MRI diagnosis of partial or complete, anterior or posterior, reducible displacement of the articular disk (stage I) is based on the relative orientation of the disk and the condyle and on the malposition of the posterior band of the disk in relation to the longitudinal condylar axis (Fig. 13.10 a, b). Anterior disk displacement is defined as the position of the posterior band of the disk in front of the condyle, especially if anteriorly displaced relative to the longitudinal condylar axis. To ascertain disk mobility one has to examine the disk in a minimum value of two positions. Reducibility of an articular disk corresponds by definition to ventrocaudal sliding of the condyle.

**Table 13.4.** MRI staging of internal derangement of the TMJ in 53 patients. (Prospective study)

| Stage | n | Definition | Morphologic features |
|---|---|---|---|
| I | 5 | Anterior/posterior disk displacement, reducible | Normal disk morphology, normal signal |
| II | 19 | Disk displacement, reducible, with deformation | With/without effusion in joint space |
| III | 10 | Disk displacement, irreducible, with deformation | With/without effusion, disk adhesion, narrowed joint space |
| IV | 10 | Osteoarthrosis and severe disk deformation | Degenerative cortical changes, articular/cartilaginous erosion, condylar destruction, thinning of intermediate band of disk |
| V | 6 | Disk rupture/perforation, severe osseous degenerative changes | Osteophytosis, remodelling |
| VI | 3 | Disk resorption, avascular necrosis, osteochondritis dissecans | Subcortical sclerosis of the condyle |

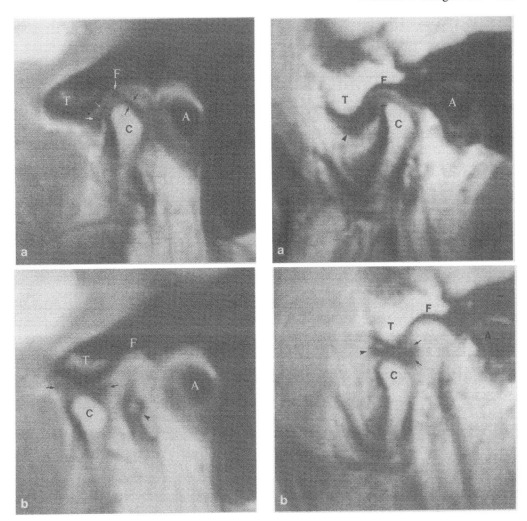

**Fig. 13.10 a, b.** Right TMJ: Internal derangement stage I. *A*, auditory canal; *C*, condyle; *F*, mandibular fossa; *T*, articular tubercle
**a** Plain sagittal MRI (SE, 1000/28). Mouth closed. The anterior disk displacement is determined by the position of the posterior band of the disk in front of the condyle
**b** Plain sagittal MRI (SE, 1000/28). Mouth open. Complete reduction of the disk

**Fig. 13.11 a, b.** Right TMJ: internal derangement stage II. *A*, auditory canal; *C*, condyle; *F* mandibular fossa; *T*, articular tubercle
**a** Plain sagittal MRI (SE, 1000/28). Mouth closed. Anterior position of a deformed disk
**b** Plain sagittal MRI (SE, 1000/28). Mouth open. The reducible articular disk is corresponding to the ventrocaudal sliding of the condyle. In relation to the mandible the movements of both structures are synchronous

In relation to the head of the mandible the coordinate movements of both structures are synchronous; the articular disk is always repositioned during mouth opening.

In stage II of internal derangement, the reducible disk displacement has led to changes in disk shape such as deformation with fibrillation, elongation, compression and shortening of the (disk) meniscus (Fig. 13.11 a, b).

In addition to the nonphysiologic changes in disk shape, MRI shows signal changes that can be interpreted as representing mesenchymal degenerative processes inside the articular disk. All forms of irreducible disk displacement belong to stage III (Fig. 13.5), which is diagnosed by failure of the disk to move relative to the condyle when the mouth is opened and closed. Often, a disk adhesion in the superior joint space is identified as the cause of functional disturbance.

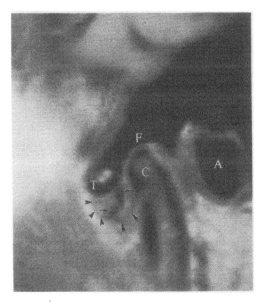

**Fig. 13.12.** Right TMJ in a 39-year-old man: internal derangement stage V. Plain sagittal MRI (SE, 1000/26). Wide, anteriorly completely displaced disk (disk rupture) with effusion in the upper and lower joint compartments. Condylar malposition and osseous destruction at the articulating surface of the condyle
*Arrows,* anterior/posterior bands of disk; *arrowheads,* joint capsule; *A,* external auditory canal; *C,* condyle; *F,* mandibular fossa; *T,* tubercle

Stage IV is distinguished by osseous changes indicative of arthropathy, with degenerative deformations at the condyle and the articular surfaces of the temporal bone. These changes in form and structure are combined with regenerative processes such as osteophytosis and positive and negative remodeling.

Stage V internal derangement of the TMJ is determined by morphologic changes of the articular disk and increasing osseous destruction. Condylar malpositioning and disk compression cause further thinning of the already thin intermediate zone of the articular disk and eventually perforation of the disk. The interrupted disk shows a loss of continuity from the posterior band of the disk to its attachment at the bilaminar zone (Figs. 13.12, 13.13).

In stage VI one can see increased condylar deformation with avascular necrosis at the joint surfaces and subcortical sclerosis. This process shows up on MRI as lower signal intensity of the spongiosa of the mandibular head. After partial or complete resorption of the articular disk the progress of internal derangement of TMJ shows increasing craniomandibular dysfunctions such as restriction of lower jaw movement, crepitation, asymmetric contractions of the masticatory muscles and unphysiologic lower jaw movements [3, 8, 13, 17, 21, 27, 28].

### 13.4.4 Hypermobility of the Mandibular Condyle

On physiologic opening of the lower jaw the condyle slides to the lowest point of the articular tubercle. The maximum physiologic opening of the mouth is about 40 mm interincisal distance (Figs. 13.14, 13.15).

When the condyle slides into a sub- or pretubercular position, this is termed subluxation and can be uni- or bilateral. Clinically this diagnosis is verified by the typical terminal joint clicking that appears when the condyle-disk complex passes the articular tubercle.

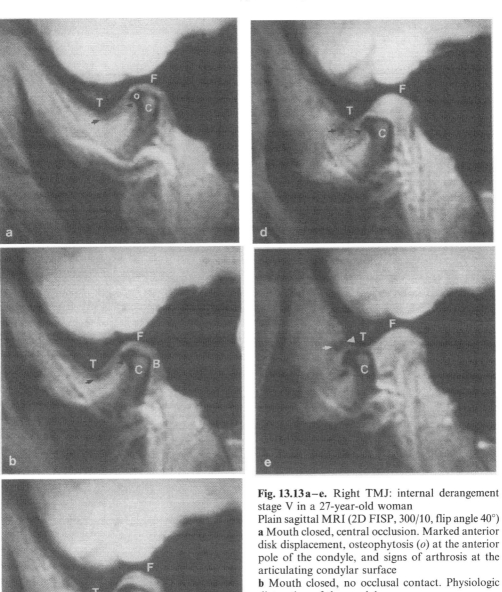

**Fig. 13.13a–e.** Right TMJ: internal derangement stage V in a 27-year-old woman

Plain sagittal MRI (2D FISP, 300/10, flip angle 40°)

**a** Mouth closed, central occlusion. Marked anterior disk displacement, osteophytosis (*o*) at the anterior pole of the condyle, and signs of arthrosis at the articulating condylar surface

**b** Mouth closed, no occlusal contact. Physiologic distraction of the condyle

**c** Abduction 0.5 cm. Disk compression during the translation movement of the condyle

**d** Abduction 1.5 cm. Subtubercular disk position and disk movement in front of the condyle

**e** Abduction 3 cm. Pretubercular disk position, functional disk detachment, no identifiable attachment of the meniscus to the bilaminar zone

*Thin arrow,* anterior band of disk; *double arrow,* posterior band of disk; *arrow, arrowhead,* joint capsule; *C,* condyle; *T,* articular tubercle; *F,* mandibular fossa; *b,* bilaminar zone

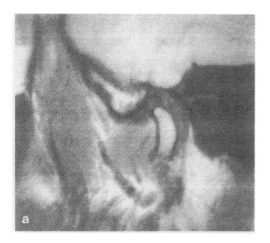 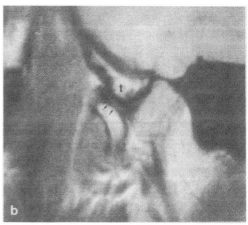

**Fig. 13.14a, b.** Left TMJ in a 29-year-old woman: hypermobility of condyle
**a** Plain sagittal MRI (SE, 1000/28). Mouth closed. Normal biconcave configuration and position of disk

**b** Plain sagittal MRI (SE, 1000/28). Mouth open (interincisal distance 25 mm). Hypermobility of the condyle anterior to the apex of the tubercle (*t*). The dorsal portion of the condyle (*arrows*) forms the abnormal articulating surface

**Fig. 13.15a–e** see p. 221

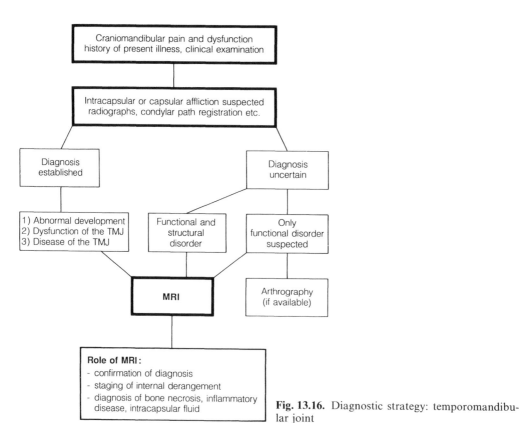

Craniomandibular pain and dysfunction
history of present illness, clinical examination

Intracapsular or capsular affliction suspected
radiographs, condylar path registration etc.

Diagnosis
established

Diagnosis
uncertain

1) Abnormal development
2) Dysfunction of the TMJ
3) Disease of the TMJ

Functional and
structural
disorder

Only
functional disorder
suspected

MRI

Arthrography
(if available)

**Role of MRI:**
- confirmation of diagnosis
- staging of internal derangement
- diagnosis of bone necrosis, inflammatory disease, intracapsular fluid

**Fig. 13.16.** Diagnostic strategy: temporomandibular joint

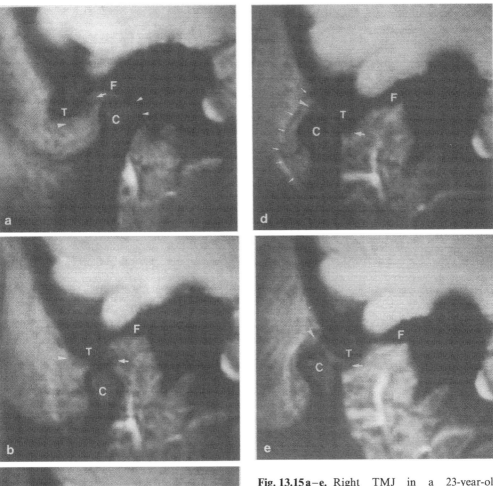

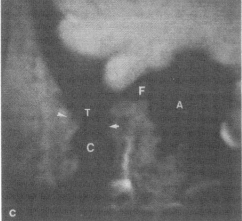

**Fig. 13.15 a–e.** Right TMJ in a 23-year-old woman: hypermobility of condyle. Plain sagittal MRI (2D FISP, 300/10, flip angle 40°)

**a** Mouth closed, no occlusal contact. Posterior displacement of the condyle, low signal of the disk structure, the condyle touches the dorsal border of the mandibular fossa (*small arrowheads*), relative anterior disk displacement with reduction

**b** Abduction 1.0 cm. Unphysiologic coordinating condylar movement with subtubercular condylar position, abnormal translation phase

**c** Abduction 2.0 cm. Unphysiologic rotation movement of the condyle

**d** Abduction 3.0 cm. End of translation movement, pretubercular position of the disk-condyle complex with creased joint capsule (*small arrows*)

**e** Abduction 4.0 cm. Abnormal rotation movement.

*Large arrow,* posterior band of disk; *large arrowhead,* anterior band of disk; *C,* condyle; *F,* mandibular fossa; *T,* articular tubercle; *A,* external auditory canal

Flaccidity of the joint capsule, or rather of the ligaments, and muscular discoordination of the superior and inferior head of the lateral pterygoid muscle have been suggested as causes.

Luxation of the TMJ, whether uni- or bilateral, is a trismus which appears during maximum opening movements, often with simultaneous laterotrusion towards the opposite side of the affected joint. Together with the disk, the condyle slides over the articular tubercle to ventral and is fixed by the muscular tract of the mandibular adductors in a position in front of and above the articular tubercle, so that spontaneous reposition, and in consequence closure of the mouth, is no longer possible (Fig. 13.15). The lower jaw is now located in a protrusional position. If this dislocation occurs repeatedly it is called habitual luxation.

Condylar hypermobility can be suspected clinically in the presence of extreme excursion movements of the lower jaw or maximum mouth opening of more than 50 mm interincisal distance with active reposition of the condyle [7, 10, 16, 21, 22].

The diagnostic strategy outlined in Fig. 13.16 is recommended for MRI of the temperomandibular joint.

### References

1. Burnett KR, Davis CL, Read J (1987) Dynamic display of the temporomandibular joint meniscus using "fast scan" MR imaging. Am J Roentgenol 147:959–627
2. Carlsson GE, Öberg T (1974) Remodelling of the temporomandibular joints. Oral Sci Rev 6:53–86
3. Cirbus MT, Gmilach MS, Beltron J, Simon L (1987) Magnetic resonance imaging in conforming internal derangement of temporomandibular joint. J Prosthet Dent 57:488
4. Drace JE, Enzmann D (1990) Defining the normal temporomandibular joint: closed, partially open and open mouth MR imaging of asymptomatic subjects. Radiology 177:67  71
5. Farrar WB, McCarty WL (1982) A clinical outline of temporomandibular joint diagnosis and treatment. Normandie, Montgomery
6. Frahm J, Hasse A, Matthaei D (1981) Rapid threedimensional MR imaging using the FLASH technique. Comput Assist Tomogr 10:980 ff
7. Hansson T, Honee W, Hesse J (1990) Funktionsstörungen im Kausystem. Hüthig, Heidelberg
8. Helms CA, Vogler JB, Morish RB Jr, Goldman SM, Lapra RE, Proctor E (1984) Temporomandibular joint internal derangements: CT diagnosis. Radiology 152:459
9. Jarheim TA, Kolbenstredt A (1984) High resolution computed tomography of the osseous temporomandibular joint: some normal and abnormal appearances. Acta Radiol Diagn Stockh 25:465–469
10. Laskin DM (1969) Etiology of the pain-dysfunction syndrome. J Am Dent Assoc 79:147–153
11. Juniper RP (1987) The pathogenesis and investigation of TMJ dysfunction. Br J Oral Maxillofac Surg 25:105–112
12. Katzberg RW (1989) Temporomandibular joint imaging. Radiology 170:297–307
13. Katzberg RW, Keith DA, Guralnich WC, Manzione JV (1983) Internal derangemet and arthritis of TMJ. Radiology 146:107–112
14. Katzberg RW, Bessette RW, Tallents RH, Plewes DB, Manzione JV, Schenk JF, Foster TH, Hart HR (1986) Normal and abnormal temporomandibular joint: MR imaging with surface coil. Radiology 158:183–189
15. Larheim TA, Smith HJ, Aspestrand F (1990) Rheumatic disease of the temporo-mandibular joint. MR imaging and topographic manifestations. Radiology 175:527–531
16. Laskin DM, Bloch S (1986) Diagnosis and treatment of myofacial pain-dysfunction (MPD) syndrome. J Prosthet Dent 56:75–84
17. Manzione JV, Katzberg RW, Brodsky GL, Seltzer SE, Mellins HZ (1984) Internal derangements of temporomandibular joint: diagnosis by direct sagittal computed tomography. Radiology 150:105
18. Mills TC, Ortendahl DA, Hylton NM, Crooks LE et al. (1987) Portial flip angle MR imaging. Radiology 162:531–539
19. Mohl ND (1988) The temporomandibular joint. In: Mohl ND, Zarb GA, Carlsson GE, Rugh JDA (eds) Textbook of occlusion. Quintessence, Chicago
20. Öberg T, Carlsson GE, Fajers CM (1971) The temporomandibular joint. A morphologic study on a human autopsy material. Acta Odontol Scand 29:349
21. Palacios E, Valvassori GE, Shannon M, Reed CF (1990) Magnetic resonance of the temporomandibular joint. Thieme, Stuttgart
22. Randzio J, Fischer-Brandies E (1986) Augmentation of the articular tubercle in treatment of chronic recurrent temporomandibular joint luxations. A preliminary case report. Oral Surg 61:19

23. Riediger D (1980) Zur Ätiologie und Pathogenese der Kiefergelenksankylose. In: Schuchardt K, Schwenzer N (eds) Erkrankungen des Kiefergelenks. Stuttgart (Fortschritte der Kiefer- und Gesichtschirurgie, vol 25)
24. Schellhas KP, Wilkes CH (1989) Temporomandibular joint inflammation: comparison of MR fast scanning with T1- and T2-weighted imaging techniques. AJNR 10:589–594
25. Syrjänen SM (1985) The temporomandibular joint in rheumatoid arthritis. Acta Radiol Diagn (Stockh) 26 (Fasc. 3) S:235–234
26. Vogl T, Kellermann O, Randzio J, Kniha H, Requardt H, Tiling R, Lissner J (1988) Ergebnisse der Kernspintomographie des Temporomandibulargelenkes mittels optimierter Oberflächenspulen. Fortschr Röntgenstr 1489:502

27. Vogl T, Eberhard D, Randzio J, Schmidt O, Lissner J (1991) KST Diagnostik des Internal Derangement des Kiefergelenkes. Radiologe 31:537–544
28. Westesson PL, Bronstein SL, Liedberg J et al. (1985) Internal derangement of the temporomandibular joint: morphologic description with correlation to joint function. Oral Surg Oral Med Oral Pathol 59:323–331
29. Wilk RM, Walford LM (1987) Multislab 3 DFT magnetic resonance imaging in temporomandibular joint imaging. Society of Magnetic Resonance in Medicine, New York, p 139
30. Wright DM, Moffett BC (1974) The postnatal development of the human temporomandibular joint. Am J Anat 141:235–249

# 14 Three-Dimensional MRI

Over the past few decades the development of new radiologic techniques such as CT and MRI has significantly improved the capabilities of diagnostic imaging in the head and neck. The usefulness of these modalities, however, is restricted by the hitherto necessary sequential observation of individual two-dimensional slices. Surgeons and clinicians often have difficulty in mentally transforming series of two-dimensional slices into the three-dimensional topography. There has therefore been great interest in attempts to develop a new technique that offers the possibility of visualizing the third dimension. Such a technique could revolutionize diagnostic imaging, especially in view of its potential applications in the planning of surgery and radiotherapy. Another promising field of application is 3D-MRI-guided laser therapy.

Only few reports on clinical trials of 3D MRI in patients suffering from head and neck lesions have been published. Three-dimensional visualization of the structures in this area is especially difficult due to the complex topography. 3D MRI is an ideal method of evaluating the spread of the lesion and assessing the relation between the lesion and the surrounding tissues (Fig. 14.1).

## 14.1 Principles

### 14.1.1 Equipment and Sequences

We have examined patients using two different MRI devices with field strengths of 1 T and 1.5 T. A 25-cm-diameter head coil was used in both cases. It has proven best to start the examination with a standard 2D plain T1-weighted SE sequence. Depending on the lesion, a T2-weighted sequence may be infor-

mative. A T1-weighted sequence with the contrast medium Gd-DTPA (0.1 mmol/kg) should be performed in patients with lesions that can be expected to enhance. On completion of the 2D part of the examination, 3D MRI is performed and the 3D data cube is transferred to a separate workstation or to an integrated unit. For the 3D measurement the standard 3D gradient pulse sequence 3D FLASH, a flow-compensated 3D FLASH sequence, or the fast T1-weighted turbo-FLASH sequence called MPRAGE (magnetization prepared rapid gradient echo) can be used. The optimal parameters for the different sequences are listed in Table 14.1.

### 14.1.2 Value of Different Sequences

In all cases the 3D-Flash results are compared with those of the SE sequences. Attention is paid to the characteristics of the lesions and to

**Table 14.1.** MRI sequences used in the 3D technique

|  | 1 tesla | 1.5 tesla |
|---|---|---|
| Sequence | 3D FLASH | 3D Turbo-FLASH MPRAGE |
| Parameters |  |  |
| TR | 40 ms | 10 ms |
| TE | 15 ms | 4 ms |
| Flip angle | 40° | 15° |
| Matrix | 256 × 256 | 256 × 256 |
| Partitions | 128 | 128 |
| Slice thickness | ≥ 0.8 mm | ≥ 1.2 mm |
| 3D reconstruction mode | Voxel-man Ray tracing | |
| Apparatus | Workstation | Integrated unit |

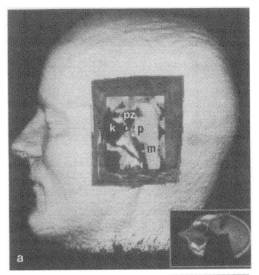

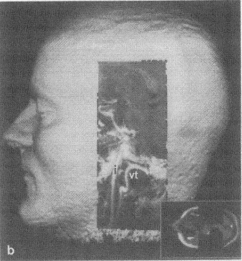

**Fig. 14.1 a, b.** Topography of the middle skull base in a 3D reconstruction using the window technique
**a** Plain sagittal MRI (3D turbo-FLASH, 1.5 T). Exact delineation of the sphenoid sinus (*k*). Visualization of brainstem and pons (*p*), prepontine cistern (*pz*), medulla oblongata (*m*), mesencephalon, and clivus. Caudally, the nasopharynx and soft palate are demonstrated
**b** Plain sagittal MR angiography (3D turbo-FLASH, 1.5 T). Display of vascular structures in an enlarged window. Documentation of the exact course of the internal carotid artery (*i*) and vertebral artery (*vt*)

their demarcation from surrounding tissues. Comparison of the contrast to noise ratio (C/N) of the T1- and T2-weighted SE sequences and the 3D gradient sequences FLASH and MPRAGE reveals that the SE technique has a higher diagnostic value. The 3D turbo-FLASH sequence, however, reduces the difference in C/N for muscle/fat and even eliminates it for CSF/white matter (Fig. 14.2).

The new technique, however, has the advantage of presenting information in three dimensions in relation to the surface of the head. Thus, despite having no additional diagnostic value, it is valuable for the planning of surgery or radiotherapy.

Among the 3D sequences, the best C/N is offered by the turbo-FLASH MPRAGE sequence (Fig. 14.3). The susceptibility of Turbo-FLASH to motion artifacts is reduced because the examination time is shorter. Thus, MR images can be produced with high spatial resolution and excellent T1-weighted contrast characteristics.

### 14.1.3 Value of Gd-DTPA

Before the 3D examination all patients have to undergo a standard 2D examination. Depending on the initial findings, the contrast medium Gd-DTPA may be used. On the same basis, the 3D examination can be performed either with or without the contrast agent. In the majority of the lesions, especially near the skull base, Gd-DTPA offers better demarcation of the tumor by shortening T1 and enhancing the signal intensity.

> A standard 2D SE examination is necessary for diagnosis. The subsequent 3D examination can be conducted with or without contrast medium. For optimal contrast and high spatial resolution the 3D Turbo-FLASH sequence is recommended.

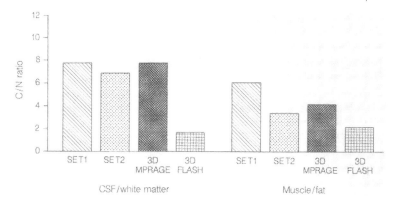

**Fig. 14.2.** Contrast to noise ratio (*C/N*): 2D v 3D sequences. Field strength 1.5 T

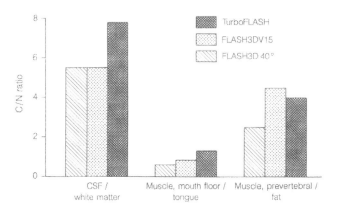

**Fig. 14.3.** Contrast to noise ratios with three different 3D techniques

## 14.2 Skull Base, Face, and Neck

In tumors affecting the skull base, face, and neck, 3D images visualizing the lesion and its relation to the surrounding tissues can be obtained from any projection (Fig. 14.5). The topographic relations of anatomic structures and the surface are displayed using the window-technique as shown in Fig. 14.1. In our group the clinical value of our improved 3D-imaging method was examined in 57 patients with various tumors such as metastases, meningiomas, neuromas, glomus tumors, paranasal sinus tumors, adenomas, and hemangiomas (Table 14.2). The tumor's relation to the internal carotid artery and the jugular vein, demonstrated by the 3D reconstruction

technique, is of particular diagnostic significance. The topographic detail of the sinus system, the nasopharynx, and the muscles is also relevant for diagnosis (Fig. 14.4) and is demonstrated clearly by the 3D technique due to the slice thickness of only 1–2 mm. Penetration of a maxillary sinus carcinoma into the subarachnoidal space is also shown using this technique, along with infiltration of the sphenoid sinus and the tumor's relationship to the internal carotid artery.

Neuromas, e.g., hypoglossal neuromas (see Fig. 6.13), can be delineated and their relations to muscles, vessels, and spinal cord precisely depicted, permitting evaluation of their course along the nerve. 3D reconstructions of meningiomas also offer excellent accuracy of

**Table 14.2.** Tumors of the skull base in 57 patients examined using 3D techniques

| Middle skull base | | Frontal skull base | |
| --- | --- | --- | --- |
| Tumor | n | Tumor | n |
| Neuroma | 5 | Carcinoma | 14 |
| acoustic | | frontal sinus | |
| hypoglossal | | maxillary sinus | |
| glossopharyngeal | | nasal cavity | |
| Meningioma | 2 | Sarcoma | 2 |
| sphenoid sinus | | Mesenchymal tumor | 2 |
| others | | Others | 11 |
| Glomus tumor | 6 | | |
| Mesenchymal tumor | 5 | | |
| Others | 10 | | |

Field strengths and apparatus: 1T, Magnetom 42 ($n = 18$); 1.5 T, Magnetom 63 SP ($n = 39$).

detail, enabling exact demarcation of the tumor from the clivus or the lesser wing of the sphenoid bone. The beneficial effect of contrast medium is shown by the 3D reconstruction of a sphenoid meningioma (Fig. 14.5). The vascularization of the lesion is evaluated by comparing images obtained before and after administration of the contrast agent Gd-DTPA. In 80% of the skull base tumors there is a significant increase in signal intensity. Especially in the neuromas, parotid adenomas (Fig. 14.6), and glomus tumors, the lesion is clearly delineated after Gd-DTPA. The enhancement in carcinomas of the maxillary sinus is sufficient to visualize the infiltration and topography of the lesion.

However, the inner structure of lesions in the region of the oropharynx can not be depicted with complete clarity by means of T1-weighted 3D imaging. These structures are shown well using the SE technique.

There are differences in extractable information among conventional 2D images, original 3D slices and 3D-reconstructed images. We investigated the depiction of tumor margins, tumor spread, and vascular relation. Tumor margins and tumor spread were shown more clearly in the 2D sequences, but the vascular relations can be judged slightly better from the original 3D data.

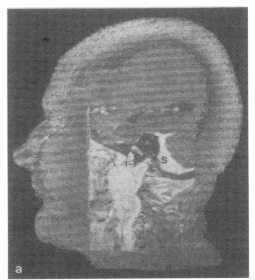

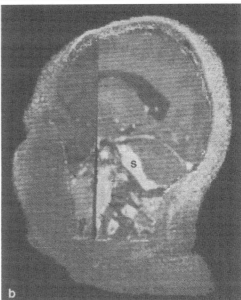

**Fig. 14.4 a. b.** Meningioma of the jugular foramen: 3D reconstructions
**a** Sagittal MRI (3D FLASH, 1 T) with Gd-DTPA
**b** Coronosagittal view (3D FLASH, 1 T) with Gd-DTPA. The lesion, measuring $7 \times 3$ cm, exhibits high signal intensity after administration of contrast medium (*arrows*). The tumor extends from the superior jugular bulb to the level of the mandible. No evidence of intracranial infiltration. Contrast medium shows enhancement of the sigmoid sinus (*s*)

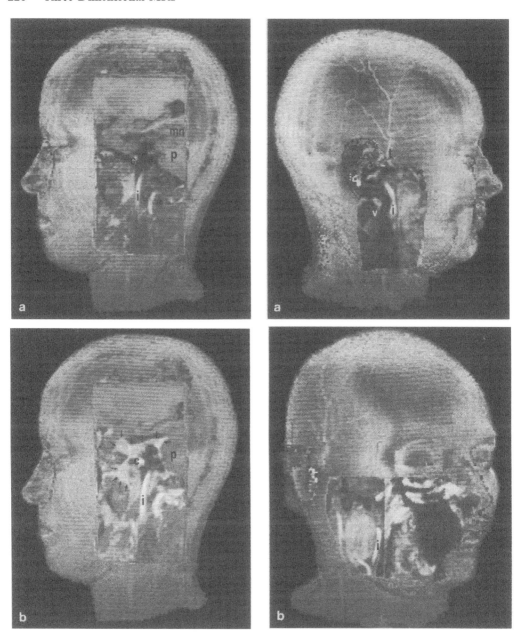

**Fig. 14.5. a, b.** Meningioma of the sphenoid sinus: 3D reconstructions
**a** Plain (3D FLASH, 1 T). The tumor is not exactly demarcated from the surrounded tissue. Topographic relations to the internal carotid artery (*i*), mesencephalon (*mn*), clivu (*c*) and brainstem (*p*)
**b** Gd-DTPA (3D FLASH, 1 T). After administration of Gd-DTPA, significant enhancement of the tumor. Visualization of the anterior, posterior, and caudal parts of the tumor (*arrows*)

**Fig. 14.6 a, b.** 3D reconstructions
**a** Sagittal view (3D FLASH, 1 T) with Gd-DTPA. Pleomorphic adenoma of the parotid gland (3 × 4 cm) originating from the deep medial lobe: In 3D reconstructions the tumor shows high inhomogeneity in signal intensity after Gd-DTPA. Its relationship to the internal carotid artery (*i*), superficial temporal artery (*t*) and jugular vein (*v*) is exactly demonstrated
**b** Parasagittal view (3D FLASH, 1 T) with Gd-DTPA. The tumor's relationship to the internal carotid artery (*i*) is depicted clearly

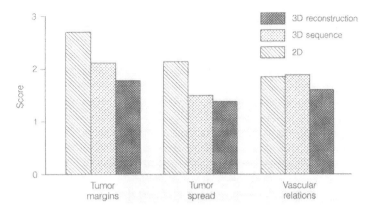

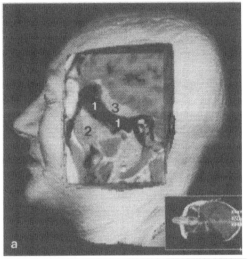

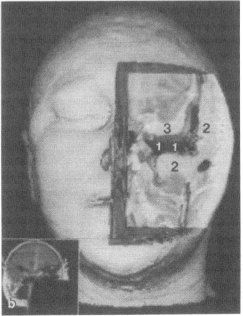

**Fig. 14.7.** Qualitative results: 3D v 2D MRI

**Fig. 14.8a, b** (*right*). Ossifying fibroma: 3D reconstructions
**a** Sagittal view (3D Turbo-FLASH, 1.5 T) with Gd-DTPA.
**b** Coronal view (3D Turbo-FLASH, 1.5 T) with Gd-DTPA. Visualization of the structures in the area of the tumor, close to the skull base. The ossifying parts are of homogeneous low intensity (*1*). The soft tissue part of the tumor is of high intensity (*2*). A concomitant inflammatory reaction of the meninges is visible (*3*)

All in all, the resolution and with it the interpretable information, is reduced in the 3D reconstruction process.

3D MRI is most useful for lesions close to the skull base, where it has significant advantages concerning topography and evaluation of the surrounding structures (Fig. 14.8a, b). The 3D technique is very helpful in the planning of surgery in this anatomically intricate area.

The usefulness of 3D MRI for preoperative planning is demonstrated by the example in Fig. 14.9. A patient with a left infratemporal leiomyosarcoma was examined using the 3D turbo-Flash technique. The lateral 3D image (Fig. 14.9a) gives an excellent impression of the tumor's extent, showing an enhancing, infiltrating mass in the infratemporal and retromaxillary region and the temporal lobe. Caudally one can appreciate the infiltration of the parapharyngeal region, and dorsally the tumor extends to the parotid space.

The coronal views (Fig. 14.9b, c) confirm the diagnosis. Additionally, the extension of the tumor towards the medial retroorbital region

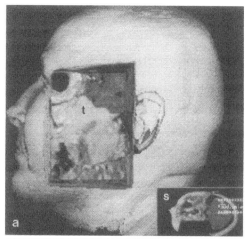

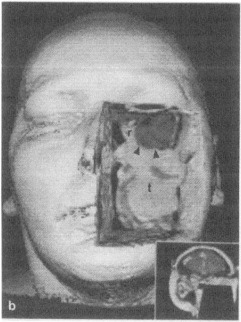

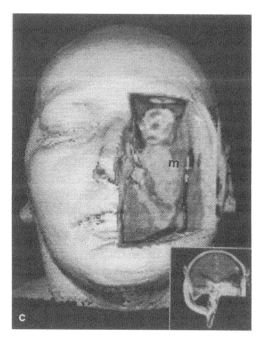

**Fig. 14.9a–c.** Retromaxillary and infratemporal leiomyosarcoma: 3D reconstructions
**a** Sagittal view (3D Turbo-FLASH, 1.5 T) with Gd-DTPA. The outline, infiltration and extension of the tumor (*t*) are visualized. An additional scout view (*s*) shows the depth of intersection in a transversal slice

**b** Coronal view (3D Turbo-FLASH, 1.5 T) with Gd-DTPA. This view shows the extension of the tumor (*t*) towards the retroorbital region (*r*) and its infiltration of the temporal lobe (*arrowheads*)
**c** Coronal view (3D Turbo-FLASH, 1.5 T) with Gd-DTPA. The tumor is seen to infiltrate the mandible (*m*) and the temporomandibular joint

is visualized and the infiltration of the optic nerve or the optic foramen is detected. Figure 14.9c especially shows the tumor's infiltration and encasement of the mandible and its head. All these 3D MRI findings are consistent with the patient's complaints of visual disturbances, weakness of vision of the left eye, and pain in the left temporomandibular joint on chewing.

## 14.3 Technique and Prospects

The advantages offered by 3D reconstruction have already been exploited clinically in disciplines such as orthopedics (hip joints), neurosurgery (brain tumors), craniofacial surgery (dysmorphologies) [1–3] and angiography. The usefulness of the 3D technique based on CT in the preoperative planning of craniofacial tumor resection has been mentioned in the literature [4]. The clinical potential of 3D MRI is just as promising as that of 3D CT, but several problems have limited its development. The loss of information caused by transferring the 128 slices into a special 3D display can be reduced, however, by further advances in software and hardware.

The 3D examination is performed with and/or without the contrast medium Gd-DTPA, depending on the lesion. The duration of the complete (MR) examination is about 1 hour. After the examination the acquired data are reconstructed three-dimensionally. The size and depth of the window in the 3D head surface showing the lesion are determined interdisciplinarily. A series of 3D reconstructions in which the depth of the window varies yields information on the extent and infiltration of the lesion. The reconstructed images are saved and viewed by the surgeon before and during (the planning stage of) surgery. Extensive preliminary investigations have shown that the size and orientation of the window are decisive parameters of the 3D image. The larger the window, the better the evaluability of the structures of interest and the surrounding tissue. However, topographic reference points such as nose, cheek, and eyes are lost when a large window is selected. Therefore the width of the window should be chosen for each patient individually, depending on the location

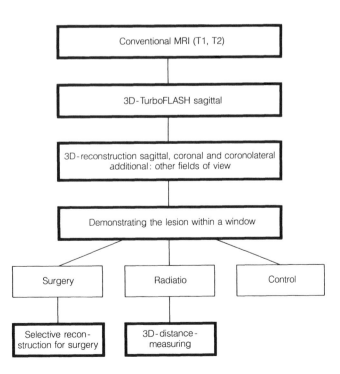

**Fig. 14.10.** Diagnostic strategy: 3D head reconstruction

and extent of the lesion, to ensure optimal diagnostic value of this technique (Fig. 14.10). The principal indications for the 3D reconstruction method are lesions of the skull base and the face, where 3D imaging is particularly advantageous in evaluating the topography. Due to the high risk of skull base surgery all possible diagnostic modalities should be used, but 3D reconstruction should not be seen only in this light, but rather as a useful diagnostic technique supplementing existing methods. With reduction of the duration of the examination and simplification of the reconstruction process 3D MRI could come into its own as a planning modality for surgery and radiotherapy. A further important step will be T2-weighted FLASH sequences to improve the sensitivity and specificity of this fast imaging procedure.

The clinical value of 3D MRI in the head and neck has to be verified interdisciplinarily in the context of ongoing research.

## References

1. Marsh JL, Vannier MW (1989) Three-dimensional surface imaging from CT scans for the study of craniofacial dysmorphology. J Craniofac Gen et Dev Biol 9:61–75
2. Schad LR, Boesecke R, Schlegel W, Hartmann GH, Sturm V, Strauss GL, Lorenz WJ (1987) Three dimensional image correlation of CT, MR and PET studies in radiotherapy treatment planning of brain tumors. J Comput Assist Tomogr 11(6):948–954
3. Takahashi H, Takagi A, Sando I (1989) Computer-aided three-dimensional reconstruction and measurement of the round window and its membrane. Otolaryngol Head Neck Surg 101(5): 517–521
4. Zinreich SJ, Mattox DE, Johns ME, Holliday MJ, Kennedy DW, Price JC, Quinn CB, Kashima HK (1988) 3D CT for cranial, facial and laryngeal surgery. Laryngoscope 98:1212–1219
5. Vogl T, Wilimzig C, Assal J, Grevers G, Lissner J (1992) 3D MR imaging with Gd-DTPA in head and neck lesion. European Radiology 2 (in press)
6. Vogl T, Wilimzig C, Grevers G, Laub G, Lissner J (1991) 3D Rekonstruktionen bei Raumforderungen im Kopf-Halsbereich. RÖFO 3, 152:253–258

# 15 Clinical Application of Magnetic Resonance Angiography

Hitherto Doppler ultrasound and conventional angiography or digital subtraction angiography (DSA) have been the methods of choice for the evaluation of supraaortic vessels. The new technique of magnetic resonance angiography (MRA) now offers the ability to image vessels with a bigger field of view than Doppler ultrasound and allows the visualization of vessels in a cine mode, yielding additional information [1–19].

Although conventional angiography and DSA are still the gold standard for the imaging of vessels in the head and neck, MRI is gaining importance in this respect. MRA, the latest offshoot of MRI, employs flowing blood itself as a "physiologic contrast medium", thus dispensing with potentially allergenic contrast medium and ionizing radiation. MRA is a noninvasive technique bearing no risks for the patient and can be easily added to routine MRI with negligible increase in acquisition time, providing the radiologist and clinician with further information about vessels and soft tissue at a single setting.

So far MRA can replace X-ray angiography or DSA only to a certain extent, due to software and hardware limitations. Further modifications of these restricting factors may not only improve the quality of MRA but also expand MRI's role in the diagnosis of vascular pathology.

In the head and neck, the best MRA results are provided by 3D FISP (fast imaging with steady-state precession) and by 2D and 3D FLASH (fast low-angle shot) sequences. Sequence selection depends on flow velocity in the vessel. MRA is performed with the head coil or the Helmholtz surface coil, depending on the region of interest (ROI). The original MRA data set is then processed using a max-imum-intensity projection (MIP) algorithm, displaying only vessels.

## 15.1 Selective Arterial MRA

### 15.1.1 Technique and Indications

The imaging of arterial structures in the head and neck region can be accomplished with time-of-flight sequences or with conventional SE sequences (Table 15.1). SE sequences provide higher S/N, reduce artifacts due to gross patient motion, and delineate vessel boundaries precisely. Nevertheless, visualization of vessels with this kind of sequence is possible only if a long enough segment of the vessel lies within the imaging slice. Another disadvantage is that selective arterial MRA can not be performed. SE sequences should be preferred to GE sequences for the evaluation of lesions involving vessel borders because they allow exact delineation of vessel wall from vessel lumen (Table 15.2) [7, 8, 12].

GE sequences are, expressed simply, SE sequences that lack the second 180° RF pulse, so that a single RF pulse produces the MR signal. Therefore wash-out effects produce negligible signal loss and flowing blood appears bright. In contrast to SE sequences, the S/N depends on the flip angle ($\alpha$) and on the TR. Signal reduction or signal loss is primarily caused by changes in flow dynamics, e.g., in aneurysms, large fields of view, or high blood velocities. Special GE sequences used for MRA are 3D FISP and 2D/3D FLASH sequences, which allow vessel visualization in a 3D volume and, after postprocessing with MIP, display the vessel without soft tissue and permit MR cineangiography.

**Table 15.1.** Recommended parameters and planes for MRA of the head and neck. (From [12])

| Sequence | Plane | TR (ms) | TE (ms) | Flip angle | Slice thickness (mm) | Remarks |
|---|---|---|---|---|---|---|
| SE | Axial<br>Coronal<br>Sagittal | 500–3000 | 22–90 | | 3–10 | |
| GE (3D FISP) | Axial<br>Coronal<br>Sagittal | 22–40 | 7–13 | 15–35° | 40–200 | One or two saturations |
| GE (2D FLASH) | Axial<br>Coronal | 25 | 8–10 | 30–60° | 3–10 | One or two saturations<br>Slice gap: −0.3 to −0.2 mm |

**Table 15.2.** Value of time-of-flight MRA sequences for the depiction of supraaortic vascular structures

| Sequence | Arterial system | Venous system | Vessel borders |
|---|---|---|---|
| SE | 2 | 2 | 2 |
| 3D FISP | 3 | 2 | 1 |
| 2D FLASH | 2 | 3 | 1 |

Image quality: 1, adequate; 2, good; 3, excellent.

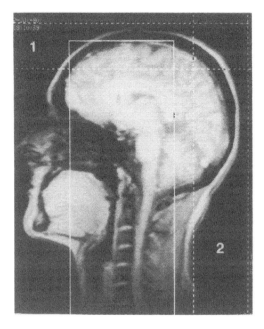

**Fig. 15.1.** Plain sagittal MRI (SE, 200/15). Example of the location of presaturation pulses (*1, 2*) and imaging volume for arterial MRA (*white lines*)

For arterial MRA with fast blood flow a 3D FISP sequence is used with the following parameters: 40/7, α 15°, slice thickness 10–200 mm, 32–64 3D partitions and one acquisition. Average measurement time is 8–11 min. The plane of examination can be sagittal with two parallel slabs, each covering one carotid artery, coronal, or, especially for the circle of Willis, axial. The venous flow is eliminated by one or two saturation pulses above the imaging volume, which are normally placed over the superior sagittal sinus and the confluens (Fig. 15.1). The 3D FISP sequence allows excellent depiction of intracranial arteries in the axial plane or gives an overview of the internal and external carotid arteries in the coronal plane. A double-slab 3D FISP sequence in the sagittal plane allows exact evaluation of the carotid bifurcation. The advantage of this technique over conventional X-ray angiography is that both carotids are visualized and can be compared [14].

> *3D FISP*
> TR/TE: 40/7, α: 15°
> Partitions: 32–64
> Slice thickness: 10–200 mm
> Matrix: 256 × 256
> – Fast blood flow
> – Axial: circle of Willis
> – Coronal: overview of carotid arteries
> – Sagittal: two slabs, each covering one carotid

For visualization of slower blood flow, especially in the branches of the external carotid artery, 2D FLASH sequences are used with the following parameters: 25/10, α 60°, 30–53 slices, thickness 3–10 mm, distance factor −0.25.

A major indication for arterial MRA of the head and neck is vessel displacement or compression due to expansive tumor growth. Patients with tumors and suspected involvement of vascular structures are first examined with conventional MRI. MRA is then performed before administration of contrast medium in order to avoid superimposition of contrast medium enhancement of soft tissue on MIP reconstruction angiograms [2]. Other indications are vessel pathology itself, such as aneurysms, stenoses, and glomus caroticum tumors. Again, MRA follows conventional MRI. The evaluation of type and extent of vascular pathology may, in some cases, be severely hampered by altered blood flow. This often leads to overestimation of the extent of a lesion, especially in the grading of stenoses. As for intracranial aneurysms, MRA is able to depict aneurysms as little as 3 mm in diameter but fails to visualize thrombosed aneurysms and underestimates the size of aneurysms with turbulent flow. These problems can be overcome by including conventional SE images and reviewing the original MRA data set.

## 15.1.2 Normal Topography

Arterial MRA of the head and neck yields excellent anatomic resolution, especially for intracranial arteries. These are best visualized employing a 3D FISP sequence in either the axial or the coronal plane. In order to increase spatial resolution, slab thickness should be kept as low as possible. There follows a brief summary of arteries that can be depicted by selective arterial MRA.

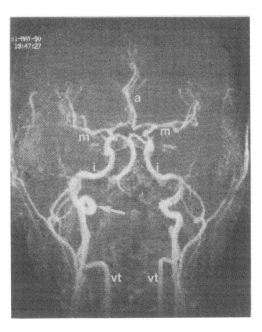

**Fig. 15.2.** Plain coronal MRI (3D FISP, 40/7, α 15°). Demonstration of coiling of the right internal carotid artery (*arrow*). Excellent delineation of the anterior cerebral (*a*), middle cerebral (*m*), internal carotid (*i*), and vertebral (*vt*) arteries

### 15.1.2.1 Intracranial Arteries

The *internal carotid artery* can be subdivided into five segments: the cervical, the petrosal, the precavernous, the intracavernous, and the supraclinoid. The cervical segment reaches from the bifurcation to the base of the skull and is usually straight, but may be kinked (23%) or coiled (9%) (Fig. 15.2). The petrosal segment extends from the base of the skull to the apex of the petrous bone and consists of a vertical and a horizontal portion. The precavernous segment begins at the apex of the petrosal bone, just above the foramen lacerum, and ends at the lateral lower border of the dorsum sellae. The intracavernous segment reaches from there to the anterior clinoid process. The supraclinoid segment begins just after the passage through the dura and ends at the bifurcation into the anterior and middle cerebral arteries. The supraclinoid segment gives off three arteries, of which only two, the ophthalmic artery and the posterior communicating artery, are visualized on arterial MRA, and then only in some cases due to the slow blood flow and the small vessel diameter. The posterior communicating artery connects the internal carotid artery to the posterior cerebral artery. A small dilatation at the origin of the posterior communicating artery is noted in some cases. This is referred to as an infundibulum if its size does not exceed 3 mm, but has to be considered as an aneurysm if larger than 3 mm [1, 11].

The *anterior and middle cerebral arteries* are classified according to Fischer [11]. The anterior cerebral artery is divided into five segments: A1, the segment between the internal carotid artery and the anterior communicating artery; A2, the ascending segment with inferior curvature; A3, the ascending segment with superior curvature; A4, the frontal retrograde segment; A5, the parietal retrograde segment. Lindgren [11] describes segment A1 alone as the anterior cerebral artery and segments A2–A5 as the pericallosal artery. The middle cerebral artery is also divided into five segments: M1, sphenoidal; M2, sylvian; M3, opercular; M4, area of angular gyrus; M5, diverging terminal branches [1, 11].

The *posterior cerebral artery* originates at the bifurcation of the basilar artery in the interpeduncular fossa; the origin is variable in location because of the variable length of the basilar artery. Abnormal origin of the posterior cerebral artery from the internal carotid artery may be found, in which case it is also referred to as the primitive trigeminal artery. The *basilar artery* gives origin to several vessels, of which MRA is able to visualize two: the anterior inferior cerebellar artery and the posterior inferior cerebellar artery.

### 15.1.2.2 Arteries of the Neck and Face

In the region of the face, 2D FLASH sequences have to be employed due to the slower blood flow. Contrast medium should not be administered because the mucosa in the oral and nasal cavities would be enhanced. The external carotid artery originates from the common carotid artery at the superior

border of the thyroid cartilage and gives rise to two groups of branches directed anteriorly and posteriorly. The anteriorly directed branches include the superior thyroid, lingual, facial and maxillary arteries. The posteriorly directed group includes the posterior auricular, occipital and ascending pharyngeal arteries [1]. The last-named is not detected by MRA.

The visualization of vessels in the neck and face is often difficult due to gross patient motion and hardware limitations (coil design). Nevertheless, MRA provides excellent additional information about vascular structures in these areas.

### 15.1.3 Pathological Findings

#### 15.1.3.1 Skull Base

Arteries of the skull base are examined employing an axial 3D FISP sequence with a small slice thickness of 70–96 mm in order to increase spatial resolution (Figs. 15.3, 15.4). This sequence provides an excellent anatomic resolution of intracranial vessels. In the evaluation of MR angiograms of intracranial vessels, MIP should be calculated for two planes to improve differential diagnosis.

Vascular lesions found in this region include aneurysms or stenoses and vessel compression (Fig. 15.5) or displacement due to tumor growth. Patients with large intracranial tumors can also be examined with 3D MRI (Fig. 15.6). The contrast medium Gd-DTPA can be administered but does not improve the resolution of MRA or the evaluation of vessel pathology. In the case of tumors, however, contrast medium allows exact delineation of the mass and the adjacent vessels on MIP angiograms.

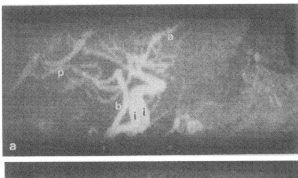

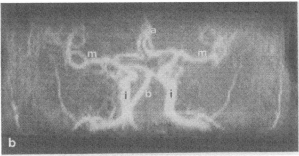

**Fig. 15.3 a, b** (*above*). Plain axial MRA (3D FISP, 40/7, α 15°). Normal findings on selective arterial MRA of the intracranial vessels and circle of Willis
**a** Rotation of the projection to coronal > sagittal: −10°. This projection allows an exact delineation of the basilar (*b*), internal carotid (*i*), anterior cerebral (*a*), and posterior cerebral (*p*) arteries
**b** Rotation of the projection to dorsal. Depiction of the basilar (*b*), internal carotid (*i*), anterior cerebral (*a*), and middle cerebral (*m*) arteries

▷

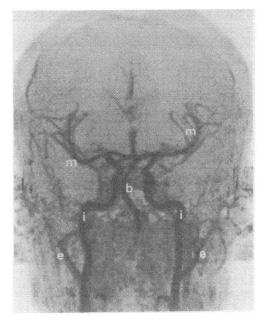

**Fig. 15.4.** Plain coronal MRA (3D FISP, α 15°). Arterial MRA in a negated MIP angiogram with normal findings of the intracranial vessels. This projection mode displays images comparable to those of DSA. *e*, External carotid artery; *i*, internal carotid artery; *b*, basilar artery; *m*, middle cerebral artery

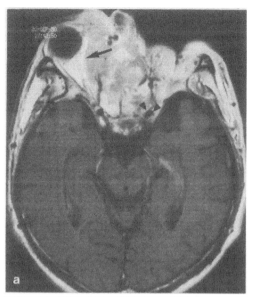

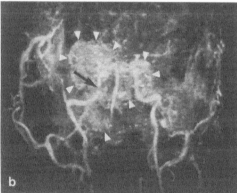

**Fig. 15.5a, b.** Leiomyosarcoma of the face, stenosis of the left internal carotid artery
**a** Axial MRI (SE, 700/15) with Gd-DTPA. Enhancement of the lesion. Infiltration of the right orbit (*arrow*) and compression of the left internal carotid artery (*arrowheads*)
**b** Coronal MRA (3D FISP, 40/7, α 15°) with Gd-DTPA. Demonstration of a stenosis of the left internal carotid artery (*arrow*) and visualization of the tumor (*arrowheads*)

### 15.1.3.2 Face and Neck

The MRA examination of vascular structures of the face is complicated by the slower intraarterial blood flow and gross patient motion. The 2D FLASH sequence provides the best evaluation of vessels in this region. Slice orientation should be perpendicular to the vessels to avoid signal loss. Pathologies in this area mainly concern vessel displacement or compression due to tumor growth. Further, lesions like aneurysms or glomus tumors of the carotid artery can be found which require exact interpretation of flow phenomena in MR angiograms. Possible pitfalls can be overcome by considering the original MRA data set as well as SE images and MIP projections (Fig. 15.7). The administration of contrast medium should be avoided due to the enhancement of the mucosa in the oral and nasal cavity that would be superimposed on vascular structures on MIP angiograms.

## 15.2 Selective Venous MRA

### 15.2.1 Technique and Indications

Venous MRA requires the employment of sequential flow-compensated 2D FLASH sequences due to the slower blood flow in veins. Similar to the 3D FISP sequences, the 2D FLASH sequence obtains a series of images which are then processed to create a projection angiogram (25/10, α 30°, 53 slices with a thickness of 3 – 5 mm and a distance factor of –0.2, causing overlapping of 20%). The slice orientation has to be perpendicular to the vessel in order to avoid signal loss due to increasing saturation of blood within one slice.

**Table 15.3.** Indications for MRA

| | |
|---|---|
| Aneurysms | Alternative to DSA and CT with contrast medium |
| Sinus thrombosis | Alternative to DSA and CT with contrast medium |
| Follow-up | Method of choice |
| Vessel stenosis | Alternative to DSA |
| Arteriovenous malformations | Alternative to DSA |
| Dissection | Method of choice |

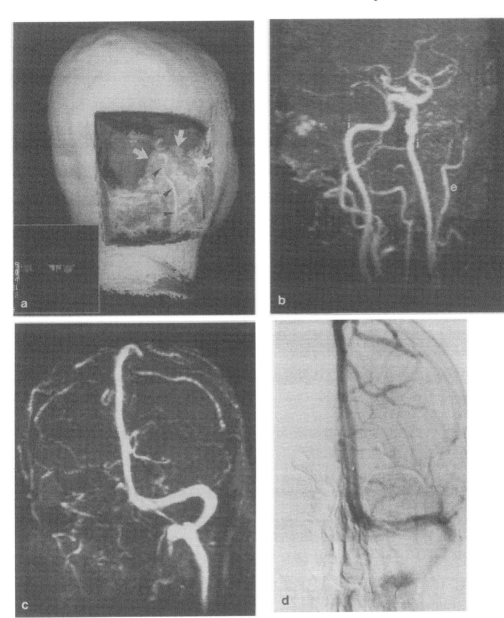

**Fig. 15.6a–d.** Sarcoma of the skull base
**a** 3D sagittal MRI (MPRAGE, 10/4, α 15°) with Gd-DTPA: dorsolateral window. The window allows evaluation of the extent of the lesion (*arrows*) and depicts the course of the internal carotid artery through the tumor (*arrowheads*)
**b** Plain coronal MRA (3D FISP, 40/7, α 15°). Arterial MRA depicts the intracranial vessels and also visualizes the external carotid artery (*e*). *i*, Internal carotid artery
**c** Plain coronal MRA (2D FLASH, 25/10, α 60°). Venous MRA reveals an occlusion of the right transverse sinus due to expansive tumorous growth
**d** Coronal venous DSA confirms the diagnosis on venous MRA: occlusion of the right transverse sinus

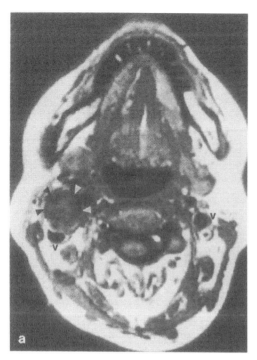 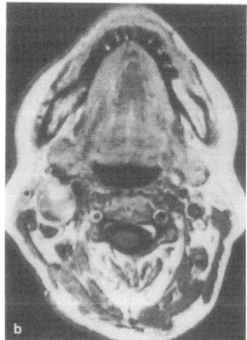

**Fig. 15.7 a–f.** Aneurysm of the right internal carotid artery
**a** Plain axial MRI (SE, 700/15). Depiction of a lesion with sharp margins on conventional plain MRI (*arrowheads*). Note the displacement of the internal jugular vein (*v*) to dorsal

**b** Axial MRI (SE, 700/15) with Gd-DTPA. Inhomogeneous enhancement of the lesion after contrast medium administration, caused by altered intravascular flow. **c–f** see p. 241

The overlapping of 20% increases spatial resolution and reduces progressive saturation of blood flow through an imaging slice. Venous MR angiograms are obtained by employment of an additional RF saturation pulse below the imaging slices, eliminating arterial blood flow.

---

*2D FLASH*
25/10, α 30°
30–53 slices, thickness: 3–10 mm
Distance factor: −0.3 to −0.2
Matrix: 256 × 256
Slice orientation: perpendicular to vessels
– Slow blood flow
– External carotid artery
– Intracranial sinus system
– Jugular vein

---

An alternative to the 2D FLASH sequence is the 3D FLASH sequence, which can be employed for the imaging of small intracranial veins. This technique requires contrast medium injection and an altered MIP algorithm in order to eliminate subcutaneous fatty tissue. Indications for venous MRA are vessel displacement, vessel occlusion, sinus thrombosis, and arteriovenous malformations (Table 15.3). Like arterial MRA, venous MRA is performed mainly after conventional SE imaging and before contrast medium administration. Problems in evaluation of venous lesions may arise from altered flow dynamics. Furthermore, a new sinus thrombosis is visualized with high signal intensity on MRA, imitating vessel perfusion. Conventional SE images help to avoid misinterpretation of MRA in these cases.

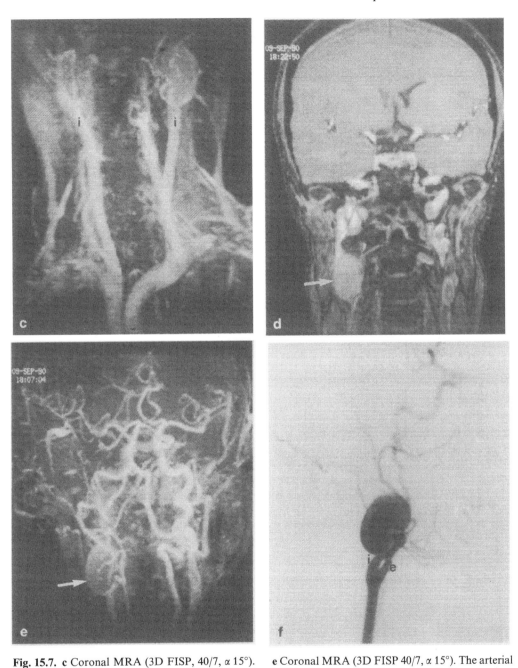

**Fig. 15.7. c** Coronal MRA (3D FISP, 40/7, α 15°). Exact depiction of an aneurysm of the internal carotid artery (*i*) on arterial MRA, employing the Helmholtz surface coil (view from posterior)
**d** Coronal MRA (3D, FISP 40/7, α 15°). Excellent delineation of the lesion (*white arrow*) in the 3D data set acquired with the head coil. The course of the vessel can be exactly evaluated with these images

**e** Coronal MRA (3D FISP 40/7, α 15°). The arterial MRA, employing the head coil, allows an evaluation of the location of the aneurysm (*white arrow*) to the vessels of the skull base, including intracranial portions
**f** Arterial DSA of the right internal carotid artery. The DSA findings correlate with the diagnosis of arterial MRA: depiction of an aneurysm of the right internal carotid artery (*i*). *e*, External carotid artery (With the kind permission of Prof. Dr. Pfeiffer, Munich)

### 15.2.2 Normal Topography

The intracranial venous sinus system can be subdivided anatomically into three main groups according to venous drainage: the superior, the anterior, and the posterior. The superior group drains into the great vein of Galen, the anterior group drains into the petrosal sinuses, and the posterior group drains into the transverse sinuses. MRA visualizes the whole intracranial sinus system and the superior part of the internal jugular vein in a single setting. The venous blood is drained via the superior sagittal sinus and the straight sinus to the confluens, whence it flows via the transverse sinus and the sigmoid sinus to the superior jugular bulb. The cavernous sinus drains via the superior or inferior petrosal sinus to the transverse or sigmoid sinus (Fig. 15.8).

### 15.2.3 Pathologic Findings

The pathologic findings on venous MRA correspond in the majority of cases to the findings of conventional X-ray angiography or DSA. The most common pathology is sinus thrombosis, which can effect only segments of a sinus or may involve the whole sinus (e.g., the superior sagittal sinus). MRA visualizes thrombus as a total signal void of the sinus involved (Fig. 15.9). A fresh sinus thrombosis shows up with high signal intensity, simulating vessel perfusion. Important for differential diagnosis are absent sinuses or altered flow velocity with the resulting signal void.

Venous pathology in the head and neck usually involve the superior jugular bulb. For this reason exact assessment of the size and location of the bulb with venous MRA is important, particularly for differential diagnosis, as

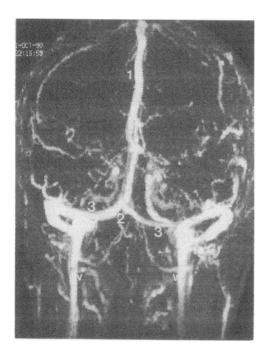

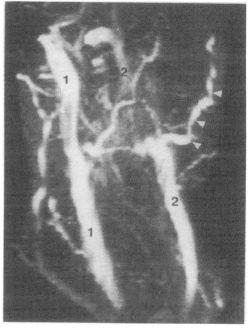

**Fig. 15.8.** Plain coronal MRA (2D FLASH, 25/10, α 60°). Venous MRA of the intracranial sinus system with normal findings. Visualization of the superior sagittal sinus (*1*), the confluens (*2*), the transverse sinuses (*3*), and both jugular veins (*v*)

**Fig. 15.9.** Plain coronal MRA (2D FLASH, 25/10, α 60°). Venous MRA of the jugular veins in the region of the neck, showing normal perfusion of the right jugular vein (*1*) and an occlusion of the left jugular vein (*2*). Note the collateral perfusion (*arrowheads*) of the distal portions of the occluded vessel

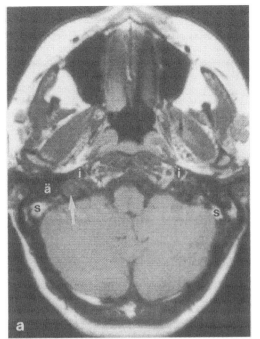

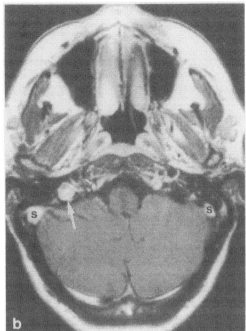

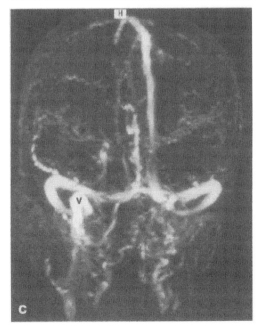

**Fig. 15.10 a–c.** Sjögren's syndrome, cranial position of right superior jugular bulb
**a** Plain axial MRI (SE, 700/15). Visualization of a soft tissue lesion with a diameter of approximately 1 cm in the area of the right superior jugular bulb (*arrow*) adjacent to the external acoustic meatus (*ä*), sigmoid sinus (*s*), and internal carotid artery (*i*)
**b** Axial MRI (SE, 700/15) with Gd-DTPA. Obvious enhancement of the lesion (arrow), with sharp margins, and of the sigmoid sinus (*s*) after contrast medium administration. Possible diagnoses are intravascular glomus tumor or cranial bulb
**c** Coronal MRA (2D FLASH, 25/10, α 60°) with Gd-DTPA. Venous MRA reveals normal perfusion of the jugular bulb and the sigmoid sinus. This excludes an intravascular glomus tumor and confirms the diagnosis of a cranially located superior jugular bulb

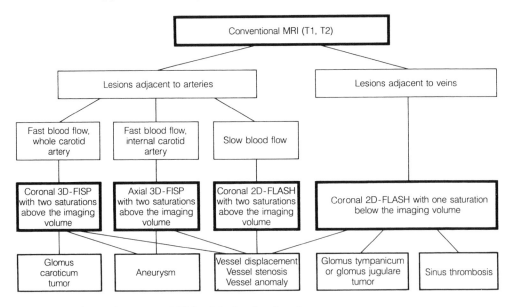

**Fig. 15.11.** Diagnostic strategy: MRA of the head and neck

SE sequences after administration of contrast medium often reveal atypical enhancement which can not be distinguished from tumor infiltration. A common variation is more cranial location of the jugular bulb (Fig. 15.10), a clinically irrelevant vessel anomaly.

The second most common indication for venous MRA is a tumor of the glomus jugulare or glomus tympanicum. Venous MRA visualizes the draining veins and the tumor's topographic relation to adjoining structures such as the sigmoid sinus, the superior jugular bulb, and the internal jugular vein. Feeding arterial vessels can not be detected, even with employment of selective arterial MRA.

*References*

1. Abrams HL (1983) Abrams angiography, vol I, 3rd edn. Vascular and interventional radiology. Little, Brown, Boston, pp 231–314
2. Anderson C, Saloner D, Tsuruda J et al. (1990) Artefacts in maximum-intensity-projection display of MR angiograms. AJR 154:623–629
3. Bongartz G, Vestring T, Fahrendorf G, Peters PE (1990) Einsatz schneller Sequenzen bei der kraniozerebralen MR-Diagnostik. Fortsch Röntgenstr 153(6):669–677
4. Brown DG, Riederer SJ, Jack CR et al. (1990) MR-angiography with oblique gradient-recalled echo technique. Radiology 176:461–466
5. Creasy JL, Price RR, Presbrey T et al. (1990) Gadolinium-enhanced MR-angiography. Radiology 175:280–283
6. Dumoulin CL, Souza SP, Walker MF, Wagle W (1989) Three dimensional phase contrast angiography. Magn Reson Med 9:139–149
7. Edelman RR, Hesselink JR (1990) Clinical magnetic resonance imaging. Saunders, Philadelphia, pp 110–182
8. Edelman RR, Mattle HP, Atkinson DJ, Hoogewoud HM (1990) Magnetic resonance angiography. In: Cardiovascular imaging. American Roentgen Ray Society, Categorial Course Syllabus, pp 51–60
9. Edelman RR, Wentz KU, Mattle HP et al. (1989) Intracerebral arteriovenous malformations: evaluation with selective MR-angiography and venography. Radiology 173:831–837

0. Ehricke H-H, Laub G (1990) Integrated 3D display of brain anatomy and intracranial vasculature in MR imaging. J Comput Assist Tomogr 14(6):846–852

1. Krayenbühl H, Yarargil MG (1979) Zerebrale Angiographie für Klinik und Praxis, 3rd edn. Thieme, Stuttgart, pp 38–241

2. Lissner J, Seiderer M (1990) Klinische Kernspintomographie, 2nd fully revised edn. Encke, Stuttgart, pp 59–83, 570–607

3. Marchal G, Bosmans H, Van Fraeyenhoven L et al. (1990) Intracranial vascular lesions: optimization and clinical evaluation of three dimensional time of flight MR-angiography. Radiology 175:443–448

4. Masaryk TJ, Modic MT, Ruggieri PM et al. (1989) Three-dimensional (volume) gradientecho imaging of the carotid bifurcation: preliminary clinical experience. Radiology 171:801–806

5. Nadel L, Braun IF, Kraft KA, Fatouros PP, Laine FJ (1990) Intracranial vascular abnormalities: value of MR phase imaging to distinguish thrombus from flowing blood. AJNR 11:1133–1140

16. Peters PE, Bongartz G, Drews C (1990) Magnetresonanzangiographie der hirnversorgenden Arterien. Fortschr Röntgenstr 152(5):528–533

17. Sevick RJ, Tsuruda JS, Schmalbrock P (1990) Three-dimensional time-of-flight MR angiography in the evaluation of cerebral aneurysms. J Comput Assist Tomogr 14(6):874–881

18. Siemens (1990) Angiography Numaris II/Version A 2.1, Edition 05/1990: Magnetom SP User Guide. Siemens AG, Erlangen, FRG

19. Suryan G (1951) Nuclear resonance in flowing liquids. Proc Indian Acad Sci Sect A 33:107

20. Vogl T, Balzer JO, Juergens M et al. (1992) MR-Angiographie für die Tumordiagnostik in der Kopf-Hals Region: Untersuchungstechnik und klinische Ergebnisse. RÖFO (in press)

21. Vogl T, Balzer JO, Juergens M et al. (1992) Neurovaskuläre Magnetresonanzangiographie: Technik, Ergebnisse, Indikationen. MMW (in press)

22. Vogl T, Balzer JO, Stemmler J et al. (1991) MR-Angiographie bei neuropädiatrischen Fragestellungen: Technik und klinische Ergebnisse. RÖFO (in press)

# 16 Magnetic Resonance Spectroscopy

## 16.1 Technical Considerations

### 16.1.1 Introduction

Magnetic resonance imaging for the diagnosis of tumors of the head and neck is characterized by high sensitivity but sometimes low specificity. Therefore great expectations have been raised by the development of high-resolution in vivo magnetic resonance spectroscopy (MRS). While MRI is based on the proton density and the relaxation times of the tissue under investigation, MRS allows determination of the molecular linkage of several atoms [9]. The purpose of spectroscopy is to evaluate the frequency of the different molecular bonds containing a given atom in the region of interest. In vivo spectroscopy investigations have established typical spectra for different types of normal or pathologic tissues.

### 16.1.2 Basic Physics of MRS

#### 16.1.2.1 The Spin of a Nucleus

Protons and neutrons, the building blocks of the nucleus of an atom, possess angular momentum or spin. When placed in a strong external magnetic field, nuclear spins precess about the main magnetic field at a rate proportional to the field strength $B_0$

$$v = \frac{\gamma * B_0}{2\pi}$$

where $v$ is the precessional or Larmor frequency and $\gamma$ is the gyromagnetic ratio, a constant for the nucleus of interest.
Spin can be envisioned as a top with positive charges whirling over its surface. The moving charge generates a small magnetic field which gives the nucleus polarity (+ or −, north or south). When spins are grouped together in pairs, as in nuclei with even atomic mass and atomic number, the magnetic field component is cancelled, resulting in a net spin of zero, but in nuclei with odd atomic mass or atomic number, spin is retained.

The rotating electrons in a molecule placed in a strong external magnetic field produce a small magnetic field oriented against the external field. This causes a partial shielding from the external field in certain regions of the molecule and thus leads to a slight change of the local magnetic field in some atoms of this molecule (Fig. 16.1). Therefore the Larmor frequency $v$ of such atoms can be described by the following equation:

$$v = \frac{\gamma * B_{local}}{2\pi} = \frac{\gamma * B_0}{2\pi} *(1-\sigma)$$

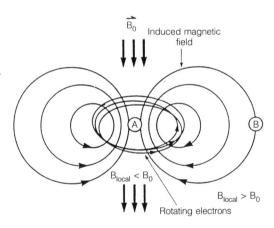

**Fig. 16.1.** Influence of the induced magnetic field on the magnetic induction $B_{local}$ at the atoms $A$ and $B$. The induced magnetic field is caused by rotating electrons, which are created by the main magnetic field $B_0$

## 16.1.2.2 Chemical Shift

The local magnetic field varies slightly at any given position within a molecule due to the strength of chemical bonds, the size of atoms, the number of local electrons, and the nearness of spins in space. These small differences in the local magnetic field slightly alter the precise resonant frequency which will be absorbed by a given atom. The net result is a shifting of the nuclear magnetic resonance (NMR) over a wider band of frequencies, or chemical shift range. The degree of shift is characteristic of the type of bond in which the nucleus is involved.

The graph or plot of signal intensity vs frequency is known as the NMR spectrum. The amplitude of the signal, or resonance, is directly proportional to the number of atoms which respond at a particular RF frequency, and the position of each signal in the frequency direction is known as its chemical shift.

### 16.1.3 Field Strength

In MRS the highest sensitivity and peak dispersion are achieved at the maximum field strength possible. Although small-bore 12-T systems are available commercially and are used in many laboratories, the highest operating field strength for clinical whole-body imaging has been 2 T. However, this does not represent a severe limitation, as most of the MRS information can be gained at 1.5 T, although improvements in S/N and peak dispersion are obtained at 2 T.

### 16.1.4 Appropriate Nuclei

Nearly half of the elements in the periodic table possess spin and can, therefore, be used for MRS. However, certain nuclei are more difficult to study than others, and some are practically useless for spectroscopy. The four principal isotopes used in MRS are listed in Table 16.1.

**Table 16.1.** The four principal isotopes used in MRS

| Nucleus | MR frequency (MHz/T) | Natural isotopic abundance (%) | Relative sensitivity |
|---------|---------|---------|---------|
| $^1$H | 42.58 | 99.98 | 1 |
| $^{19}$F | 40.06 | 100 | 0.834 |
| $^{13}$C | 10.70 | 1.108 | 0.016 |
| $^{31}$P | 17.24 | 100 | 0.066 |

## 16.1.4.1 Hydrogen-1

The $^1$H spectra of all organs show two predominant peaks which originate from the protons in water and fat molecules. These two signals can even be detected on MRI. The resonances of metabolites of greater biochemical interest, such as lactate, phosphocreatine, and amino acids, are more difficult to obtain. The reasons for this are their low concentration (<50 mmol/kg) compared to water (ca. 40 mol/kg) and the necessary homogeneity of the magnetic field because of the relatively small frequency range of the resonances. Recently developed MRS sequences allow localized optimization of magnetic field homogeneity in the volume of interest [3]. Three slices oriented perpendicular to each other that contain the volume of interest are stimulated using slice-selective pulses. The advantage of this technique is that localized spectral information can be obtained with a single transmitter pulse. Water-suppressed localized proton MRS using stimulated echoes has been successfully employed to detect metabolites in the human brain in vivo [2]. The resonances that can be identified include those of acetate, N-acetyl aspartate, γ-amino butyrate, glutamine, glutamate, aspartate, creatine and phosphocreatine, choline-containing compounds, taurine, and inositols.

Tumor studies have shown changes in the distribution of choline, N-acetyl aspartate, and lactate [6].

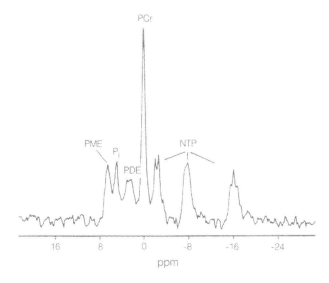

**Fig. 16.2.** $^{31}$P spectra of healthy neck muscle acquired using a 50-mm surface coil at 1.5 T. It is possible to differentiate the resonance of the following metabolites: phosphomonoester (*PME*), inorganic phosphate (*Pi*), phosphodiester (*PDE*), phosphocreatine (*PCr*), and nucleoside triphosphate (*NTP*)

### 16.1.4.2 Carbon-13

The two main advantages of $^{13}$C over $^1$H are its wide chemical shift range (200 ppm vs 10 ppm) and the fact that the large water resonance which is normally present in vivo $^1$H spectra is not detected. The disadvantages include the low natural abundance of $^{13}$C, making it more difficult to observe in a short amount of time.

### 16.1.4.3 Fluorine-19

The high sensitivity of fluorine to the MRS technique and the fact that its normal concentration in the body is effectively zero make it possible to obtain a series of $^{19}$F spectra quickly without interference from other biologic compounds. In vivo metabolism of the anticancer drug 5-fluorouracil to fluoro-b-alanine can be observed by means of $^{19}$F spectroscopy.

### 16.1.4.4 Phosphorus-31

Because of its physical, chemical and physiologic properties, $^{31}$P is especially suitable for in vivo investigations. In an in vivo spectrum of healthy muscle tissue it is possible to differ-

entiate the peaks of phosphomonoester (PME), inorganic phosphorus (Pi), phosphodiester (PDE), phosphocreatine (PCr), and nucleoside triphosphate (NTP) (Fig. 16.2). Since the position of PCr in the spectrum is independent of pH value, it is used as a reference point for the chemical shift. PME consists of precursors of membrane biosynthesis (mainly phosphorylcholine and phosphorylethanolamine) and sugar phosphates. The three NTP peaks mainly consist of ATP, which coincides with the resonances of ADP and NAD(H). Differentiation of these peaks is possible only in high-resolution in vitro spectra.

### 16.1.5 Calculation of pH

The spectral position of inorganic phosphate depends on the $H_2PO_4^-/HPO_4^{2-}$ ratio and therefore on the pH value. For this reason, chemical shift of Pi can be used in $^{31}$P studies for precise calculation of the pH.

### 16.1.6 Examples of Localization Techniques

Clinical in vivo studies require a localization method sufficient to define the measurement volume. Recently, techniques have been de-

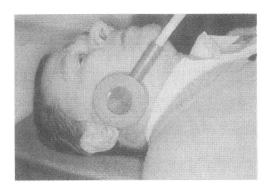

**Fig. 16.3.** The 50-mm surface coil for $^{31}$P spectroscopy

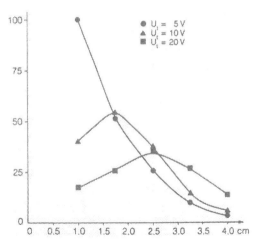

**Fig. 16.4.** The 50-mm surface coil: diagram of relative sensitivity (*ordinate*) at transmitter amplitudes of 5, 10, and 20 V. At a transmitter amplitude ($V_t$) of 5 V the sensitivity is highest directly under the coil

veloped to select hemispheric, cubic, or any other volumes of interest in one, two, or three dimensions. Even spectroscopic imaging with low resolution is possible.

#### 16.1.6.1 Surface Coils

Because the volumes of interest are usually located superficially, the surface coil technique with its good S/N is suitable for examinations of the neck. The surface coil is centered upon the ROI (Fig. 16.3). Usually, the possibility of matching the coil to the resonance frequency of $^{31}$P (25 MHz at 1.5 T) and protons (63 MHz at 1.5 T) allows it to be used for both spectroscopy and imaging. The sensitive volume of the coil depends on the selected transmitter amplitude. To determine the suitable parameters for different tumor locations, the depth profile of sensitivity is evaluated using a phantom at different transmitter amplitudes (Fig. 16.4). The diagram allows adaption of the sensitive volume to different tumor locations.

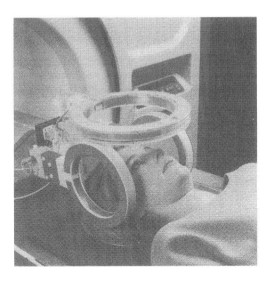

**Fig. 16.5.** Combination coil for $^{1}$H imaging (horizontal Helmholtz coils and $^{31}$P spectroscopy (vertical Helmholtz coils)

#### 16.1.6.2 Image Selected In Vivo Spectroscopy

Ordidge et al. [7] designed a technique to select cubic volumes through the analysis of NMR signals from eight measurements, which results in coaddition of NMR data from within the cube and cancellation of signals from all external regions. This technique is usually applied in clinical $^{31}$P MRS with a combination coil for proton imaging and phosphorus spectroscopy (Fig. 16.5). The sequence parameters of the MRS are selected according to the location of the region of interest determined by the previous imaging. The present design of RF coils and RF amplifiers allows in vivo $^{31}P$ MRS at volumes of about 64 cm$^3$ with this technique.

### 16.1.7 MRS Investigation Procedure

#### 16.1.7.1 Imaging

In clinical MRS studies, imaging of the ROI is necessary for the precise application of the surface coil, or for the selection of the appropriate parameters in other localization techniques. Most modern MRS coils can be set to the resonance of the spectroscopy nucleus as well as to $^1H$, or are combination coils, so that high-quality imaging and spectroscopy are possible without changing the patient's position.

#### 16.1.7.2 Shimming

The MRS examination requires a very homogeneous magnetic field. The optimization, so-called shimming, is done by changing the currents in the gradient coils. Homogeneity is indicated by a decrease in FID (free induction decay) level or by line broadening of the water peak in a proton spectrum. Shimming can be done manually or by means of automatic routines.

#### 16.1.7.3 Spectroscopy

The spectroscopy itself is the accumulation of one or several FIDs. The averaging of several FIDs improves the S/N and is usually necessary in in vivo studies because of the low sensitivity of nuclei and the small voxel size. The measurement duration depends on the number of FIDs and the repetition time.

#### 16.1.7.4 Processing and Analysis of the Spectra

Filtering with a gaussian or an exponential function reduces the noise component of the FID. Fourier transformation from the time into the frequency domain is the carried out, and phase and baseline correction is done. The spectrum is usually evaluated using a least-squares procedure, which determines chemical shift, T2 relaxation time, and the relative area of the peaks caused by the corresponding metabolites.

## 16.2 Clinical Spectroscopy of the Head and Neck

The head and neck region is characterized by a high incidence of tumors with unclear histology. Hitherto, reliable differentiation between malignant and nonmalignant histologies has been possible only via biopsy. Therefore great expectations are placed on in vivo MRS as a noninvasive technique for the analysis of questionable tissue.

To evaluate the clinical potential of this method, investigators at the University of Munich performed several studies of head and neck tumors with in vivo $^{31}P$ MRS. The goal of these investigations was to establish the appropriate measurement technique for tumors at different locations, to find out whether different types of tumors have characteristic phosphorus spectra, and to examine the applicability of MRS to therapy planning and to the checking of the response to treatment in oncology. Two different localization methods were used according to the location of the ROI. Superficial ROIs were analyzed by surface coils with adjusted transmitter amplitudes, while in the other cases the ISIS technique [7] was employed.

**Table 16.2.** Pretherapeutic MRS studies: concentrations of metabolites in tumor tissue relative to normal muscle

| Histology | PME | Pi | PDE | PCr | NTP | pH |
|---|---|---|---|---|---|---|
| 1. Synovial sarcoma recurrence | ▲▲ | ▲ | ▲▲▲ | ▼▼▼ | – | 7.21 |
| 2. Squamous cell carcinoma | ▲▲▲ | ▲ | ▲▲▲ | ▼▼▼ | ▲ | 7.26 |
| 3. Squamous cell carcinoma | ▲▲▲ | – | ▲▲▲ | ▼▼▼ | ▼▼▼ | 7.35 |
| 4. Squamous cell carcinoma | ▲ | ▲ | ▲▲▲ | ▼▼▼ | ▲▲ | 7.16 |
| 5. Squamous cell carcinoma recurrence | ▲▲▲ | ▲ | – | ▼▼ | ▼ | 7.16 |
| 6. Squamous cell carcinoma | ▲ | ▲ | ▲ | ▼▼▼ | – | 7.33 |
| 7. Squamous cell carcinoma | ▲▲▲ | ▼ | ▲▲▲ | ▼▼▼ | – | 7.28 |
| 8. Squamous cell carcinoma | ▲ | ▲ | – | ▼▼▼ | – | 7.26 |
| 9. Squamous cell carcinoma | ▲▲ | ▲ | ▲ | ▼▼▼ | – | 7.30 |
| 10. Squamous cell carcinoma | ▲ | ▲ | ▲▲ | ▼▼▼ | – | 7.26 |
| 11. Tuberculosis | ▲ | ▲ | ▲ | ▼▼ | ▼ | 7.10 |
| 12. Chronic inflammation | ▲▲ | – | ▲ | ▼▼ | ▼ | 7.16 |
| 13. Hodgkin's lymphoma | ▲ | – | – | ▼▼▼ | ▲ | 7.16 |
| 14. High-grade-lymphoma | ▲ | – | ▼ | ▼▼ | ▲▲▲ | 7.26 |

| – | Increase/decrease of the concentrations for less than 1% of the spectrum. |
|---|---|
| ▲–▼ | Increase/decrease of the concentrations for more than 1% of the spectrum. |
| ▲▲–▼▼ | Increase/decrease of the concentrations for more than 4% of the spectrum. |
| ▲▲▲–▼▼▼ | Increase/decrease of the concentrations for less than 8% of the spectrum. |

### 16.2.1 Examination by Means of Surface Coils

Twenty-five patients with many different malignant and nonmalignant lesions underwent examination with surface coils. The most frequent histology was squamous cell carcinoma, which was found in 12 cases (Table 16.2).

#### 16.2.1.1 Carcinoma and Sarcoma

Figure 16.6 shows the recurrence of a *parietal synovial sarcoma*. Both T1- and T2-weighted sequences revealed a region of increased signal intensity in the center of the tumor. In comparison with MRI findings 3 months previously, considerable tumor expansion was obvious. The subtraction image after administration of contrast medium showed lower enhancement in the necrotic center of the tumor than in the periphery (Fig. 16.6a). The tumor spectrum determined at a transmitter amplitude of 5 V (Fig. 16.6b) showed some significant differences from healthy muscle tissue (Fig. 16.6c).

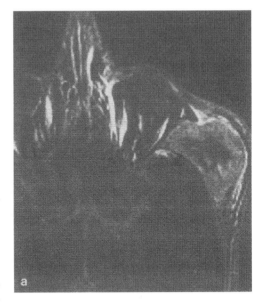

**Fig. 16.6a–d.** Recurrence of a synovial sarcoma near the left orbit
**a** Axial MRI (SE, 500/23) with Gd-DTPA: subtraction image. Limited accumulation of Gd-DTPA in the center of the tumor showing low vascularization corresponding to necrosis
**b–d** see p. 252

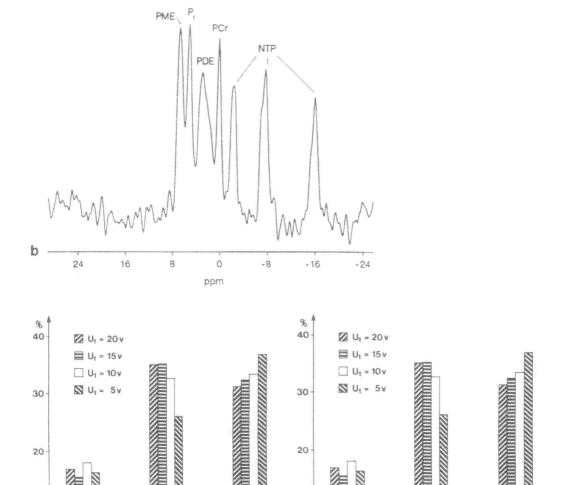

**Fig. 16.6. b** $^{31}$P spectrum of the tumor ($U_t = 5$ V)
**c** Spectroscopically measured concentrations of
metabolites in the tumor (*hatched columns*) and in
muscle tissue (*white columns*)

**d** Dependence of the metabolite concentrations on
the transmitter amplitude ($U_t$). The 5-V spectrum
(mostly superficial tissue) is typical for tumor, the
20-V spectrum (deep-lying measurement volume) is
characteristic for brain tissue

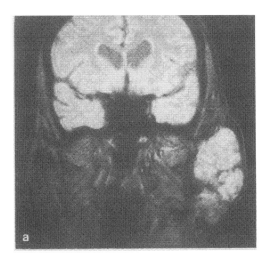

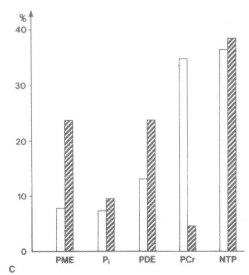

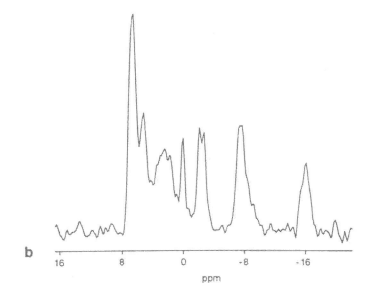

**Fig. 16.7 a–c.** Carcinoma of the parotid gland
**a** Coronal MRI (FLASH, 500/17, α 40°). The high signal intensity of the parotid gland in this GE sequence allows exact differentiation from the surrounding soft tissues

**b** $^{31}$P spectrum of the tumor
**c** Spectroscopically measured metabolite concentrations in tumor (*hatched columns*) and muscle tissue (*white columns*)

The fit procedure demonstrated a doubling of the PME and PDE concentrations, 35% increase in Pi, and a 75% decrease in PCr. The pH was slightly higher (7.21) than in muscle (7.12). To demonstrate the influence of the transmitter amplitude on the sensitive volume, in addition to tumor localization at 5 V, measurements were made at 10, 15, and 20 V. The fit routine showed that an increase of the amplitude was accompanied by a continuous tendency away from concentrations typical for tumors toward the kind of spectrum usually obtained from brain tissue (high PDE, low Pi, low NTP) (Fig. 16.6d).

The next case presented had a large *carcinoma of the parotid gland* accompanied by multiple metastases to the neck lymph nodes (Fig. 16.7). MRI showed an infiltrating tumor of heterogeneous structure and signal intensity, particularly in the FLASH sequence (Fig. 16.7a). The subtraction images after administration of contrast medium showed a high degree of Gd-DTPA enhancement, an indication of a high metabolic rate and little necrosis. The $^{31}$P spectrum (Fig. 16.7b) showed an enormous peak of PME (+208%), elevated PDE (+83%), and a nearly complete loss of the PCr peak (−75%) (Fig. 16.7c) in the tumor. The pH was calculated to be 7.26.

Twelve patients with lymph node metastasis of *squamous cell carcinoma* were studied using MRI and spectroscopy. The least-squares fits of the spectra showed that there are some significant differences between tumor and muscle tissue (Fig. 16.8). In all cases but one there was an elevation of PME by an average of 74% (maximum +250%). PDE was also elevated, but not as much as PME, the values ranging from unchanged to nearly double (average 48%). Similar changes were observed in Pi: a slight decrease was seen in one case, whereas in another case it was nearly double (+86%). Furthermore, contrast medium studies suggested that there may be a correlation between the elevation of Pi and the degree of tumor necrosis.

For example, in one case where extremely inhomogenous Gd-DTPA enhancement was found on MRI, pretreatment spectroscopy showed an elevation of Pi of 86%, whereas in

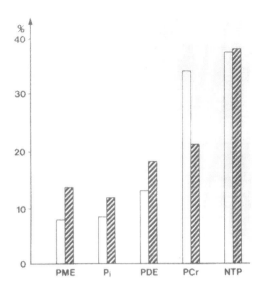

**Fig. 16.8.** Squamous cell carcinoma: metabolite concentrations in tumor (*hatched columns*) and muscle tissue (*white columns*)

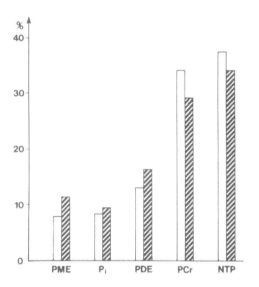

**Fig. 16.9.** Tuberculosis of cervical lymph nodes: metabolite concentrations in tumor (*hatched columns*) and muscle tissue (*white columns*)

another tumor of the same histologic subtype a decrease of Pi (−25%) was accompanied by a large and homogeneous accumulation of contrast medium. Since it decreased significantly in all tumors, PCr proved to be the most reliable indicator of tumor activity. The largest decrease was observed in two cases of tumors of the base of the tongue with widespread lymph node metastases. The NTP concentrations in the tumors were similar to those in muscle.

### 16.2.1.2 Benign Tumor

The spectrum obtained from a patient suffering from *tuberculosis* with lymph node involvement showed slightly raised Pi, PME, and PDE levels (Fig. 16.9). PCr ($-14\%$) and NTP ($-9\%$) were slightly decreased, and the calculated pH (7.10) did not differ from that of healthy tissue.

In another benign tumor, this time a *chronic inflammation of the submandibular gland*, the spectrum did not differ significantly from spectra obtained from malignant lesions (Fig. 16.10). The concentration of PME was $+116\%$, while the PCr level was lower ($-19\%$). The other metabolites remained practically unchanged.

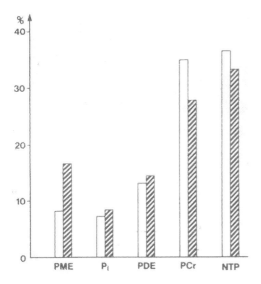

**Fig. 16.10.** Chronic inflammation of the submandibular gland: metabolite concentrations in tumor (*hatched columns*) and muscle tissue (*white columns*)

### 16.2.1.3 Lymphoma

Figure 16.11 shows data from a patient who had extensive enlargement of the lymph nodes adjacent to the sternocleidomastoid muscle. Histological studies revealed a Hodgkin's lymphoma. MRI studies before treatment showed enormous enlargement of the deep cervical lymph nodes with high signal intensity in the T1- and T2-weighted images. In a FLASH sequence with a flip angle of 40°, the contrast to surrounding soft tissue was better (Fig. 16.11 a). Subtraction images after administration of Gd-DTPA revealed homogeneous enhancement, indicating high metabolic activity in the tumor. Figure 16.11 b shows the $^{31}P$ spectrum of the involved lymph nodes. Quantification by least-squares fit revealed an increase in PME ($+40\%$) and a decrease in PCr ($-25\%$). The concentrations of Pi and PDE and the pH were slightly higher than in muscle tissue (Fig. 16.11 c).

The spectral characteristics of another patient with a lymphoma were similar, except for a large increase in NTP ($+32\%$).

### 16.2.2 Examination by Means of ISIS

An alternative localization technique commonly used in head and neck spectroscopy is ISIS [7]. In the University of Munich study, 10 patients with intracranial tumors (meningioma, astrocytoma, neuro- or glioblastoma or deep-lying squamous cell carcinoma) underwent investigations using this method. Figure 16.12 a shows the coronal MRI image of a patient with a large *oligodendroglioma*. After Gd-DTPA administration, strong enhancement was seen on the tumor border but none in the center. Spectra were obtained from normal brain tissue and from the tumor voxel. The spectrum obtained from the tumor tissue (Fig. 16.12 b) showed a considerable increase in PME ($+54\%$) and Pi ($+67\%$) compared with the normal brain spectrum (Fig. 16.12 c), with its characteristic high PDE and low Pi levels.

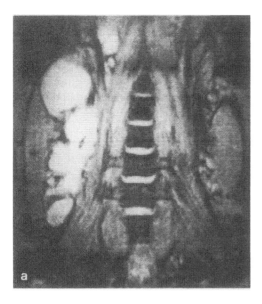

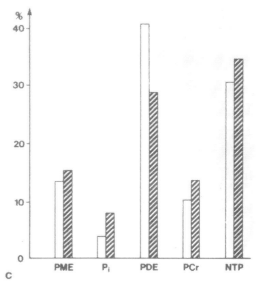

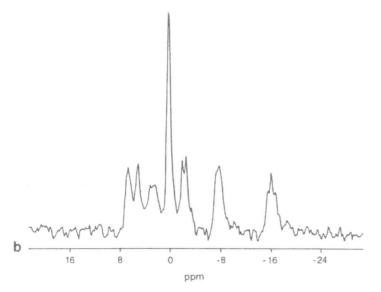

**Fig. 16.11 a–h.** Hodgkin's lymphoma with involved lymph nodes next to the sternocleidomastoid muscle

**a** Coronal MRI (FLASH, 500/17, α 40°). High signal intensity of the enlarged lymph nodes
**b** $^{31}$P spectrum of the enlarged lymph nodes
**c** Metabolite concentrations in tumor (*hatched columns*) and muscle tissue (*white columns*)

**d** Schedule of MRS, MRI, and chemotherapy ▷
**e** Coronal MRI (FLASH, 500/17, α 40°): same slice as in **a**. Obvious regression of the enlarged lymph nodes during 6 weeks of chemotherapy
**f** Decrease of tumor volume during chemotherapy
**g, h** Change in concentrations of PME and PCr during chemotherapy. ●——● Involved lymph node; □——□ muscle tissue

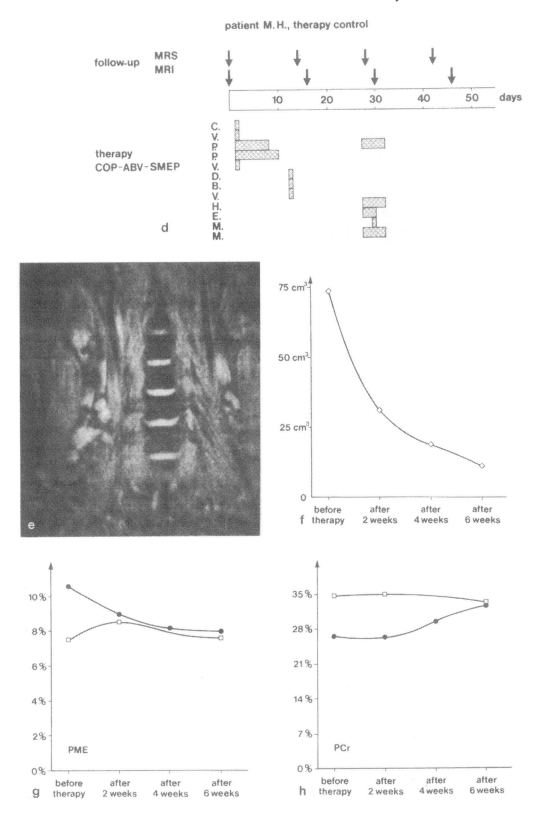

d

e

f

g    PME

h    PCr

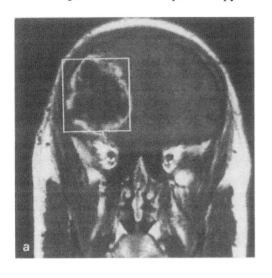

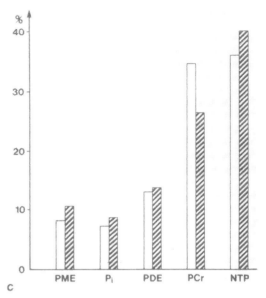

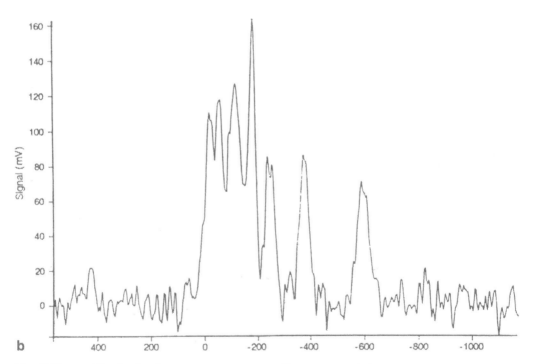

**Fig. 16.12 a–c.** Oligodendroglioma
**a** Coronal MRI (FLASH, 500/17, α 40°) with Gd-DTPA. Marked peripheral enhancement, no enhancement in center of tumor

**b** $^{31}$P spectrum of the tumor
**c** Spectroscopically measured metabolite concentrations in tumor (*hatched columns*) and muscle tissue (*white columns*)

### 16.2.3 Follow-Up Studies During Therapy

In five patients, follow-up studies were carried out during radio- or chemotherapy (Table 16.3).

A patient with an *esthesioneuroblastoma* located in the right maxillary sinus underwent radiotherapy at a dose of 60 Gy. Spectra were obtained immediately before therapy and after 1, 2, and 4 weeks. The shape of the volume that was measured was adapted to the alterations in the tumor volume. The quantitative analysis of the spectra revealed decreases in PME, Pi, and NTP and rises in PDE and PCr. In a case of *squamous cell carcinoma*, follow-up studies were done during radiotherapy. The considerable shrinking of the tumor was accompanied by a significant increase in PME and a decrease in Pi. PDE remained practically unchanged during the first week but showed a large increase after 2 weeks. An increase of NTP that lasted for 1 week was seen in the region 2 days after the start of therapy. The large inherent error in the pH calculation prevents a reliable interpretation of the single investigation carried out.

In three cases of *lymphoma* (Table 16.3) the influence of chemotherapy was studied by MRS. The common result in all patients was that the tumor spectra became similar to the muscle spectra while the tumor was shrinking.

This effect is probably caused by the changing relation between tumor and surrounding tissue and is responsible for the difficulties in long-term follow-up studies of tumors which shrink rapidly during therapy.

## 16.3 Discussion

The differences we observed between tumor and muscle spectra are consistent with the results of in vivo and in vitro studies carried out by other groups [4, 8]. Tumor growth is characterized by increased concentrations of PME and Pi and a large decrease in PCr. As yet, we have seen no reliable relation between tumor histology and $^{31}$P spectra, while most groups have reported quite a good correlation between spectra and the metabolic state of the tumor, particularly the degree of vascularization. E. J. Hall [5] discriminates between three types of tumor cell with respect to their proximity to vascular capillaries. Within about 10 cell layers of a capillary, the tumor cells are sufficiently well supplied with oxygen and nutrients to sustain aerobic respiration and are able to eliminate toxic waste products efficiently. Beyond these aerobic cells are layers of cells that are hypoxic but still viable. Regions of the tumor most distant from vascular capillaries consist of anoxic necrotic cells. The

**Table 16.3.** Follow-up studies with $^{31}$P-MRS

| Histology | PME | Pi | PDE | PCr | NTP | pH |
|---|---|---|---|---|---|---|
| Squamous cell carcinoma | | | | | | |
| – before therapy | – | ▲▲▲ | ▲ | ▼▼▼ | ▲ | 7.25 |
| – after 2 days | – | ▲▲ | – | ▼▼▼ | ▲▲▲ | 7.38 |
| – after 1 week | ▲ | ▲▲ | ▲ | ▼▼▼ | ▲▲▲ | 7.40 |
| – after 2 weeks | ▲ | ▲ | ▲▲▲ | ▼▼▼ | ▼ | 7.21 |
| Hodgkin's lymphoma | | | | | | |
| – before therapy | ▲ | – | – | ▼▼▼ | ▲ | 7.16 |
| – after 2 weeks | ▲ | – | ▲ | ▼▼▼ | ▲▲ | 7.13 |
| – after 4 weeks | ▲ | ▼ | ▲ | ▼ | – | 7.12 |
| – after 6 weeks | – | – | ▼ | – | ▲ | 7.14 |
| High-grade lymphoma | | | | | | |
| – before therapy | ▲ | – | ▼ | ▼▼ | ▲▲▲ | 7.26 |
| – after 2 weeks | – | ▲ | ▲ | ▼▼ | ▲ | 7.21 |

Symbols: see Table 16.2.

spectra from such cells show an intense Pi signal and a very small residual PME peak. A comparison of the Pi concentrations measured and the MR images of the patients in our study confirms those results [10, 11]. This fact may be useful in radiotherapy of malignancies, since MRS allows hypoxic cells with low radiosensitivity to be detected. Administration of radiosensitizers in these cases may improve the effect of therapy.

The initial expectation that it would be possible to evaluate tumor histology by $^{31}$P spectroscopy can not be confirmed. The differences within groups of similar histology are too high. Errors may have been caused by inadequate definition of the volume to be measured, which would result in spectra supposedly from tumor tissue in fact to some extent deriving from the surrounding soft tissue. Our observation of a relation between the decrease in PCr and tumor size suggests that the PCr originates exclusively from the muscle surrounding the tumor. Previous follow-up studies during chemotherapy in animals and humans have mainly shown a decrease in high-energy phosphates (PCr, NTP) and an increase in pH and Pi. These effects are confirmed by our follow-up studies, although the rapidly decreasing tumor volume prevents exact comparison of the spectra. We assume that the progressive approach of the metabolite concentrations in the tumor spectra to the muscle values is mainly due to a decrease in the tumor-to-muscle ratio during therapy in the sensitive volume of the coil. Therefore, in future, only tumors which are not expected to change in size during therapy, should be evaluated in long-term follow-ups.

As a result of our studies, we can confirm that there is a significant difference between spectra of head and neck tumors and healthy tissue. Although no relation between histology and spectra was found, it is possible to evaluate the vascularization and metabolic state of the tissue by $^{31}$P spectroscopy. Possible clinical applications of $^{31}$P spectroscopy in the neck region may be detection of tumor growth, individual tailoring of therapy according to the metabolic state, and evaluation of the effects of treatment.

## 16.4 Prospects

Most of spectroscopy's problems result from its relative insensitivity. Spectroscopists have attempted to overcome this technical limitation in two ways: by using higher field strength magnets to increase the available signal, and by improving techniques to make spectroscopy at 1.5 T more sensitive and efficient. Preliminary reports indicate that the spectra generated by 4-T devices are a major improvement over those obtained at lower field strengths. Along with greater spectral resolution, the increased signal strength obtained at 4 T allows both acquisition times and voxel size to be reduced. The higher costs and heightened safety concerns, however, impose practical restrictions on the application of these magnets in clinical research [1].

### References

1. Egerter DE (1989) Is MR spectroscopy ready for prime time? Diagn Imaging. September: 127–146
2. Frahm J, Bruhn H, Gyngell ML, Merboldt KD, Hänicke W, Sauter R (1989) Localized high-resolution NMR spectroscopy using stimulated echoes: initial applications to human brain in vivo. Magn Reson Med 9:79–93
3. Frahm J, Merboldt KD, Hänicke W (1987) Localized proton spectroscopy using stimulated echoes. J Magn Reson 72:502
4. Griffiths JR, Cady E, Edwards RHT, McCready VR (1983) 31-P-NMR studies of human tumor in situ. Lancet i:1435–1436
5. Hall EJ (1987) Radiobiology for the radiologist. Harper & Row, New York
6. Luyten PR, Heindel W, Herholz K, Marien AJH, van Gerwen PHJ, den Hollander JA, Friedmann G, Heiss W-D (1990) 1H NMR spectroscopic imaging and positron emission tomography of patients with intracranial tumors. European Congress of NMR in Medicine and Biology. Strasbourg, 2–5 May 1990, Book of abstracts 94
7. Ordige RJ, Connelly A, Lohman JAB (1986) Image-selected in vivo spectroscopy (ISIS). A new technique for spatially selective NMR spectroscopy. J Magn Reson 66:283–294
8. Semmler W (1988) Monitoring tumor response to chemotherapy in patients with 31-P-MR spectroscopy. Symposium on Positron Emission Tomography and Magnetic Resonance

Spectroscopy in Oncology, Heidelberg. Book of abstracts:15

9. Vogl T, Peer F, Reimann V, Holtmann S, Rennschmid C, Weber H, Hahn D, Lissner J (1989) In-vivo 31P-Magnetresonanz-Spektroskopie und MRI bei Patienten mit oberflächlich gelegenen Tumoren. Fortschr Röntgenstr 1:58–65

10. Vogl T, Peer F, Schedel H, Reimann V, Holtmann S, Rennschmid C, Sauter R, Lissner J (1989) 31P-Spectroscopy of head and neck tumors – surface coil technique. Magn Reson Imaging 7:425–435

11. Vogl T, Rennschmid C, Sauter R, Holtmann S, Schedel H, Peer F, Lissner J (1988) 31P in-vivo spectroscopy of human tumors with image guided technique (ISIS). Tumor Diagn Therapy 9:168–169

# 17 Conclusions

The unique topography of the head and neck makes it a region where imaging techniques play a crucial part in investigations. A multitude of different tissue structures and sense organs which often simultaneously control physiologic processes and movements are crowded into a confined space. The particular task of imaging methods in the head and neck is to detect tumors and determine their extent. The innovations of MR technology, such as in vivo spectroscopy, need to be investigated to establish their potential applications for diagnosis of head and neck lesions. Within the framework of a research project, a total of more than 1000 patients with masses in this region were prospectively examined using MRI and other imaging modalities. The aim of the study was to optimize the MRI examination technique as well as to assess its diagnostic value. For lesions of the skull base, MRI exhibited sensitivity of 100% and specificity of 96%, significantly better than all other imaging methods. These outstanding results, however, are based on strict interdisciplinary selection of patients according to their clinical symptoms and radiologic signs. Clinical symptoms in the region of the internal auditory meatus, the inner ear, and the cerebellopontine angle constitute an absolute indication for MRI with the paramagnetic contrast medium Gd-DTPA.

By means of diagnostic scores and assessment by three independent investigators, it was shown that MRI yields more information than other modalities in tumors of the pharynx, oral cavity, and neck. This applies to primary diagnosis, checking the response to therapy, and detection of recurrences. Clinical examination and endoscopy remain the primary methods for investigation of the pharynx and neck. For a tumor of stage pT1 no imaging procedure is necessary, but MRI should be used to help plan the treatment of all higher stage tumors.

Tissue differentiation on MRI has to be improved by using in vivo $^{31}$P spectroscopy for tumor diagnosis. Various studies before and during therapy have yielded new information on the metabolism of tumors.

Altogether, the results of studies on the value of MR techniques in the head and neck represent the basis for a new diagnostic concept in this region. The role of these new imaging methods will be established in close cooperation with the clinical disciplines. The essential conclusions are:

1. MRI should be the imaging method in the case of clinical suspicion of masses in the internal auditory canal, cerebellopontine angle, and skull base.
2. The combination of endoscopy and MRI represents the optimal diagnostic strategy for tumors of the pharynx and oral cavity.
3. $^{31}$P spectroscopy allows for the first time, in vivo investigation of the phosphorus metabolism of tumors. A higher concentration of membrane phosphates is characteristic for malignant tumors.
4. Studies during both radiotherapy and chemotherapy show the potential of MRI for checking the response of tumors to treatment.
5. New techniques such as three-dimensional reconstruction and MR angiography will broaden the application of MR methods.

# Subject Index

**H.-M. Hoogewoud,** Fribourg;

**G. Rager,** University of Fribourg;

**H.-B. Burch,** Fribourg, Switzerland

# Computed Tomography, Anatomy, and Morphometry of the Lower Extremity

With contributions by P. Cerutti and G. Rilling

1990. XI, 124 pp. With a comparative CT and anatomical atlas containing 48 plates consisting of 123 sep. illus., and 12 further figs. Including morphometry and 3D graphic software on a 5.25" floppy disk for IBM PCs and compatibles.
Hardcover. ISBN 3-540-51002-8

This book presents completely up-to-date information on CT imaging of the lower extremity. It includes an atlas correlating new, high-resolution CT scans with identical thin anatomical slices covering the lower extremity from the crista iliaca to the planta pedis. Additional figures, including CT arthrograms of the hip, knee and ankle, depict the anatomy in detail. The technique and clinical relevance of CT measurements especially in orthopedic surgery is also clearly explained. Of special interest is the new method developed by the authors for assessing the coverage of the femoral head. The special morphometry software and a 3D program allowing representation in space make it possible to precisely and accurately measure the coverage with normal CT scans of the hip. The software runs on IBM PCs and compatibles and is on the floppy disk delivered with the book.

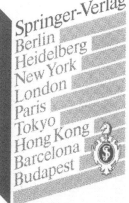

Springer-Verlag
Berlin
Heidelberg
New York
London
Paris
Tokyo
Hong Kong
Barcelona
Budapest

**M. Osteaux, K. de Meirleir, M. Shahabpour,**
University of Brussels (Eds.)

# Magnetic Resonance Imaging and Spectroscopy in Sports Medicine

With contributions by numerous experts

Foreword by H. G. Knuttgen

1991. XVI, 199 pp. 144 figs. in 244 sep. illus. Hardcover
ISBN 3-540-52548-3

Magnetic resonance represents a major diagnostic advance in sports medicine. It is a new and totally non-invasive method that demonstrates sport injuries to cartilage, ligaments, tendons and fine bone texture with an unrivalled clarity. Similarly, MR spectroscopy is a novel and fascinating tool for the in vivo dynamic study of muscle metabolism.

The main part of the book focuses on the proven clinical indications, contributions and semiology of MRI in sports medicine, especially with regard to the osteo-articular system. The knee, the joint most commonly injured by athletes and best exemplifying the spectacular assets of MRI, is thoroughly discussed and abundantly illustrated.

The book gives a short introduction to the technical and physical aspects of MRI. It also includes a discussion of MRI in clinical research and the study of sport physiology, namely in sports cardiology and muscle physiology.

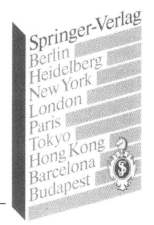

Springer-Verlag
Berlin
Heidelberg
New York
London
Paris
Tokyo
Hong Kong
Barcelona
Budapest

2735754R00157

Printed in Great Britain
by Amazon.co.uk, Ltd.,
Marston Gate.